Advances in Renal Cell Carcinoma Research

Advances in Renal Cell Carcinoma Research

Edited by **Barbara Mayer**

New Jersey

Published by Foster Academics,
61 Van Reypen Street,
Jersey City, NJ 07306, USA
www.fosteracademics.com

Advances in Renal Cell Carcinoma Research
Edited by Barbara Mayer

International Standard Book Number: 978-1-63242-036-7 (Hardback)

Printed in the United States of America.

Contents

Preface

The purpose of the book is to provide a glimpse into the dynamics and to present opinions and studies of some of the scientists engaged in the development of new ideas in the field from very different standpoints. This book will prove useful to students and researchers owing to its high content quality.

The area of renal cell cancer has experienced tremendous resurgence. This book provides a synopsis of latest research and innovative ideas for the future in this rapidly changing field, which encompasses medicine, surgery, radiation oncology, basic science, pathology, radiology, and supportive care. The book encompasses tumor and molecular biology, surgery mechanisms, radiation therapy, challenges in the treatment of renal carcinoma, oxidative stress and steroids receptors in carcinoma. The objective was to present a detailed account that would act as a credible source for scientists and clinicians; and interpret the domain for trainees in surgery, medicine, radiation oncology and pathology. This book targets clinicians, scientists and professionals who have interest in renal cell cancer.

At the end, I would like to appreciate all the efforts made by the authors in completing their chapters professionally. I express my deepest gratitude to all of them for contributing to this book by sharing their valuable works. A special thanks to my family and friends for their constant support in this journey.

Editor

Part 1

Surgery

1

Gasless Single Port Surgery for Renal Cell Carcinoma: Minimum Incision Endoscopic Surgery

Kazunori Kihara, Yasuhisa Fujii, Satoru Kawakami,
Hitoshi Masuda, Fumitaka Koga, Kazutaka Saito,
Noboru Numao, Yoh Matsuoka and Yasuyuki Sakai
Department of Urology, Graduate School,
Tokyo Medical and Dental University
Japan

1. Introduction

Advances in minimally invasive urologic surgery have accumulated rapidly in recent years with the advent of laparoscopic and robot-assisted surgeries (Clayman, 1991; Guillonneau, 1999; Dasgupta, 2009; Lee, 2009). The procedures for renal cell carcinoma (RCC), radical nephrectomy and partial nephrectomy are among those that have benefited from such innovation. Both laparoscopic surgery and robot-assisted surgery have markedly reduced the invasiveness of surgeries compared to conventional open procedures; laparoscopic surgery is characterized by the use of endoscopy, insufflation with carbon dioxide (CO_2) gas, and insertion of instruments from several trocar ports, while robot-assisted surgery also incorporates stereovision and state-of-the-art movable instruments.

At present, both branches of surgery focus mainly on further minimizing postoperative scarring by performing surgery via a single site (Figure 1) (Ponsky, 2008; Raman, 2008; Kommu, 2009; Kaouk, 2009; Han, 2011). There are currently two major obstacles to achieving the goal of minimally invasive urologic surgery, namely, the necessity of CO_2 insufflation and the high cost of the equipment. The purpose of this chapter is to present a surgery for RCC which can be performed through single-port access, under gasless conditions, and using low-cost equipment (Fig. 1). This form of surgery, which we call minimum incision endoscopic surgery (MIES) or gasless laparoendoscopic single port surgery (GasLESS), has been under development in our department since 1998; techniques have been developed for almost all urological organs (Kihara, 2002, 2004, 2007, 2009a, 2009b, 2010a, 2010b; Kageyama, 2004; Koga, 2007; Saito, 2010). MIES was certified as advanced surgery by the Japanese government in 2006, and was first covered in the Japanese universal health insurance system in 2008 (Kihara et al., 2009a). Here, we will describe the methods and results of MIES-radical nephrectomy and MIES-partial nephrectomy for RCC and discuss its advantageous features that are not associated with other forms of laparoscopic or robot-assisted surgery.

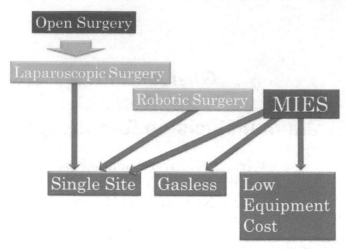

Fig. 1. Three characteristics which are currently important goals in minimally invasive urologic surgery: a single site, a gasless procedure and a low equipment cost. MIES: minimum incision endoscopic surgery.

2. Outline of procedures

2.1 Outline of minimum incision endoscopic surgery (MIES)

An outline of procedures is provided in Figure 2. 1) A minimal incision is made which will serve as a single port and permit extraction of the target specimen. 2) Through this port, a wide working space is made by separating the anatomical plane extraperitoneally; this opening is maintained with special retractors rather than gas insufflation. 3) An endoscope and all other instruments are inserted through the port. 4) Surgeons enjoy the benefits of endoscopy, especially the availability to all participants of magnified images from the beginning to the end of the operation, while the supplemental view with the naked eye remains visible through the port with stereovision and panoramic vision (Figure 3). Three dimensional high-vision endoscope is also being used at present. The size of the port can be tailored to the patient's situation before or during the operation for safety and proper practice, although this is rarely necessary. The multiple options for images and the possibility of modifying the size of the single port may mitigate technical demand and avoid patient selection. Patient position (lateral or supine) can be selected according to each patient's situation or tumour location. The operation is performed without CO_2 gas, without trocar ports, basically without antimicrobial prophylaxis, with an intact peritoneum and with minimal disposable instruments.

2.2 Representative specimen extractions

Representative extractions of various specimens are depicted. All operations were performed extraperitoneally: i) radical nephrectomy via a lumbar port in the lateral position (Figure 4), ii) radical nephrectomy through a paramedian port in the supine position (Figure 5), iii) partial nephrectomy of T1 RCC via a lumbar port (Figure 6) and iv) partial nephrectomy of T2 RCC via a lumbar port (Figure 7) .

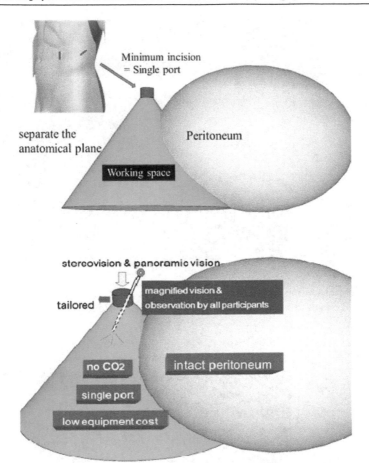

Fig. 2. Outline of the MIES procedures.

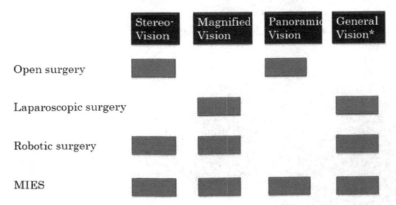

Fig. 3. Image availability in minimally invasive surgeries. *: images are available to all participants.

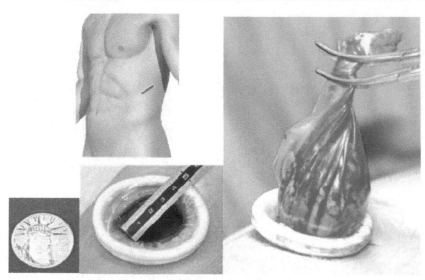

Fig. 4. Radical nephrectomy through a single lumbar port less than 4cm in diameter in the lateral position. To keep the wound open and protect it, an Alexis wound retractor® is typically used.

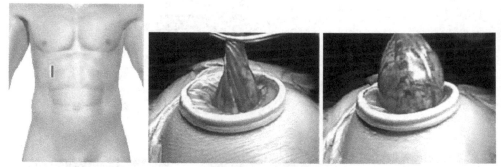

Fig. 5. Radical nephrectomy through a paramedian port in the supine position, performed extraperitoneally.

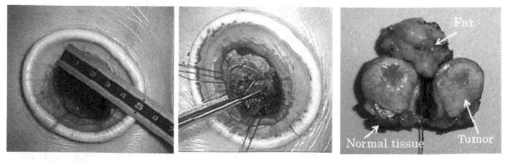

Fig. 6. Partial nephrectomy of T1 RCC via a lumbar port.

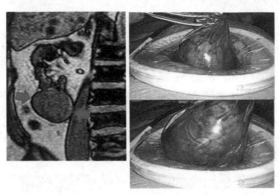

Fig. 7. Partial nephrectomy of T2 RCC through a lumbar port.

3. Methods

An outline of the technique, entitled "MIES-radical nephrectomy and MIES-partial nephrectomy", has been previously reported (kihara, 2009a, 2010a) and presented in the video library of the European Association of Urology (EAU) (Kihara, 2009b, 2010b). At our hospital, MIES-radical nephrectomy has been performed regularly over the last few years for large T1b-T3 RCC and for RCC in dialysis patients, while MIES-partial nephrectomy is performed for most (lately more than 85%) cases of T1a RCC. MIES-partial nephrectomy is typically performed without renal ischemia at our hospital to preserve renal function to as great a degree as possible.

3.1 MIES-radical nephrectomy

A lumbar or paramedian retroperitoneal approach is used. The latter approach is mainly selected when the patient has severe cardiovascular or respiratory disturbances or a large tumour adjacent to the renal pedicle. Antimicrobial prophylaxis is not used.

3.1.1 Lumbar retroperitoneal approach

After the induction of general anaesthesia, the patient is placed in the flank position over the break of the table. An incision just large enough to narrowly permit extraction of the kidney with perinephric fat, usually 3.5-6 cm, is made obliquely forward following the line of the 12th rib (Figure 4). After splitting the muscles, incising the transversalis fascia and moving the flank pad aside, the lateroconal fascia is exposed. During this procedure a small portion of the distal edge of the 12th rib may be removed if necessary. After opening the lateroconal fascia, separation is performed between the fascia of the psoas muscle posteriorly and Gerota's fascia anteriorly. During this separation procedure, the ureter can be readily identified medially. Next, an Alexis wound retractor ® is set up and the single port is prepared (Figure 4). Separation along the posterior Gerota's fascia allows immediate access to the renal artery and vein. The renal artery is circumferentially mobilized, then doubly ligated and divided (Figure 8). Next, the renal vein is freed, doubly ligated and divided. The ureter, which was identified previously, is freed as low as possible and then ligated and divided.

After the wide separation along the posterior Gerota's fascia, a similar separation is performed along the anterior Gerota's fascia, allowing immediate access to the adrenal gland. Next, the perinephric fat is transversely divided at the level of transection of the ureter and subsequently between the adrenal gland and the kidney by retracting the kidney downward with a retractor. The adrenal gland is usually preserved, but when necessary it can be removed along with the kidney. After confirming the complete isolation of the kidney with perinephric fat by passing a tube around the perinephric fat, the specimen is extracted through the single port using a Flexible catcher®. Before the wound is closed, the operative field is washed thoroughly with saline, and the subcutaneous tissue is washed again with saline before epidermal suture to avoid the need for prophylactic antimicrobial agents.

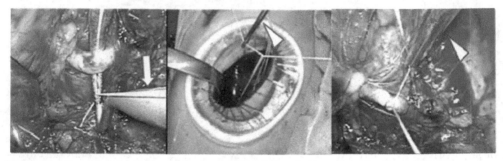

Fig. 8. Ligation of the renal artery using a Thread Pass® (arrow) and a Knot Slide® (arrowhead).

3.1.2 Paramedian retroperitoneal approach

This approach is the same as the lumbar retroperitoneal approach described above except in the following points. The patient is placed in the supine position under general anaesthesia. An incision just large enough to narrowly permit extraction of the kidney with perinephric fat is made downward on the pararectal line, 1-2 cm below the rib (Figure 5). By incising the anterior and posterior sheaths of the rectus muscle while preserving the muscle, the transversal fascia is exposed. The fascia is bluntly pushed downward off the transversal muscle to allow access to the flank pad on the lateroconal fascia. Next, the lateroconal fascia is opened and the anterior Gerota's fascia is separated medially to allow immediate access to the renal vein and artery.

After division of the renal artery and vein, wide separation along the anterior and posterior Gerota's fascia is performed. The kidney with the perinephric fat is freed from the surrounding tissue and extracted as described above, in the section on the translumbar retroperitoneal approach (Figure 5).

3.2 Partial nephrectomy

Partial nephrectomy using an MIES technique is typically performed without renal ischemia at our hospital. In some cases, such as when the tumour is adjacent to the renal pedicle, clamping of the renal vessels is performed as necessary. Either the lumbar retroperitoneal approach or the paramedian retroperitoneal approach is selected. Antimicrobial prophylaxis is not used unless the collecting system is opened.

Regardless of approach, the procedures are similar to those used in radical nephrectomy until the exposure of Gerota's fascia. After setting up the single port, separating the posterior and anterior Gerota's fascias from the surrounding tissue, and holding them back with an Alexis wound retractor®, the tumour is located within the perinephric fat by means of ultrasound (Figure 9). The surface of the kidney is exposed at some distance from the tumour, and the exposure is then extended to near the tumour.

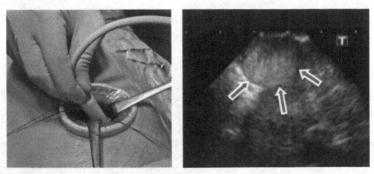

Fig. 9. Identification of the tumour using ultrasound.

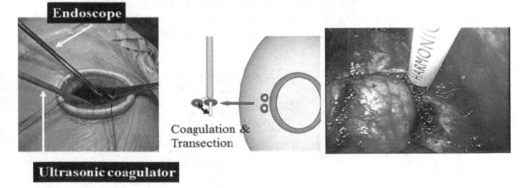

Fig. 10. Coagulation of the normal tissue around the tumour.

Using an ultrasonic coagulator, the normal tissue adjacent to the tumour is penetrated and coagulated (Figure 10). When coagulations around the tumour are completed, the tissue between coagulations is coagulated and transected. Using a suction tube, the coagulated normal tissue is shaped into the form of a pedicle connected to the tumour (Figure 11). The pedicle is tied with a rubber tape or a silk thread, with which the tumour is gently pulled up (Figure 11). After the operative field is filled with saline, the bottom of the tumour in the pedicle is identified with ultrasound. The tumour, its bottom and its transected region can be checked and the line to be transected is now identified (Figure 11).

According to the line identified, the normal tissue neighbouring the bottom of the tumour is transected using a coagulator as soon as the distance between the bottom and the collecting system is large enough. When the bottom is near the collecting system, the pedicle is transected little by little while the tissue is sutured on the calyx side. Finally, the target specimen is freed and extracted through the single port (Figure 12). Immediately after the specimen is extracted, it is split in half and the margin of the tumour is evaluated (Figure 6). When the margin seems too small, a situation which arises very rarely, adjacent normal tissue can be additionally coagulated or resected. The remaining bed is coagulated by means of an argon laser or pasted with coagulating paste, if necessary, and is carefully confirmed to be bloodless (Figure 6). Then the perinephric fat is repaired to cover the kidney defect. Before the wound is closed, the operative field is washed with 2000 ml of saline so that prophylactic antibiotics are not required. Finally, the skin is closed with an epidermal suture (Figure 12).

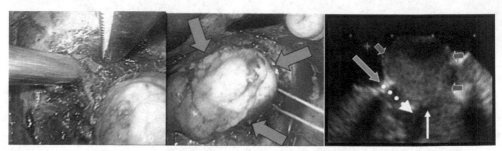

Fig. 11. Ensuring that the normal tissue beneath the tumour is clear. Transection of the normal tissue beneath the tumour is performed under ultrasound guidance. White dotted arrow, the line to be transected; blue arrow, transected normal tissue; red arrow, tumour; white arrow, bottom of the tumour.

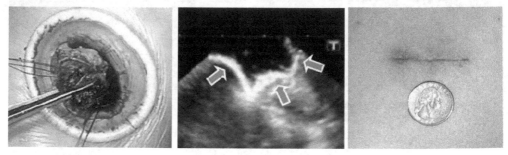

Fig. 12. Extraction of the tumour (left), remaining defect of the kidney (centre) and post-operative scar compared with a quarter (right).

3.3 Instruments

All instruments are inserted through a single port. Since this single port, usually 3-6 cm in diameter, is larger than the trocar ports typically used in laparoscopic surgery, larger instruments can be used which are not only less costly but also reusable. Representative instruments are cited. To keep the wound open as well as to protect it, an Alexis wound retractor® is usually used, but it is not always essential (Figure 4). To maintain the working space, original PLES retractors® are inserted (Figure 13). Haemostasis ligation is often achieved by means of two original devices, the Thread Pass® and the Knot Slide®, which allow easy ligation through the single port (Figure 14). A metal suction tube is useful both to clean up the operative field and to separate the anatomical plane. Transection is often performed with a reusable ultrasonic coagulation device inserted through the port. To extract the kidney, an inexpensive original Flexible catcher® is used (Figure 15). All of the original devices mentioned here are commercially available and relatively inexpensive. For radical nephrectomy, only two of the required devices are disposable, the Flexible catcher® and the Alexis wound retractor®, and both of these are inexpensive, so that the overall cost of equipment is low. For partial nephrectomy, a Sonosurg® reusable ultrasonic coagulator can be used (Figure 16).

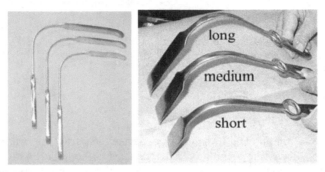

Fig. 13. Original PLES retractor®.

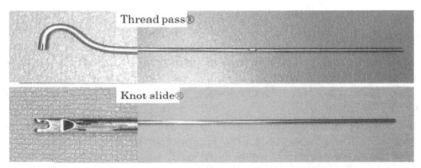

Fig. 14. Original devices for ligation: Thread Pass® and Knot Slide®. Ligation is often used for haemostasis and can be performed easily with these devices through the single port.

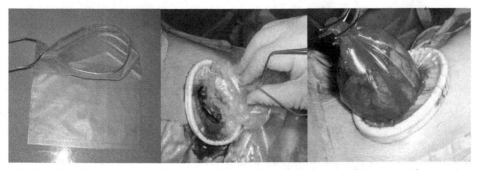

Fig. 15. The Flexible Catcher®, the original inexpensive catcher used to extract the specimen.

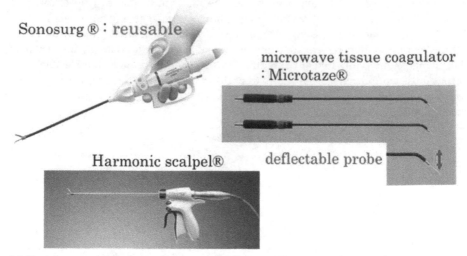

Fig. 16. For tissue coagulation and transection , especially in partial nephrectomy, a Sonosurg® reusable ultrasonic coagulator, a disposable Harmonic scalpel®, or a Microtaze® deflectable microwave tissue coagulator are used depending on the situation.

4. Results

4.1 Radical nephrectomy

The results of the initial 80 consecutive cases, performed by a small group of surgeons between August 1998 and June 2003, have been presented previously (Kihara et al., 2004). The results of 50 more recent consecutive cases, treated between 2009 and 2011, which were performed by a larger group of surgeons (including many inexperienced ones) are presented here. Patient age ranged from 35 to 85 years (mean 64). The duration of the operation was 186 min (range, 114 to 349). The median estimated blood loss was 229 ml (range, 2 to 1500). One patient subsequently received a blood transfusion. A complication arose during a single operation, namely, a small injury to the pleura which was repaired with a suture during the operation.

On the first postoperative day, oral feeding was possible in 90% of cases, and walking more than 100 m was possible in 92%. Within two postoperative days, discharge was possible for 86%. No complications ≥ grade 3a according to the Clavien–Dindo classification were observed postoperatively. The rate of surgical site infection was 4% though no antimicrobial prophylactic agents were used. All infections were successfully treated by administrating antibiotics.

Oncological outcomes of treatment for pT1-T2 RCC by means of this procedure at our hospital are as follows (Iimura et al., 2008): in 154 consecutive cases between 1998 and 2006, five-year overall survival, five-year recurrence-free survival and five-year cancer-specific survival were 95%, 91% and 96%. No local recurrence has been observed since 1998, when this procedure was introduced.

4.2 Partial nephrectomy

Between 2000 and 2011, over 150 cases of renal tumour underwent MIES-partial nephrectomy. In this chapter, we present the surgical outcomes of recent 50 consecutive cases treated between January 2009 and August 2010. Eight surgeons, including several who were inexperienced, performed these operations. The 50 cases consisted of 14 females and 36 males with a median age of 57 years (range, 36 to 79). Preoperative clinical T stage was T1a in 45 cases (90%), T1b in 3 (6%) and T2 in 1 (2%), and the median tumour size was 2.3 cm (range, 1.2 to 8.0). The location of tumour was peripheral in 37 cases (74%), central (a tumour contacting the renal sinus) in 12 (24%) and hilar (a tumour contacting the hilar vessels) in 1 (2%). The indication of partial nephrectomy was imperative in 2 cases (4%, chronic kidney disease and previous history of nephrectomy, respectively) and elective in the remaining 48 (96%).

In all cases but one, which was a central T1b tumour, partial nephrectomy was completed without clamping the hilar vessels. The median operation time was 234 min (range, 128 to 382). The median estimated blood loss was 210 ml (range, 0 to 2274). One case (2%) required allogeneic blood transfusion. No intraoperative complications were encountered.

On the first postoperative day, 47 patients (94%) resumed oral feeding. Patients were typically allowed to begin walking on the second postoperative day, when 43 patients (86%) were able to walk 100 m or farther. The median postoperative day on which the drainage tube was removed was 3 (range, 1 to 20). By postoperative day 3, 38 patients (76%) had recovered to such a degree that they no longer required inpatient care. Surgical site infection was observed in 2 cases (4%), both of which were successfully treated by administrating antibiotics. Major postoperative complications of Clavien–Dindo grade 3 or greater were observed in 2 cases (4%); both cases required retroperitoneal drainage under local anaesthesia (Clavien grade 3a) for urine leakage and retroperitoneal abscess, respectively.

Pathological examination revealed that 41 tumours (82%) were RCC while the remaining 9 (18%) were benign. Although 5 (12%) of the 41 RCC patients had a positive surgical margin as determined microscopically, tumour tissues at the margin underwent thermal denaturation applied via an ultrasonic or a microwave coagulating device. To date, none of 150 cases including these 50 patients has experienced local disease recurrence. As for renal function of the 50 cases, the median % decrease in eGFR 3 months after the operation was 5.9%.

5. Advantageous features of MIES

CO_2 gas insufflation is associated with various risks, including hypertension, hypotension, hypercapnia, pulmonary embolism, decrease of pulmonary compliance and subcutaneous emphysema (See et al., 1993; Alberto et al., 2008); these arise mainly due to the effects of insufflation on the cardiovascular, respiratory and renal systems, although clinical problems rarely arise from careful anaesthesia. Gasless surgeries, such as this operation, can reduce the above risks and might prove especially helpful in operations on aged patients who often have concurrent cardiovascular, respiratory and renal disturbances. As the global population has aged, the number of aged patients has shown rapid increase lately. A high but fortunately subclinical rate of cardiac CO_2 embolism has been reported in laparoscopic radical prostatectomy for prostate cancer which usually occurs in aged men (Hong et al.,

2010); gasless surgery could reduce this rate. From the standpoint of global warming, furthermore, a reduction in the amount of CO_2 emitted from the hospital would be welcomed. In addition, MIES is associated with a low equipment cost similar to that associated with open surgery, because neither expensive disposable instruments nor robotic assistance is necessary, and with a low admission cost similar to that associated with laparoscopic surgery, because the procedure is minimally invasive which results in earlier discharge from the hospital. For cases of T4 RCC, advanced-stage RCC invading neighbouring organs, this surgery can be modified by extending the incision as necessary. Other common modifications are described below.

5.1 Radical nephrectomy for dialysis patients

It is well known that dialysis patients have high rates of RCC. Since dialysis patients usually have various concurrent conditions, especially of their cardiovascular or respiratory systems, and often undergo bilateral radical nephrectomy due to bilateral cancers (Sakura et al., 2007), the gasless nature of MIES is preferable for these patients as it reduces the risks of complications in the above systems. The retroperitoneal approach permitted by MIES is also helpful in that it reduces the likelihood of adhesion of the peritoneum, since some of these patients undergo peritoneal dialysis. The option to use the supine position in MIES is beneficial in that it reduces the risk of shunt obstruction. Finally, the low cost of MIES may also be helpful to the patients, given the high cost of dialysis.

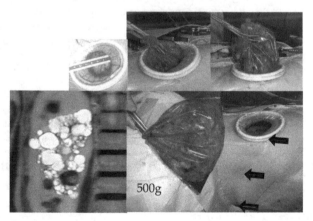

Fig. 18. Radical nephrectomy of a dialysis patient via a port 4 cm in diameter who had previously undergone partial resection of the liver. The arrows indicate the postoperative scar. The weight of the specimen extracted was 500g. CT scan shows ACDK, acquired cystic disease of the kidney, with RCC.

5.2 Modification of MIES for carcinoma of the renal pelvis

Carcinoma of the renal pelvis is considered a renal tumour and is sometimes difficult to distinguish from RCC. In other words, differential diagnosis between invasion of carcinoma of the renal pelvis into the renal parenchyma and RCC is occasionally not possible. In such cases, this procedure can be modified to allow two-port access for en-bloc extraction of the kidney and ureter (Figure 19); this is described in the EAU video library (Saito et al., 2010). The kidney is isolated and extracted through a flank port while still connected with the ureter, as in MIES-radical nephrectomy, and is immediately analyzed to determine the presence of urothelial carcinoma or RCC. When urothelial carcinoma is highly suspected, the table is rotated from a lateral position to a semioblique position, and the distal ureter with the bladder cuff is isolated through a paramedian port about 3 cm in diameter in the lower abdomen. Thereafter, the specimen is extracted en bloc through the flank port and the paramedian port is used for drainage.

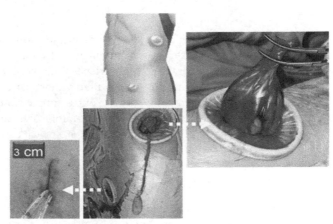

Fig. 19. MIES-total nephroureterectomy. See the text for details.

5.3 Preservation of renal function

It is essential in renal surgery to avoid the postoperative development of chronic kidney disease (Yokoyama et al., 2011a). In our analysis of 219 patients who underwent MIES-radical nephrectomy, 54 developed chronic kidney disease within 2 postoperative years. Univariate and multivariate analyses revealed that age, presence of diabetes mellitus, and preoperative estimated glomerular filtration rate were independent predictors of its development (Yokoyama et al., 2011b). Partial nephrectomy is recommended, if possible, for patients with the abovementioned risks. In order to preserve renal function insofar as it is possible during the operation, it is best to avoid clamping the renal vessels and using CO_2 insufflation which may cause compression of the renal vein. Recently, the rate of clampless MIES-partial nephrectomy at our hospital has been above 95%.

5.4 No usage of antimicrobial prophylaxis

Antimicrobial prophylaxis is associated with several negative effects, including drug-induced complications of major organs, possible introduction of drug-resistant bacteria and high cost. MIES has several features that may help reduce the incidence of infectious complications: a minimal incision, wound protection provided by the Alexis® wound retractor and completion of procedures without insertion of fingers. We prospectively evaluated the incidences of surgical site infection (SSI) after MIES for renal and adrenal tumours in the absence of antimicrobial prophylaxis (Yoshida et al., 2007; Kijima et al.,

2011). In 301 patients, the incidences of superficial SSI and deep SSI were very low, 1.3% and 0.7%, respectively. All perioperative infections were successfully treated by administrating antimicrobial agents.

Antimicrobial prophylaxis is fundamentally not necessary in MIES-radical nephrectomy or MIES-partial nephrectomy in which the urinary tract is not opened during the operation. After stopping the routine usage of antimicrobial prophylaxis, the incidence of drug-resistant bacterial infection has markedly decreased at our ward (unpublished data).

5.5 Limitations of MIES

The limitations of MIES are due to the insertion of all instruments, including the endoscope, through a small single port. It is necessary to be familiar with the handling of the instruments used in the operation. Nevertheless, inexperienced surgeons become able to deliver results similar to those of high-volume surgeons within a short period (Kihara et al., 2010a). It may be attributed to the fact that this surgery offers four visions as described above (Figure 2), and can be modified to accommodate the operator's level of experience by extending the incision as necessary. More than 2000 MIES for urological cancers have been safely performed up to now in our hospital.

6. Spread of MIES

In Japan, several regulatory requirements must be met to perform MIES, but at present more than 70 major hospitals meet these requirements, and this number is increasing year by year. This surgery has been introduced worldwide, in such places as Europe, the US, China, Korea and Brazil. MIES-radical nephrectomy, MIES-partial nephrectomy and MIES-nephroureterectomy have been cited in the video library of EAU (Kihara, 2009b, 2010b; Saito et al., 2010), and textbooks on this technique have been published in China (Kihara, 2003, 2010c).

7. MIES in the near future

The two-dimensional endoscope is being replaced by a three-dimensional endoscope in our hospital, in which case direct supplemental visualization through the port for stereovision is unnecessary. As for the size of the port, it has already been reduced to just over 2 cm in diameter for a small specimen such as the adrenal gland. The console presently used for robotic surgery may become more compact to the point of being useable as a head mount. Depending on the economic situation involved, MIES could be modified into a gasless single-port (2 cm if necessary) and conomical robotic (non-console) surgery.

8. Conclusion

MIES for RCC has several unique characteristics including its gasless nature, single-port access, the use of the retroperitoneal approach, no usage of prophylactic agents, no clamping of the renal vessels and a relatively low equipment cost. MIES shows that low invasiveness similar to that in laparoscopic surgery can be achieved in surgery for RCC without gas insufflation and without expensive disposable instruments and expensive machines.

Future work will integrate the surgical techniques described here with new devices, and perhaps robots (non-console), to fulfil additional needs in the field of surgery for urological cancers.

9. References

Alberto, R.; Bollens, R. & Cohen, B.E. (2008). Fundamentals of laparoscopic surgery. In: *Manual of laparoscopic urology*, Springer-Verlag, pp. 3-17, ISBN 978-3-540-74726-0, Berlin, Germany

Clayman, R.V.; Kavoussi, L.R.; Soper,N.J.; Dierks, S.M.; Darcy, M.D.; Long,S.R.; Roemer, F.D.; Pingleton, F.D. & Thomson, P.G. (1991). Laparoscopic nephrectomy. *N. Engl. J. Med.*, Vol.324, No.19, pp. 1370-1371

Dasgupta, P. & Kirby, R.S. (2009). Outcomes of robotic assisted radical prostatectomy. *Int. J. Urol.*, Vol.16, No.3, pp. 244-248

Guillonneau, B. & Vallancien, G. (1999). Laparoscopic radical prostatectomy: initial experience and preliminary assessment after 65 operations. *Prostate*, Vol.39, No.1, pp. 71-75

Han, W.K.; Kim, D.S.; Jeon, H.G.; Jeong, W.; Oh, C.K.; Choi, K.H.; Lorenzo, E.I. & Rha,K.H. (2011). Robot-assisted laparoendoscopic single-site surgery: partial nephrectomy for renal malignancy. *Urology*, Vol.77, No.3, pp. 612-616

Hong, J.Y.; Kim, W.O. & Kil, H.K. (2010). Detection of subclinical CO2 embolism by transesophageal echocardiography durilng laparoscopic radical prostatectomy. *Urology*, Vol.75, No.3, pp. 581-584

Iimura, Y.; Kihara, K.; Saito, K.; Masuda, H.; Kobayashi, T. & Kawakami, S. (2008). Oncological outcome of minimum incision endoscopic radical nephrectomy for pathologically organ confined renal cell carcinoma. *Int. J. Urol.*, Vol.15, No.1, pp.44-47

Kageyama, Y.; Kihara, K.; Kobayashi, T.; Kawakami, S.; Fujii, Y.; Masuda, H.; Yano, M. & Hyochi, N. (2004). Portless endoscopic adrenalectomy via a single minimum incision by retroperitoneal approach: Experience with initial 30 cases. *Int. J. Urol.* Vol.11, No.9, pp. 693-699

Kaouk, J.H. & Goel, R.K. (2009). Single-port laparoscopic and robotic partial nephrectomy. *Eur. Urol.*, Vol.55, No.5, pp. 1163-1169

Kihara, K.; Kageyama, Y.; Kobayashi, T.; Okuno, T.; kawakami, S.; Hayashi, T.; Masuda, H.; Suzuki, M.; Hyouchi N. & Arai G. (2002). *Portless endoscopic urological surgery*. Igaku-shoin, ISBN 4-260-13356-X, Tokyo, Japan (Japanese & English)

Kihara, K.; Kageyama, Y.; Kobayashi, T. ; Okuno, T.; Kawakami, S.; Hayashi, T.; Masuda, H.; Suzuki, M.; Hyouchi N. & Arai G. (2003). *Portless endoscopic urological surgery*. Liaoning Science and Technology Publishing House, pp. 10-185, ISBN 7-5381-3988-5, Liaoning, China (Chinese)

Kihara, K.; Kageyama, Y.; Yano, M.; Kobayashi, T.; Kawakami, S.; Fujii, Y.; Masuda, H. & Hyochi, N. (2004). Portless endoscopic radical nephrectomy via a single minimum incision in 80 patients. *Int. J. Urol.*, Vol.11, No.9, pp.714-720

Kihara, K. (2007). *Ilustrated minimum incision endoscopic urological surgery*. Igaku-shoin, pp. 1-130, Japanese, ISBN 978-4-260-00481-7, Tokyo, Japan (Japanese)

Kihara, K.; Kawakami, S.; Fujii, Y.; Masuda, H. & Koga, F. (2009a). Gasless single-port access endoscopic surgery in urology: minimum incision endoscopic surgery, MIES. *Int. J. Urol.*, Vol.16, No.10, pp.791-800

Kihara, K.; Kawakami, S.; Fujii, Y.; Masuda H.; Koga F. & Saito F. (2009b). Gasless single port access radical nephrectomy. *Eur. Urol. Suppl.*, Vol.8, No.4, pp. 392

Kihara, K.; Kobayashi. T.; Kawakami, S.; Fujii, Y.; Kageyama, H. & Masuda, H. (2010a). Minimum Incision Endoscopic Surgery (MIES)in Japanese Urology: Results of Adrenalectomy, radical nephrectomy and radical prostatectomy. *Aktuelle. Urol.*, Vol.41, Suppl.1, S15-S19

Kihara, K.; Tushima, S.; Kawakami, Y.; Fujii, Y.; Masuda H.; Koga F. & Saito F. (2010b). Gasless single port access ultrasound-guided clampless partial nephrectomy: MIES partial nephrectomy. *Eur. Urol. Suppl.*, Vol.9, N0.2, pp. 335-336

Kihara, K. (2010c). *Ilustrated minimum incision endoscopic urological surgery.* Guangxi Science and Technology Publishing House, pp. 1-130, ISBN 978-7-80763-578-9, Guangxi, China (Chinese)

Kijima, T.; Masuda,H.; Yoshida, S.; Tatokoro,M.; Araki, S.; Yokoyama, M.; Numao,N.; Okada,Y.; Saito, K.; Koga,F.; Fujii,Y. & Kihara,K. (2011). Antibiotic prophylaxis is not neccessary in minimally inasive surgery for renal and adrenal tumors: A prospective study of 301 consecutive patients. *J. Urol. Suppl.*, Vol.185, No.4, pp. 470-471

Koga, F.; Kihara, K.; Masuda, H.; Kageyama, Y.; Kawakami, S. & Kobayashi. T. (2007). Minimum incision endoscopic Nephrectomy for giant hydronephrosis. *Int. J. Urol.*, Vol.14, No.8, pp.774-776

Kommu, S.S.; Kaouk, J.H. & Rane, A. (2009). Laparo-endoscopic single-site surgery: preliminary advances in renal surgery. *BJU Int.*, Vol.103, No.8, pp1034-1037

Lee, R.S.; Sethi, A.S.; Passerotti, C.C.; Retik, A.B.; Borer, J.G.; Nguyen, H.T. & Peters, C.A. (2009). Robot assisted laparoscopic partial nephrectomy : a viable and safe option in children. *J. Urol.*, Vol.181, No.2, pp. 823-828

Ponsky ,L.E.; Cherullo, E.E.; Sawyer, M. & Hartke, D. (2008). Single access site laparoscopic radical nephrectomy:initial clinical experience. *J. Endourol.*, Vol.22, No.4, pp. 663-666

Raman, J.D.; Cadeddu, J.A.; Rao, P. & Rane, A. (2008). Single-incision laparoscopic surgery: initial urological experience and comparison with natural-orifice transluminal endoscopic surgery. *BJU Int.*, Vol.101, No.12, pp. 1493-14936

Saito, K.; Kihara, K.; Kawakami, Y.; Fujii, Y.; Masuda H. & Koga F. (2010). Gasless two port access total nephroureterectomy: MIES nephroureterectomy. *Eur. Urol. Suppl.*, Vol.9, No.2, pp. 335

Sakura, M.: Kawakami, S.; Masuda, H.; Kobayashi, T.; Kageyama, Y. & Kihara, K. (2007). Sequential bilateral minimum incision endoscopic radical nephrectomy in dialysis patients with bilateral renal cell carcinomas. *Int. J. Urol.*, Vol.14, No.12, pp.1109-1112

See, W.A.; Monk, T.G. & Weldon, B.C. (1993). Complications of laparoscopy. In: Clayman, R.V.; McDougall, E.M (eds). *Raparoscopic urology.* Quality Medical Publishing Inc., pp.183-206 ISBN 0-942219-41-4, St. Louis, MO, U.S.A.

Yokoyama, M.; Fujii, Y.; Iimura, Y.; Saito, K.; Koga, F.; Masuda, H.; Kawakami, S. & Kihara, K. (2011a). Longitudinal change in renal function after radical nephrectomy in Japanese patients with renal cortical tumors. *J. Urol.*, Vol.185, No.6, pp. 2066-2071

Yokoyama, M.; Fujii, Y.; Iimura, Y.; Saito, K.; Koga, F.; Masuda, H. & Kihara, K. (2011b). A nomogaram for predicting the development of chronic kidney disease within 2 years after radical nephrectomy in patients with renal cortical tumor. *J. Urol. Suppl.*, Vol.185, No.4, pp. 436

Yoshida, S.; Masuda, H.; Yokoyama, M.; Kobayashi, T.; Kawakami, S. & Kihara,K. (2007). Absence of prophylactic antibiotics in minimum incision endoscopic urological surgery(MEUS) of adrenal and renal tumors. *Int. J. Urol.*, Vol.14, No.5, pp. 384-387

2

Prognostic Impact of Perirenal Fat or Adrenal Gland Involvement in Renal Cell Carcinoma Exhibiting Venous Vascular Extension

Tetsuo Fujita, Masatsugu Iwamura, Shinji Kurosaka,
Ken-ichi Tabata, Kazumasa Matsumoto, Kazunari Yoshida and Shiro Baba
Department of Urology, Kitasato University School of Medicine
Japan

1. Introduction

Venous vascular extension is one of the aggressive tumor behaviors especially for renal cell carcinoma (RCC). It has been reported that 4% to 10% have tumor thrombus extending into the venous system among patients with newly diagnosed RCC (Marshall et al., 1970; Hoehn & Hermanek, 1983; Casanova & Zingg, 1991; Hatcher et al., 1991; Pagano et al., 1992). Compared with conservative treatment regimens, surgical resection remains the most effective treatment for these patients (Staehler & Brkovic, 2000). The mean 5-year survival rates of such patients with inferior vena cava involvement undergoing radical surgery for RCC have been reported as 32% to 64% (Neves & Zincke, 1987; Skinner et al., 1989; Montie et al., 1991; Swierzewski et al., 1994; Glazer & Novick, 1996).

Since the introduction of the tumor, node, metastasis (TNM) staging system, the pathologic stage has been considered the most important prognostic factor in RCC. According to the 2002 American Joint Committee on Cancer (AJCC) TNM staging classification (Greene et al., 2002), pT3 RCCs are subclassified into tumors invading perirenal fat and/or the ipsilateral adrenal gland (2002-pT3a), those presenting with tumor thrombus within the renal vein or the vena cava below the diaphragm (2002-pT3b) and those with vena cava thrombus above the diaphragm (2002-pT3c). This classification was very recently modified in 2009 (Edge et al., 2009), modified subclassification of pT3 RCCs are defined as tumors grossly extending into the renal vein or its segmental branches, or tumors invading perirenal and/or renal sinus fat but not beyond Gerota's fascia (2009-pT3a), those presenting with tumor thrombus within the vena cava below the diaphragm (2009-pT3b) and those with vena cava thrombus above the diaphragm or invaded the wall of the vena cava (2009-pT3c).

It has been debated that the TNM classification needs improvement in order to provide prognostic accuracy (Thompson et al., 2005; Leibovich et al., 2005; Ficarra et al., 2007). Several studies have discussed the correlation between prognosis and level of venous extension (Hatcher et al., 1991; Ljungberg et al., 1995; Tongaonkar et al., 1995; Glazer & Novick, 1996; Kuczyk et al., 1997; Staehler & Brkovic, 2000; Kim et al., 2004; Moinzadeh & Libertino, 2004). However, the prognostic impact of perirenal fat or adrenal gland involvement – based on the tumor characteristics of 2002 AJCC TNM staging classification

2002	2009
T1: Tumor 7 cm or less in greatest dimension, limited to the kidney	**T1:** Tumor 7 cm or less in greatest dimension, limited to the kidney
T1a: Tumor 4 cm or less in greatest dimension, limited to the kidney **T1b:** Tumor more than 4 cm but not more than 7 cm in greatest dimension, limited to the kidney	**T1a:** Tumor 4 cm or less in greatest dimension, limited to the kidney **T1b:** Tumor more than 4 cm but not more than 7 cm in greatest dimension, limited to the kidney
T2: Tumor more than 7 cm in greatest dimension, limited to the kidney	**T2:** Tumor more than 7 cm in greatest dimension, limited to the kidney
	T2a: Tumor more than 7 cm but less than or equal to 10 cm in greatest dimension, limited to the kidney **T2b:** Tumor more than 10 cm, limited to the kidney
T3: Tumor extends into major veins or invades adrenal gland or perinephric tissues but not beyond Gerota's fascia	**T3:** Tumor extends into major veins or perinephric tissues but not into the ipsilateral adrenal gland and not beyond Gerota's fascia
T3a: Tumor directly invades adrenal gland or perirenal and/or renal sinus fat but not beyond Gerota's fascia **T3b:** Tumor grossly extends into the renal vein or its segmental (muscle-containing) branches, or vena cava below the diaphragm **T3c:** Tumor grossly extends into the vena cava above the diaphragm or invades the wall of the vena cava	**T3a:** Tumor grossly extends into the renal vein or its segmental (muscle containing) branches, or tumor invades perirenal and/or renal sinus fat but not beyond Gerota's fascia **T3b:** Tumor grossly extends into the vena cava below the diaphragm **T3c:** Tumor grossly extends into the vena cava above the diaphragm or invades the wall of the vena cava
T4: Tumor invades beyond Gerota's fascia	**T4:** Tumor invades beyond Gerota's fascia (including contiguous extension into the ipsilateral adrenal gland)

Table 1. AJCC primary tumor staging classification of RCC

(2002-pT3a) – has not been seriously examined in patients with RCC exhibiting venous vascular extension. We hypothesized that RCC exhibiting venous vascular extension represents passive invasive features, since the low blood pressure in the renal vein allows tumors to easily extend into the venous system without aggressive characteristics, while perirenal fat or adrenal gland involvement represents active invasive features. Thus in this chapter, we describe the prognostic impact of perirenal fat or adrenal gland involvement in

Prognostic Impact of Perirenal Fat or Adrenal Gland Involvement in Renal Cell Carcinoma
Exhibiting Venous Vascular Extension

21

patients with RCC exhibiting venous vascular extension and the proposal for reclassification of the current TNM staging.

2. RCC exhibiting venous vascular extension

Forty-three patients with RCC exhibiting venous vascular extension entirely below the diaphragm were evaluated. Patients were treated by radical nephrectomy with complete resection of tumor thrombus extending into the venous system. Venous extension was defined as gross involvement. The patients included 35 males and 8 females, with median age at surgery of 62 years (range 43-82 years). The median tumor size was 8.79 cm (range 2.3-17.0 cm). The tumor site was on the right in 20 cases and on the left in 23 cases.

All patients received a preoperative evaluation that included routine blood test, chest x-rays, ultrasonography, and computerized tomography (CT), magnetic resonance imaging, or both. They then underwent radical nephrectomy with complete resection of the tumor and thrombus. Regional lymphadenectomy was performed concurrently with the radical nephrectomy. Postoperative evaluations, performed at intervals of 1 to 3 months, included blood test, chest x-rays, and CT. Bone scans were obtained when indicated. Hospital charts were retrospectively reviewed, and patient status was ascertained via office visit or telephone call to the patient.

All histological samples were reviewed by a single pathologist and were defined as tumor thrombus only or as tumor thrombus with perirenal fat or adrenal gland involvement.

Nonparametric estimates of survival were performed using Kaplan-Meier curves. Survival curves were generated based on disease-specific survival, representing patients still alive at specified intervals from the time of surgery to the date of death or the last follow-up visit. Log-rank tests were used for statistical comparisons.

Differences in identified prognostic parameters between tumor thrombus only and tumor thrombus with perirenal fat or adrenal gland involvement were analyzed using t test and chi-square test. Survival analysis regression model was assessed by Cox proportional hazards model to estimate the relative importance of the variables.

Additionally, nonparametric Kaplan-Meier survival estimates were performed to compare perirenal fat or adrenal gland involvement only (2002-pT3a), tumor thrombus only, and tumor thrombus with perirenal fat or adrenal gland involvement. The perirenal fat or adrenal gland involvement only (2002-pT3a) cohort represented 65 cases with complete resection of the tumor. Survival curves and log-rank tests were analyzed.

3. Prognostic impact of perirenal fat or adrenal gland involvement

3.1 Patient characteristics

The tumor thrombus only cohort included 21 males and 2 females (total 23 patients; 53.5%) with a median age of 61 years (range 44-78 years) and median follow-up period of 37 months (range 2-106 months). The median tumor size was 9.0 cm (range 2.3-17.0 cm); tumor site was on the right in 10 cases and on the left in 13 cases.

The tumor thrombus with perirenal fat or adrenal gland involvement cohort included 14 males and 6 females (total 20 patients; 46.5%) with a median age of 64 years (range 43-82 years) and median follow-up period of 9.5 months (range 2-45 months). The median tumor size was 8.45 cm (range 4.0-16.0 cm); tumor site was on the right in 10 cases and on the left in 10 cases.

When several parameters were analyzed for differences between tumor thrombus only cohort and tumor thrombus with perirenal fat or adrenal gland involvement cohort using t test or chi-square test, two parameters – Eastern Cooperative Oncology Group (ECOG) performance status (PS) 0 and histological grade 3 – proved statistically significant (P = 0.0329 and 0.0377, respectively; chi-square test).

Characteristic	Tumor thrombus only	Tumor thrombus with perirenal fat or adrenal gland involvement	P Value
Patients (n)	23	20	–
Follow-up period (month)			
Median	37	9.5	
Range	2-106	2-45	–
Age $ (year)			
Median	61	64	
Range	44-78	43-82	–
Mean ± SE	60.1 ± 1.9	64.3 ± 2.3	0.1673
Gender (n)			
Male	21	14	
Female	2	6	0.1180
Tumor diameter $ (cm)			
Median	9.0	8.45	
Range	2.3-17.0	4.0-16.0	–
Mean ± SE	9.0 ± 0.9	8.3 ± 0.8	0.5240
Tumor site (n)			
Right	10	10	
Left	13	10	–
ECOG PS 0 * (n)	15	6	0.0329
Initial symptom (n)	21	16	0.3929
Preoperative metastasis (n)	5	8	0.3184
Grade 3 * (n)	1	6	0.0377
pN (n)	1	5	0.0814
Clear cell (n)	21	14	0.1180
Spindle cell (n)	0	3	0.0924

KEY: ECOG PS = *Eastern Cooperative Oncology Group performance status.*
$ *Analysis assessed by* t *test.*
* *Statistically significant.*

Table 2. Patient characteristics and comparison among groups

3.2 Kaplan-Meier survival analysis

Nonparametric survival was analyzed by Kaplan-Meier survival curves, plotting both tumor thrombus only and tumor thrombus with perirenal fat or adrenal gland involvement.

Prognostic Impact of Perirenal Fat or Adrenal Gland Involvement in Renal Cell Carcinoma
Exhibiting Venous Vascular Extension

23

Mean disease-specific survival time for patients with tumor thrombus with perirenal fat or
adrenal gland involvement was 25.0 ± 4.4 (SE) months. On the other hand, mean survival
time for those with tumor thrombus only was significantly longer at 70.9 ± 9.1 (SE) months
(P = 0.0032, Fig. 1).

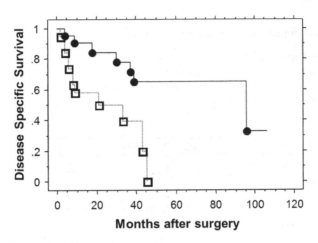

Fig. 1. Kaplan-Meier disease-specific survival after nephrectomy

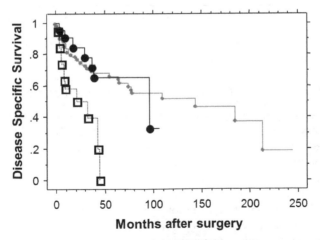

Fig. 2. Kaplan-Meier disease-specific survival after nephrectomy for those with perirenal fat
or adrenal gland involvement only (2002-pT3a)

Mean disease-specific survival time for patients with perirenal fat or adrenal gland involvement only (2002-pT3a) was longer still at 116.1 ± 12.3 (SE) months. This value is significantly longer than for those with tumor thrombus with perirenal fat or adrenal gland involvement (P = 0.0044, Fig. 2), but not statistically significant different from that for those with tumor thrombus only.

3.3 Cox proportional hazards regression analysis

Univariate Cox proportional hazards regression analysis was performed for each variable. Significantly shorter disease-specific survival after surgery was predicted by presence of perirenal fat or adrenal gland involvement (P = 0.0065), preoperative metastasis (P = 0.0025), surgical specimens positive for lymph node metastasis (P = 0.0183), and spindle cell factor (P = 0.0233).

Variable	Hazard Ratio	95% CI	P Value
Perirenal fat or adrenal gland involvement *	4.11	1.49–11.4	0.0065
ECOG PS 0	1.34	0.54–3.34	0.5303
Initial symptom	2.13	0.28–16.2	0.4639
Preoperative metastasis *	4.32	1.68–11.2	0.0025
Tumor diameter	1.03	0.90–1.17	0.6984
Grade 3	0.34	0.11–1.11	0.0732
pN *	0.30	0.11–0.81	0.0183
Clear cell	1.76	0.57–5.39	0.3248
Spindle cell *	0.16	0.03–0.78	0.0233

KEY: CI = *confidence interval; ECOG PS = Eastern Cooperative Oncology Group performance status.*
* Statistically significant.

Table 3. Univariate analysis by Cox proportional hazards model

4. Prognostic factors for RCC exhibiting venous vascular extension

Although the pathologic stage highly correlates with outcome in patients with RCC, the prognosis may vary even among tumors of the same stage. Thus, additional prognostic factors are needed. For RCCs exhibiting venous vascular extension, several investigators have described the prognostic significance of the level of venous extension (Hatcher et al., 1991; Ljungberg et al., 1995; Tongaonkar et al., 1995; Glazer & Novick, 1996; Kuczyk et al., 1997; Staehler & Brkovic, 2000). Most recent series have reported that the level of tumor thrombosis in the inferior vena cava does not significantly effect long-term survival (Kim et al., 2004; Moinzadeh & Libertino, 2004). Local tumor stage and grade are better predictors of prognosis than extent of venous involvement (Kim et al., 2004), but the most significant factors for survival in patients with RCC exhibiting venous vascular extension are still unknown.

The impact of perirenal fat or adrenal gland involvement in patients with RCC exhibiting venous vascular extension has not been seriously examined. Only the impact of perirenal fat involvement on prognosis of RCC patients has been documented (Gettman et al., 2003). On multivariate analyses, perirenal fat involvement led to a significantly worse prognosis, as did histological grade and metastasis (Gettman et al., 2003). However, perirenal fat involvement cannot be simply categorized, given the data we present here for the category of tumor thrombus with perirenal fat or adrenal gland involvement. This is the first investigation to specifically examine RCCs exhibiting tumor thrombus with perirenal fat or adrenal gland involvement and suggest that they represent a separate subcategory.

Tumor thrombus with perirenal fat or adrenal gland involvement has shorter disease-specific survival time than tumor thrombus only, or perirenal fat or adrenal gland involvement only (2002-pT3a). Tumors that are both tumor thrombus and perirenal fat or adrenal gland involvement are not the same as those that are only tumor thrombus. If patients with tumor thrombus also have perirenal fat or adrenal gland involvement, the prognosis is significantly poorer. The 5-year disease-specific survival estimate for tumor thrombus only was 65%, while that for tumor thrombus with perirenal fat or adrenal gland involvement was 0%. On univariate analyses, perirenal fat or adrenal gland involvement, preoperative metastasis, positive lymph node metastasis, and spindle cell factor were significant predictors of poor prognosis. Metastatic disease has been reported as an adverse predictor of disease-specific survival by several investigators (Neves & Zincke, 1987; Hatcher et al., 1991; Swierzewski et al., 1994; Tongaonkar et al., 1995; Nesbitt et al., 1997; Gettman et al., 2003). Generally, histological grade is identified as an independent prognostic factor in all RCCs (Méjean at al., 2003), but our results suggest histological grade does not affect survival in patients specifically having RCCs exhibiting tumor thrombus with perirenal fat or adrenal gland involvement.

5. Adrenal gland involvement in RCC

Patients with adrenal gland involvement have significantly worse survival than those with perirenal fat involvement (Han et al., 2003; Siemer et al., 2005). Direct ipsilateral adrenal gland involvement in RCC is rare, found in only 2.5% of radical nephrectomy specimens, and representing 13% of all 2002-pT3a lesions (Han et al., 2003). In this study, there were too few patients with RCCs exhibiting tumor thrombus with perirenal fat or adrenal gland involvement to allow a comparison of survival for patients with adrenal gland or perirenal fat involvement. However, previous investigators have emphasized that adrenal gland involvement should reclassified because of the worse prognosis (Han et al., 2003; Siemer et al., 2005; Fujita et al., 2008). According to the 2002 AJCC TNM staging classification (Greene et al., 2002), pT4 RCC is defined as tumor invades beyond Gerota's fascia. The median disease-specific survival for patients with ipsilateral adrenal gland involvement was significantly worse than that for tumor infiltrating only the perirenal fat and was similar to that for patients with 2002-pT4 RCCs (Han et al., 2003). The 5-year disease-specific survival probabilities have been reported 20.2% (Thompson et al., 2005) and 0% (Fujita et al., 2008). Primary adrenal carcinoma that invades the kidney is classified as pT4 disease (Ng & Libertino, 2003; Norton et al., 2005). A number of previous reports have suggested that, analogously, RCC with adrenal gland involvement should be reclassified as 2002-pT4 (Sandock et al., 1997; Han et al., 2003; Siemer et al., 2005; Thompson et al., 2005). Based on these investigations, adrenal gland involvement has been classified pT4 in 2009 AJCC TNM staging classification (Edge et al., 2009).

6. Proposal for reclassification of the TNM staging

According to a commentary by the Union Internationale Contre le Cancer (UICC) regarding continuous improvement of the TNM classification, the criteria for instituting changes include clinical relevance for assessment, treatment and outcome, presence of evidence for improved prognostic ability, and acceptance by the members of the UICC TNM committee (Gospodarowicz et al., 2004). The 2002 AJCC TNM system for patients with pT3 RCC incorporates the features of tumor thrombus, perirenal fat invasion and direct ipsilateral adrenal gland involvement (Greene et al., 2002). Several studies addressing 2002-pT3 staging have been reported and debated (Thompson et al., 2005; Leibovich et al., 2005; Ficarra et al., 2007; Fujita et al., 2008). And very recently, AJCC TNM staging classification was updated (Edge et al., 2009). However, tumor thrombus with perirenal fat or adrenal gland involvement was not well included in this modification. The prognosis of patients with tumor thrombus with perirenal fat or adrenal gland involvement was poor, as well as adrenal gland involvement which was subclassified as pT4 in 2009 AJCC TNM classification (Fujita et al., 2008; Edge et al., 2009). Reclassification will be still needed for tumor thrombus with perirenal fat or adrenal gland involvement RCCs. Reclassification of the current TNM staging system for RCCs according to the available clinical data and in accordance with the proposed process to update the staging system will render it a more powerful tool for predicting patient outcomes (Ficarra et al., 2006). The resultant staging system should be intended to give prognostic information that will allow accurate patient counseling, therapeutic selection, and surveillance (Howard & Wood, 2006). Our suggested revisions to the TNM classification represent a significant improvement in its prognostic accuracy.

7. Conclusion

The presence of perirenal fat or adrenal gland involvement in patients with RCC exhibiting venous vascular extension entirely below the diaphragm leads to a significantly poorer prognosis. Presence of perirenal fat or adrenal gland involvement is important for such cases and calls for active investigation. Additionally, reclassification will be needed for tumor thrombus with perirenal fat or adrenal gland involvement RCCs.

8. References

Casanova, G.A. & Zingg, E.J. (1991). Inferior Vena Caval Tumor Extension in Renal Cell Carcinoma. *Urologia Internationalis*, Vol.47, No.4, (no date), pp. 216-218, ISSN 0042-1138

Edge, S.B., Byrd, D.R., Compton, C.C., Fritz, A.G., Greene, F.L. & Trotti, A., III. (2009). *AJCC Cancer Staging Manual* (7th ed.), Springer, ISBN 978-0-387-88440-0, New York, United States of America

Ficarra, V. & Artibani, W. (2006). Staging System of Renal Cell Carcinoma: Current Issues. *European Urology*, Vol.49, No.2, (February 2006), pp. 223-225, ISSN 0302-2838

Ficarra, V., Novara, G., Iafrate, M., Cappellaro, L., Bratti, E., Zattoni, F. & Artibani, W. (2007). Proposal for Reclassification of the TNM Staging System in Patients with Locally Advanced (pT3-4) Renal Cell Carcinoma According to the Cancer-Related Outcome. *European Urology*, Vol.51, No.3, (May 2007), pp. 722-731, ISSN 0302-2838

Fujita, T., Iwamura, M., Yanagisawa, N., Muramoto, M., Okayasu, I. & Baba, S. (2008). Reclassification of the Current Tumor, Node, Metastasis Staging in pT3 Renal Cell Carcinoma. *International Journal of Urology*, Vol.15, No.7, (July 2008), pp. 582-586, ISSN 1442-2042

Prognostic Impact of Perirenal Fat or Adrenal Gland Involvement in Renal Cell Carcinoma
Exhibiting Venous Vascular Extension

27

Gettman, M.T., Boelter, C.W., Cheville, J.C., Zincke, H., Bryant, S.C. & Blute, M.L. (2003). Charlson Co-Morbidity Index as a Predictor of Outcome after Surgery for Renal Cell Carcinoma with Renal Vein, Vena Cava or Right Atrium Extension. *Journal of Urology*, Vol.169, No.4, (April 2003), pp. 1282-1286, ISSN 0022-5347

Glazer, A.A. & Novick, A.C. (1996). Long-term Followup after Surgical Treatment for Renal Cell Carcinoma Extending into the Right Atrium. *Journal of Urology*, Vol.155, No.2, (February 1996), pp. 448-450, ISSN 0022-5347

Gospodarowicz, M.K., Miller, D., Groome, P.A., Greene, F.L., Logan, P.A. & Sobin, L.H. (2004). The Process for Continuous Improvement of the TNM Classification. *Cancer*, Vol.100, No.1, (January 2004), pp. 1-5, ISSN 1097-0142

Greene, F.L., Page, D.L., Fleming, I.D., Fritz, A.G., Balch, C.M., Haller, D.G. & Morrow M. (2002). *AJCC Cancer Staging Manual* (6th ed.), Springer-Verlag, ISBN 978-0-387-95271-0, New York, United States of America

Han, K.R., Bui, M.H., Pantuck, A.J., Freitas, D.G., Leibovich, B.C., Dorey, F.J., Zisman, A., Janzen, N.K., Mukouyama, H., Figlin, R.A. & Belldegrun, A.S. (2003). TNM T3a Renal Cell Carcinoma: Adrenal Gland Involvement is not the Same as Renal Fat Invasion. *Journal of Urology*, Vol.169, No3, (March 2003), pp. 899-904, ISSN 0022-5347

Hatcher, P.A., Anderson, E.E., Paulson, D.F., Carson, C.C. & Robertson, J.E. (1991). Surgical Management and Prognosis of Renal Cell Carcinoma Invading the Vena Cava. *Journal of Urology*, Vol.145, No.1, (January 1991), pp. 20-24, ISSN 0022-5347

Hoehn, W. & Hermanek, P. (1983). Invasion of Veins in Renal Cell Carcinoma-Frequency, Correlation and Prognosis. *European Urology*, Vol.9, No.5, (no date), pp. 276-280, ISSN 0302-2838

Howard, G.E. & Wood, C.G. (2006). Staging Refinements in Renal Cell Carcinoma. *Current Opinion in Urology*, Vol.16, No.5, (September 2006), pp. 317-320, ISSN 0963-0643

Kim, H.L., Zisman, A., Han, K.R., Figlin, R.A. & Belldegrun, A.S. (2004). Prognostic Significance of Venous Thrombus in Renal Cell Carcinoma. Are Renal Vein and Inferior Vena Cava Involvement Different? *Journal of Urology*, Vol.171, No.2 pt 1, (February 2004), pp. 588-591, ISSN 0022-5347

Kuczyk, M.A., Bokemeyer, C., Köhn, G., Stief, C.G., Machtens, S., Truss, M., Höfner, K. & Jonas, U. (1997). Prognostic Relevance of Intracaval Neoplastic Extension for Patients with Renal Cell Cancer. *British Journal of Urology*, Vol.80, No.1, (July 1997), pp. 18-24, ISSN 0007-1331

Leibovich, B.C., Cheville, J.C., Lohse, C.M., Zincke, H., Kwon, E.D., Frank, I., Thompson, R.H. & Blute, M.L. (2005). Cancer Specific Survival for Patients with pT3 Renal Cell Carcinoma—Can the 2002 Primary Tumor Classification be Improved? *Journal of Urology*, Vol.173, No.3, (March 2005), pp. 716-719, ISSN 0022-5347

Ljungberg, B., Stenling, R., Österdahl, B., Farrelly, E., Åberg T. & Roos G. (1995). Vein Invasion in Renal Cell Carcinoma: Impact on Metastatic Behavior and Survival. *Journal of Urology*, Vol.154, No.5, (November 1995), pp. 1681-1684, ISSN 0022-5347

Marshall, V.F., Middleton, R.G., Holswade, G.R. & Goldsmith, E.I. (1970). Surgery for Renal Cell Carcinoma in the Vena Cava. *Journal of Urology*, Vol.103, No.4, (April 1970), pp. 414-420, ISSN 0022-5347

Méjean, A., Oudard, S. & Thiounn, N. (2003). Prognostic Factors of Renal Cell Carcinoma. *Journal of Urology*, Vol.169, No.3, (March 2003), pp. 821-827, ISSN 0022-5347

Moinzadeh, A. & Libertino, J.A. (2004). Prognostic Significance of Tumor Thrombus Level in Patients with Renal Cell Carcinoma and Venous Tumor Thrombus Extension. Is All T3b the Same? *Journal of Urology*, Vol.171, No.2 pt 1, (February 2004), pp. 598-601, ISSN 0022-5347

Montie, J.E., el Ammar, R., Pontes, J.E., Medendorp, S.V., Novick, A.C., Streem, S.B., Kay, R.
    Montague, D.K. & Cosgrove D.M. (1991). Renal Cell Carcinoma with Inferior Vena
    Cava Tumor Thrombi. *Surgery, Gynecology and Obstetrics*, Vol.173, No.2, (August
    1991), pp. 107-115, ISSN 0039-6087
Nesbitt, J.C., Soltero, E.R., Dinney, C.P., Walsh, G.L., Schrump, D.S., Swanson, D.A., Pisters,
    L.L., Willis, K.D. & Putnam, J.B., Jr. (1997). Surgical Management of Renal Cell
    Carcinoma with Inferior Vena Cava Tumor Thrombus. *Annals of Thoracic Surgery*,
    Vol.63, No.6, (June 1997), pp. 1592-1600, ISSN 0003-4975
Neves, R.J. & Zincke, H. (1987). Surgical Treatment of Renal Cancer with Vena Cava
    Extension. *British Journal of Urology*, Vol.59, No.5, (May 1987), pp. 390-395, ISSN
    0007-1331
Ng, L. & Libertino, J.M. (2003). Adrenocortical Carcinoma: Diagnosis, Evaluation and
    Treatment. *Journal of Urology*, Vol.169, No.1, (January 2003), pp. 5-11, ISSN 0022-5347
Norton, J.A. (2005). Adrenal tumors, In: *Cancer: Principles and Practice of Oncology* (7th ed.),
    DeVita, V.T. Jr., Hellman, S., Rosenberg, S.A. (eds.), pp. 1528-1540, Lippincott
    Williams & Wilkins, ISBN 0-781-74450-4, Philadelphia, United States of America
Pagano, F., Dal Bianco, M., Artibani, W., Pappagallo, G. & Prayer Galetti, T. (1992). Renal
    Cell Carcinoma with Extension into the Inferior Vena Cava: Problems in Diagnosis,
    Staging and Treatment. *European Urology*, Vol.22, No.3, (September 1992), pp. 200-
    203, ISSN 0302-2838
Sandock, D.S., Seftel, A.D. & Resnick, M.I. (1997). Adrenal Metastases from Renal Cell
    Carcinoma: Role of Ipsilateral Adrenalectomy and Definition of Stage. *Urology*,
    Vol.49, No.1, (January 1997), pp. 28-31, ISSN 0090-4295
Siemer, S., Lehmann, J., Loch, A., Becker, F., Stein, U., Schneider, G., Ziegler, M. & Stöckle, M.
    (2005). Current TNM Classification of Renal Cell Carcinoma Evaluated: Revising Stage
    T3a. *Journal of Urology*, Vol.173, No.1, (January 2005), pp. 33-37, ISSN 0022-5347
Skinner, D.G., Pritchett, T.R., Lieskovsky, G., Boyd, S.D. & Stiles, Q.R. (1989). Vena Caval
    Involvement by Renal Cell Carcinoma. Surgical Resection Provides Meaningful
    Long-term Survival. *Annals of Surgery*, Vol.210, No.3, (September 1989), pp. 387-394,
    ISSN 0003-4932
Staehler, G. & Brkovic, D. (2000). The Role of Radical Surgery for Renal Cell Carcinoma with
    Extension into the Vena Cava. *Journal of Urology*, Vol.163, No.6, (June 2000), pp.
    1671-1675, ISSN 0022-5347
Swierzewski, D.J., Swierzewski, M.J. & Libertino, J.A. (1994). Radical Nephrectomy in
    Patients with Renal Cell Carcinoma with Venous, Vena Caval, and Atrial
    Extension. *American Journal of Surgery*, Vol.168, No.2, (August 1994), pp. 205-209,
    ISSN 0002-9610
Thompson, R.H., Cheville, J.C., Lohse, C.M., Webster, W.S., Zincke, H., Kwon, E.D., Frank,
    I., Blute, M.L. & Leibovich, B.C. (2005). Reclassification of Patients with pT3 and
    pT4 Renal Cell Carcinoma Improves Prognostic Accuracy. *Cancer*, Vol.104, No.1,
    (July 2005), pp 53-60, ISSN 1097-0142
Thompson, R.H., Leibovich, B.C., Cheville, J.C., Lohse, C.M., Frank, I., Kwon, E.D., Zincke,
    H. & Blute, M.L. (2005). Should Direct Ipsilateral Adrenal Gland Invasion from
    Renal Cell Carcinoma be Classified as pT3a? *Journal of Urology*, Vol.173, No.3,
    (March 2005), pp. 918-921, ISSN 0022-5347
Tongaonkar, H.B., Dandekar, N.P., Dalal, A.V., Kulkarni, J.N. & Kamat, M.R. (1995). Renal
    Cell Carcinoma Extending to the Renal Vein and Inferior Vena Cava: Results of
    Surgical Treatment and Prognostic Factors. *Journal of Surgical Oncology*, Vol.59,
    No.2, (June 1995), pp. 94-100, ISSN 0022-4790

3

Laparoscopic Partial Nephrectomy – Current State of the Art

Paul D'Alessandro, Shawn Dason and Anil Kapoor

Divison of Urology, Department of Surgery McMaster University, Hamilton, Ontario, Canada

1. Introduction

Clayman et al described the first successful laparoscopic nephrectomy in 1991 [1]. Since that time, laparoscopic radical nephrectomy has become the standard of care for renal tumors. At the same time, the widespread use of contemporary imaging techniques has resulted in an increased detection of small incidental renal tumors. In efforts to avoid chronic kidney disease, the management of the small renal mass has trended away from radical nephrectomy toward nephron-conserving surgery. In 1993, successful laparoscopic partial nephrectomy (LPN) was first reported in a porcine model [2]. Winfield et al reported the first human LPN in 1993 [3]. From that time, centres around the world have developed laparoscopic techniques for partial nephrectomy through retroperitoneal and transperitoneal approaches. Classically, only small, peripheral, exophytic tumors were eligible for LPN, but larger, infiltrating tumors have been managed with LPN in more recent series [4].

Currently, partial nephrectomy is a standard of care treatment for the surgical management of localized renal tumors <4cm [5], and recommended in guidelines published by the American Urological Association [6] and European Association of Urology [7]. LPN combines the benefits of nephron-sparing surgery and laparoscopy to decrease the morbidity of partial nephrectomy.

The LPN technique has evolved significantly over the past decade such that its safety and efficacy rival those of open partial nephrectomy (OPN) and laparoscopic radical nephrectomy (LRN) techniques for tumors less than 4cm. LPN produces low overall morbidity, faster post-operative recovery, and comparable oncologic outcomes compared to other techniques.

Technical difficulty in LPN is encountered when securing renal hypothermia, renal parenchymal hemostasis, pelvicalyceal reconstruction, and parenchymal renorrhaphy by pure laparoscopic techniques. The appropriate and optimal length of warm ischemia time (WIT) remains particularly controversial. Nevertheless, ongoing advances in laparoscopic techniques and operator skills have allowed the development of a reliable technique that duplicates the established principles and technical steps underpinning open partial nephrectomy. With the advent of the da Vinci Surgical System (Intuitive Surgical, Sunnyvale, CA, USA), robot-assisted LPN (RPN) has advanced laparoscopic techniques even further. In this chapter we evaluate the role of LPN in the nephron-sparing armamentarium.

2.1 Indications and contraindications

Partial nephrectomy is performed for benign and malignant renal conditions. In the setting of malignant renal diseases, this is indicated in situations where radical nephrectomy would leave the patient anephric due to bilateral renal tumors or unilateral tumor and compromised or at risk the other side. Some investigators also defined the role of elective PN in patients with unilateral renal tumors and normal contralateral kidneys to reduce the risk of developing chronic kidney disease in the future [8].

Due to its technical limitations, LPN was initially reserved for select patients with small, peripheral, superficial, superficial, and exophytic tumors. As laparoscopic experience increased, the use of LPN was expanded to technically challenging tumors, such as tumors invading deeply into the parenchyma up to the collecting system or renal sinus, intrarenal tumors, tumors abutting the renal hilum, tumors in solitary kidneys, or tumors substantial enough to require heminephrectomies. Recent series include larger, Stage T1b tumours [9-11]; endophytic tumours near the hilum and upper pole [12]; bilateral tumors [13]; multiple ipsilateral tumors [14]; and stage T1a tumours presenting in select patients over the age of 70 [15].

General contraindications to abdominal laparoscopic surgery are applied to LPN. Specific absolute contraindications to LPN include bleeding diathesis (such as renal failure induced platelet dysfunction and blood thinners), renal vein thrombus, and aggressive locally advanced disease. Morbid obesity and a history of prior renal surgery may prohibitively increase the technical complexity of the procedure and should be considered a relative contraindication for LPN. Overall, the ultimate decision to proceed with LPN should be based on the tumor characteristics and the surgeon's skill and experience with such an approach.

2.2 Preoperative preparation

Preoperative evaluation includes routine preoperative investigations as well as a computed tomography angiogram of the abdomen to delineate renal vasculature. Renal scintigraphy is obtained if there is a question about the global renal function. Preoperative medical clearance should be obtained when there is any question of the patient's fitness for major abdominal or vascular surgery. We routinely cross-match 4 units of packed red blood cells on demand. Mechanical bowel preparation of one bottle of magnesium citrate is given the evening before the surgery, and intravenous prophylactic antibiotics are given prior to entering the operating room.

2.3 Operative technique

A substantive LPN entails renal hilar control, transection of major intrarenal vessels, controlled entry into and repair of the collecting system, control of parenchymal blood vessels, and renal parenchymal reconstruction, all usually under the pressure of minimizing warm ischemia. As such, significant experience in the minimally invasive environment, including expertise with time-sensitive intracorporeal suturing, is essential. LPN can be approached either transperitoneally (our preferred approach) or retroperitoneally based on the surgeon's experience and the tumor location. The transperitoneal approach is usually chosen for anterior, anterolateral, lateral, and upper-pole apical tumors. Retroperitoneal laparoscopy is reserved for posterior or posterolaterally located tumors. A retrospective, match-pair comparison of 105 patients who underwent either transperitoneal or retroperitoneal approaches for T1a renal masses demonstrated that both approaches provide comparable surgical and functional results [16]. Although studies report shorter operative time, decreased blood loss and shorter hospital stay with the retroperitoneal approach [16, 17], many centers prefer the transperitoneal approach for its greater working space and easy tumor accessibility[18].

After induction of general anesthesia, a Foley catheter and nasogastric tube are placed prior to patient positioning. Cystoscopy and ureteral catheter placement are performed if preoperative imaging indicates a risk of collecting system violation during resection of the lesion (a-requirement for intraparenchymal resection greater than 1.5 cm or tumor abutting the collecting system). Although many laparoscopists prefer to place their patients at a 45 to 60° angle in · the flank position, we prefer to place our patients undergoing renal surgery in the lateral flank position at 90°. This provides excellent access to the hilum and allows the bowel and spleen (on the left side) to fall off the renal hilum during procedures complicated by bowel distention.

Laparoscopic surgery is performed using a transperitoneal approach with a Veress needle, directly using the Optiview (Ethicon Endo-surgery ®) trocar system, or using the Hassan technique, to attain pneumoperitoneum. Three to four ports (including two 10-12 mm ports) are routinely placed in our technique. Exposure of the kidney and the hilar dissection are performed using a J-hook electrocautery suction probe or by using the ultrasound energy-based harmonic shears (Ethicon Endo-surgery ®) This is done by reflecting the mesocolon along the Line of Toldt, leaving Gerota's fascia intact. Mobilizing the kidney within this fascia, the ureter is retracted laterally, and cephalad dissection is carried out along the psoas muscle leading to the renal hilum. Once the tumour is localized, we dissect the Gerota's fascia and defat the kidney, leaving only the perinephric fat overlying tumor (Figure 8.1). Intraoperative ultrasonography with a Philips Entos LAP 9-5 linear array transducer (Philips ®) can be used to aid in tumor localization if it is not exophytic or if the tumor is deep into the renal parenchyma. A laparoscopic vascular clamp (Karl Storz ®) is placed around both the renal artery and the renal vein (without separation of the vessels) for hilar control in cases associated with central masses and heminephrectomy procedures, as described by Gill et al [19] (Figures 8.2-8.4).

Conversely, during a retroperitoneoscopic nephrectomy, the renal artery and vein are dissected separately to prepare for placement of bulldog clamps on the renal artery and vein individually. Mannitol may be used (0.5 g/kg intravenously) prior to hilar clamping or renal hypothermia. Resection of renal parenchyma is performed with cold scissors (Figures 8.5-8.10), and the specimen is retrieved using a 10-cm laparoscopic EndoCatch bag (US Surgical Corporation, Norwalk, Connecticut ®) and sent for frozen section analysis (sometimes with excisional biopsy from the base) to determine the resection margin status (Figures 8.17 and 8.18).

Hemostasis is accomplished using intracorporeal suturing, argon beam coagulator, and hemostatic matrix (Floseal®, Baxter, Vienna, Austria) application in a manner previously described by others (Figures 8.10-8.16) [20-23].

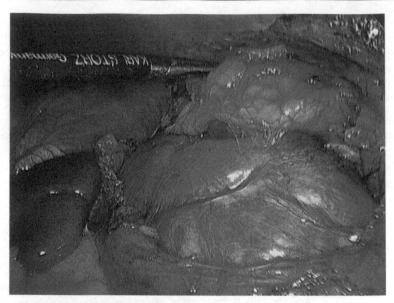

Fig. 8.1. Defatted kidney except area overlying the tumor

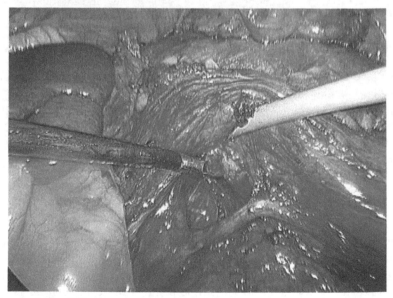

Fig. 8.2. Exposed renal hilum.

Intravenous injection of indigo carmine dye is used to delineate any collecting system violation, or retrograde injection of this dye via a ureteric catheter if it was inserted perioperatively. Any identifiable leak in the collecting system is oversewn with 4-0 absorbable sutures using the freehand intracorporeal laparoscopic technique.

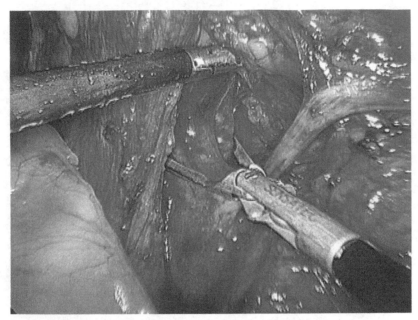

Fig. 8.3. Exposed hilum ready for clamping.

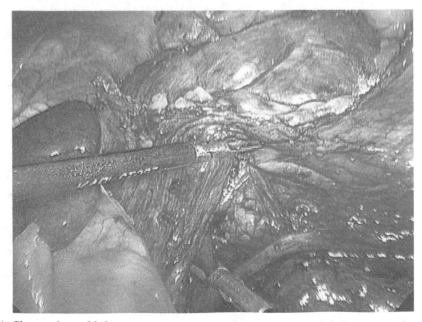

Fig. 8.4. Clamped renal hilum

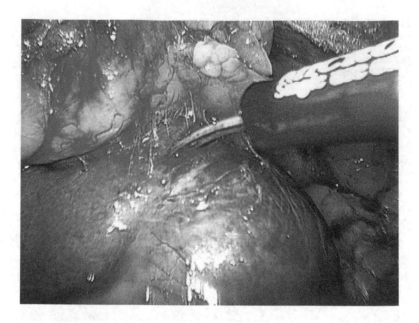

Fig. 8.5. Tumor resection using the cold scissor.

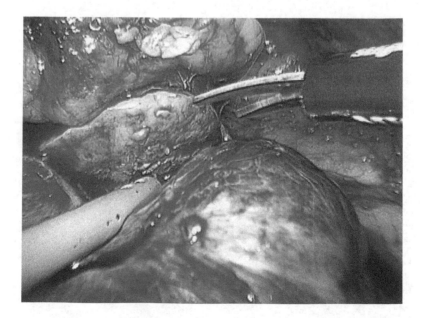

Fig. 8.6. continued tumor resection with surrounding normal parenchyma.

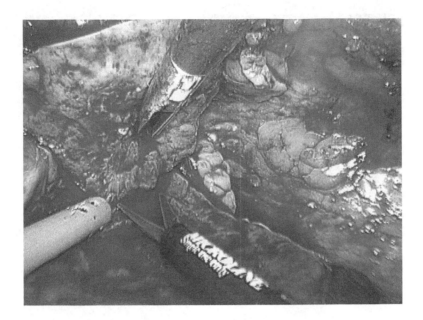

Fig. 8.7. Continued tumor resection.

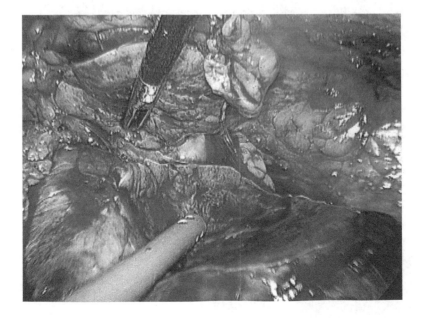

Fig. 8.8. Completely detached tumor.

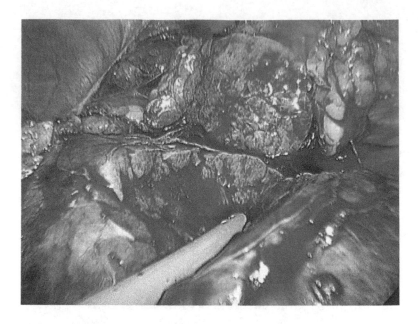

Fig. 8.9. Completely detached tumor with good surrounding parenchyma.

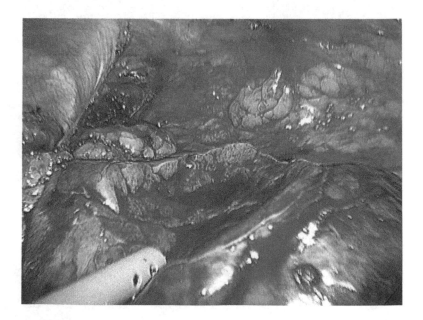

Fig. 8.10. Tumor bed.

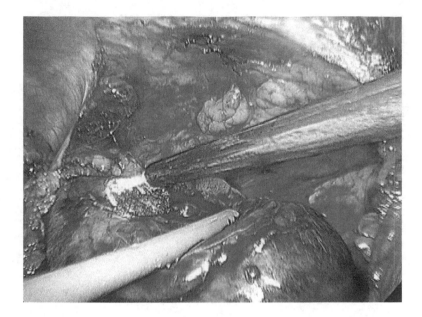

Fig. 8.11. Argon beam coagulator for bed hemostasis.

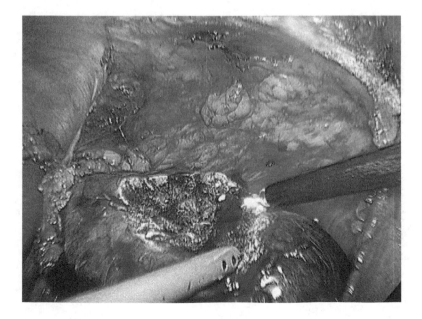

Fig. 8.12. Argon beam coagulator for bed hemostasis.

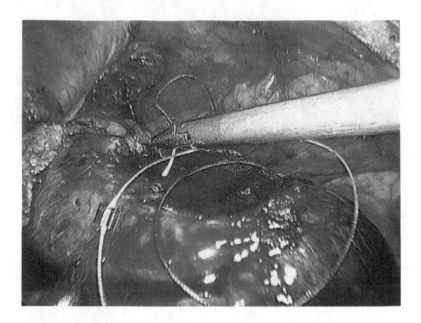

Fig. 8.13. Parenchymal intracorporeal suturing with Lapra-TY at one end.

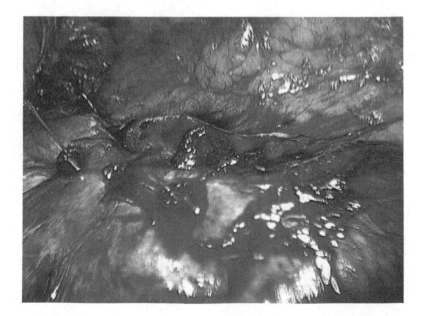

Fig. 8.14. Completed sutures with Lapra-TY on both ends.

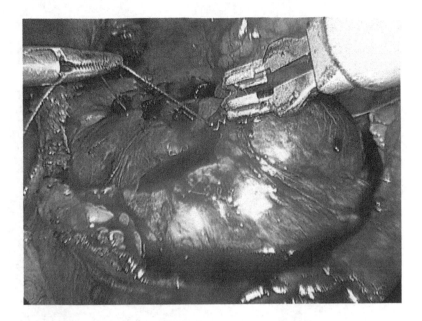

Fig. 8.15. Parenchymal suturing with Lapra-TY.

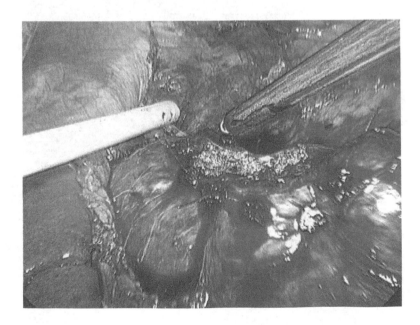

Fig. 8.16. Hemostasis with Argon beam coagulator after hilar unclamping.

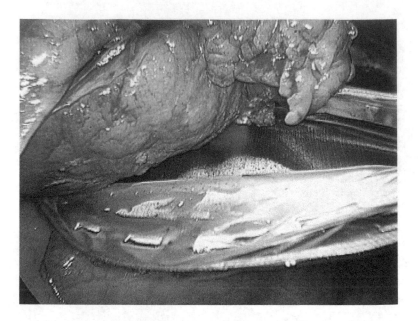

Fig. 8.17. Tumor entrapment in an Endocatch bag.

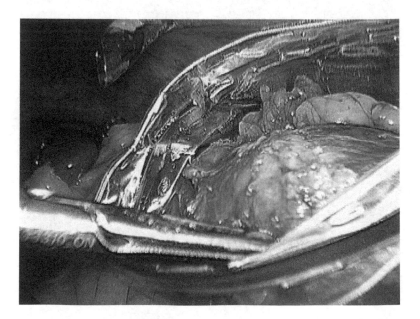

Fig. 8.18. Tumor completely entrapped.

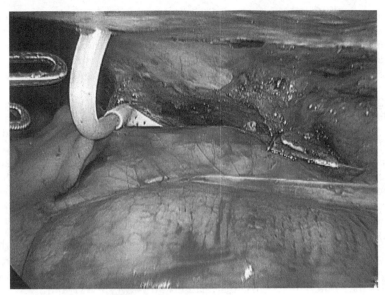

Fig. 8.19. Percutanous drain around the operated site.

If the collecting system is entered, ureteral stenting additional to a Jackson-Pratt percutanous drain placement is routinely performed (Figure 8.19). Specific figure-of-eight sutures are placed at the site of visible individual transected intrarenal vessels using a CT-1 needle and 2-0 Vicryl suture. Parenchymal closure is achieved by placing prefashioned rolled tubes or packets of oxidized cellulose sheets (Fibrillar®, Ethicon) into the parenchymal defect. Braided 2-0 absorbable sutures are used to bolster the sheets into position, and Floseal ® is applied over the operative site using a laparoscopic applicator. We perform our parenchymal repair using multiple interrupted 2-0 absorbable sutures and securing them in position using absorbable polydioxanone polymer suture clips (Lapra-TY®, Ethicon, Endosurgery). Placing one Lapra-TY clip to the end of the suture then another one to the opposite side after compressing the kidney achieves this (Figures 8.13-8.15). Surgeons can also use Hem-o-Lok ® in the place of Lapra-Ty ® for parenchymal compression, or the combination of the two for a "sliding technique".

This modification has resulted in a significant reduction of our warm ischemia time that was consumed primarily by intracorporeal suturing. Once renorrhaphy is completed, the vascular clamp is released, and the complete hemostasis and renal revascularization is confirmed. Whenever possible, the perinephric fat and Gerota's fascia is re-approximated. We extract the resected tumor along with its containing bag through a small extension of the lowermost abdominal port site incision. Laparoscopic exit under direct vision is performed once the 10-12 mm ports are closed.

3. Issues in laparoscoplc partial nephrectomy

3.1 Warm ischemia and renal hypothermia

The highly differentiated cellular architecture of the kidney is dependent on the primarily aerobic renal metabolism. As such, the kidney is acutely vulnerable to the anaerobic insult conferred by warm ischemia. The severity of renal injury and its reversibility are directly proportional to the period of warm ischemia time (WIT) imposed on the unprotected kidney. The optimal warm ischemia time remains controversial. Previous studies demonstrated that recovery of renal function is complete within minutes after 10 minutes of warm ischemia, within hours after 20 minutes, within 3 to 9 days after 30 minutes, usually within weeks after 60 minutes, and incomplete or absent after 120 minutes of warm ischemia [24-26]. A 5-year, multi-centre study of WIT in LPN vs. OPN cases (n=1800) reported that the mean WIT was 30.7 minutes and 20 minutes, respectively, in each group [27]. Though the incidence of pre-operative chronic kidney disease (CKD, defined as serum creatitine >2.0 mg/dl) was measured to be 1.6% and 6.4% in each respective group, the post-operative incidence of acute renal injury was 0.9% in both groups. Unfortunately, most classic studies of WIT used crude methods of determining renal function. More recent studies, including those that implement mercaptoacetyl triglycine (MAG3) lasix renal scintigraphy to more accurately assess kidney function, have resulted in more refined guidelines.

A series of 56 consecutive LPN cases performed by a single surgeon at a single institution, using pre-operative and post-operative MAG3-lasix renal scintigraphy, demonstrated a relationship between WIT (minutes) and renal differential function (RDF) [5]. Interestingly, the authors noted that the relationship between WIT and declining kidney function was more pronounced after 32 minutes. This suggests that within 30 minutes, focus should be on limiting resection margins, careful closure of the collecting system, and hemostasis.

Roles for cold ischemia and no ischemia have also been investigated. Also using renal scintgraphy analysis, Tatsugami and colleagues reported that, based on preoperative and postoperative analysis by renal scintigraphy of patients after OPN and LPN, cold ischemia conferred an advantage to postoperative recovery of affected renal function. The authors suggested that cold ischemia should be considered if the patient is at risk of renal function deterioration, or when warm ischemia time is expected to be >30 minutes [28]. A retrospective comparison of warm ischemia versus no ischemia during partial nephrectomy on a solitary kidney in OPN and LPN cases showed that patients with warm ischemia (median of 21 min) were more likely to develop acute renal failure (O.R. 2.1, p=0.04) and post-op GFR <15 ml/min/1.73 m^2 (OR 4.2, p=0.007) [29]. However, a surgeon selection bias was present. Patients who received warm ischemia also had significantly higher pre-op GFR and larger tumors. Even so, the authors concluded that PN without any ischemia could be considered when technically feasible.

In 2009, an expert international panel recommended that WIT be kept to <20 minutes, and that in difficult cases, cold ischemia be started immediately and should not exceed 35 minutes [30]. Currently, the debate about the appropriate and safe amount of WIT in partial nephrectomy remains unresolved. Though 30 minutes remains the acceptable limit in practice, further studies involving sophisticated means of assessing renal function may prompt changes in the future.

3.2 Hilar clamping

In LPN, clear visualization of the tumor bed is imperative. Hilar clamping achieves a bloodless operative field and decreases renal turgor. Hence, hilar clamping enhances the achievement of a precise margin of healthy parenchyma during tumor excision, suture control of transected intrarenal blood vessels, precise identification of calyceal entry followed by water-tight suture repair, and renal parenchymal reconstruction. The controlled surgical environment provided by transient hilar clamping is advantageous for a technically superior LPN. The small completely exophytic tumor with minimal parenchymal invasion may be wedge resected without hilar clamping as it would have been performed in open surgery [31, 32].

However, recent studies have demonstrated favorable results in LPN procedures conducted without hilar clamping, or by clamping only the renal artery or one of its segmental branches. Theoretically, the technique of hilar unclamping can create a less clear operative field, resulting in uncontrolled bleeding, unidentified injuries to the collecting system, and difficulty identifying the correct excisional plane. The necessity of hilar or arterial clamping becomes clear in cases where tumor resection is difficult or complex, such as tumors that are partially exophytic with a certain depth of parenchymal invasion or are large in size. A recent retrospective case series of patients who underwent LPN with or without renal artery clamping—deemed necessary when the depth of tumor invasion was greater than 50% of the renal parenchyma as seen via CT or MRI—showed that although mean operative time was longer in the clamped group (p=0.007), there were no significant differences in peri-operative or post-operative complications [33]. Groups were not evenly balanced, with the rate of malignant tumors confirmed via pathology being 18% in the non-clamped group, and 90% in the clamped group (p=0.002), suggesting. Many investigators have advocated clamping of the renal artery alone (rather than the whole pedicle. This technique facilitates precise excision, repair in a bloodless field, and continuous venous drainage to decrease venous oozing and reduce possible free-radical damage during ischemic periods. Gerber and Stockton conducted a survey to assess the trend among urologists in PN practice and found 41% of the respondents clamp the renal artery only to obtain vascular control [34]. Clamping of a segmental artery alone has also been investigated. A retrospective study at one centre has demonstrated that clamping of a single segmental artery in patients undergoing LPN for T1a or T1b tumors resulted in increased blood loss (p<0.006) and WI time (p<0.001), but equivalent post-operative complication rates, and better post-operative renal function at 3 months (p<0.001) compared to renal artery clamping [35]. It was noted, however, that the size (<3.5cm) and location (polar or posterior) of the tumor influenced the decision to attempt segmental artery clamping, suggesting that the novel technique was safe and feasible in select patients. Ultimately, clamping results in renal ischemia, and thus necessitates precise and expedient tumor excision and renal reconstruction. Although newer methods have been shown to be feasible, these should be reserved for select patients in the care of an experienced surgeon comfortable with these techniques.

4. Hemostasis

One of the essential elements in PN is to achieve secure renal parenchymal hemostasis. The classic technique for achieving hemostasis of the parenchymal vessels that are transected during LPN is precise suture ligation followed by a tight reapproximation of the renal parenchyma (renorrhaphy) over absorbable bolsters [36]. The renal hilum or the renal artery is cross-clamped to halt renal blood flow, similar to open PN. In efforts to decrease blood loss and warm ischemia, many hemostatic devices and materials have been reported. These are frequently used in combination and differ in their indication, efficacy, side-effects, equipment requirements and cost [34].

4.1 Hemostatic techniques

4.1.1 Parenchymal compression

Several techniques for achieving hemostasis by parenchymal compression have been described. These techniques are intended for achieving hemostasis in the resection of polar tumors. Circumferential compression of the kidney proximal to the tumor decreases blood flow to the resection site without requiring clamping.

Several recent human reports suggest that a clamping of the renal parenchyma without hilar clamping is feasible for hemostasis during LPN and open PN [37-41]. A clamp may be used on the parenchyma without dissection of the renal hilum. Clamping is limited to polar tumors and positioning the clamp can sometimes be challenging. Additionally, there are risks that the clamp may slip, causing hemorrhage, or that the pressure of the clamp may cause damage to the underlying parenchyma. Verhoest et al [42] report the use of a Satinsky clamp (Xomed Micro, France) in 5 patients undergoing LPN. The mean tumor diameter was 3.06 cm and all were polar. Mean operative time was 238 minutes and mean blood loss was 250 mL with no transfusions or other complications. Other authors have reported similar feasibility with a laparoscopic Nussbaum clamp (Aesculap AG, Tuttlingen, Germany ®) [43] and their own proprietary circumferential clamp [44].

Other methods of parenchymal compression have also been described. The double loop tourniquet technique consists of two U-loop strips of umbilical tape extending from a 17 Fr plastic sheath described by Gill et al [45] in a single LPN. McDougall et al [2] and Caddedu et al [46] have reported the use of a plastic cable tie for LPN in a pig model [2]. Compression with pledgeted sutures [47] and an Endoloop [48] have also been reported in pigs.

4.1.2 Argon beam coagulator

The argon beam coagulator (ABC) (CONMED, Utica, NY ®) is used for hemostasis along the surface of retained renal parenchyma in LPN. It is not used to coagulate larger blood vessels or for dissection. ABC works by conducting electrical current to tissue along a jet of inert, non-flammable argon gas. This gas blows away blood and other liquids on the tissue surface, enhancing visualization of the bleeding site as well as eliminating electric current dissipation in the blood. Smoke is also reduced as argon gas displaces oxygen. The surgeon should be aware of argon gas flow rates and pneumoperitoneum pressures in efforts to prevent tension pneumothorax[49] and gas embolism [50, 51]

Hernandez et al [52] have reported the successful use of the ABC for hemostasis in 25 canine partial nephrectomies without hilar clamping. The mean blood loss was 135 cc and mean depth of tissue necrosis was 2.4 mm. Meanwhile, Lucioni et al [53] have studied the use of the ABC as the sole hemostatic agent during 24 porcine laparoscopic heminephrectomies with hilar clamping. A higher power setting and completion nephrectomy were each required in one case to control bleeding.

Although no human trials reporting the efficacy of ABC have been reported, its use in conjunction with other methods is frequent [34].

4.1.3 Ultrasonic shears

Ultrasonic shears, also known as the *harmonic scalpel* (*Ultracision or Harmonic ACE*, Ethicon Endo-Surgery, Cincinnati, OH ®), allow for simultaneous tissue division and hemostasis. Hemostasis is achieved by a titanium blade vibrating at 55 000 Hz which achieves thermal denaturation of tissue into a coagulum. Animal and human studies by Jackman et al [54] and Tomita et al [55] respectively suggest that ultrasonic shears alone are insufficient for hemostasis of arcuate or larger vessels.

Harmon et al [32] evaluated its use in 15 patients undergoing LPN with small tumors (mean size 2.3 cm) without vascular clamping, and reported a mean blood loss of 368 ml and a mean operative time of 170 minutes. These investigators also employed an argon beam coagulator and oxidized cellulose gauze. Guillonneau et al [56] performed a nonrandomized retrospective comparison of two techniques for LPN, that is without and with clamping the renal vessels. In group 1 (12 patients) PN was performed with ultrasonic shears and bipolar cautery without clamping the renal vessels; while in group 2 (16 patients) the renal pedicle was clamped before tumor excision with a cold knife and hemostasis achieved by sutures and hemostatic mesh. All tumors but 1 were exophytic. Mean renal ischemia time was 27.3 minutes (range 15-47 minutes) in group 2 patients. Mean laparoscopic operating time was 179.1 minutes (range 90-390 minutes) in group 1 compared with 121.5 minutes (range 60-210 minutes) in group 2 (p = 0.004). Mean intraoperative blood loss was significantly higher in group 1 than in group 2 (708.3 versus 270.3 ml, p = 0.014). Surgical margins were negative in all specimens.

Ultrasonic shears are primarily useful in small peripheral lesions which may be excised without vascular occlusion. Disadvantages of ultrasonic shears used for this purpose include tissue charring, tissue adherence, and an inexact line of parenchymal incision with poor visualization of the tumor bed. They are also inadequate as a sole hemostatic agent and not recommended for larger or deeper tumors. The *harmonic scalpel* is not recommended when vascular clamping is employed as the harmonic scalpel is slower than other methods and may result in kidney damage secondary to increased warm ischemic time [56].

4.1.4 Water (hydro) jet dissection

Hydro-jet (Erbe Elektromedizia GmbH, Tubingen, Germany ®) involves using a high-pressure jet of saline to selectively dissect parenchymal tissue. Blood vessels and the collecting system are not penetrated if a 400-600 psi pressure is used [57]. Shekarriz et al have investigated this technology during LPN with hilar control in the porcine model[58] and reported a virtually bloodless field with the vessels and collecting system preserved. Moinzadeh et al [57] similarly evaluated hydro-jet assisted LPN in the calf model. Vessels were controlled with a BIClamp (Erbe Elektromedizia GmbH, Turbingen, Germany) bipolar instrument. Of 20 LPN, 18 were performed without hilar clamping and in 15 only the bipolar instrument was required for hemostasis. The mean Hydro-jet PN time was 63 minutes (range 13-150 minutes) and mean estimated blood loss was 174 ml (range 20 to 750 mL). Corvin et al [59] have also demonstrated the feasibility of Hydro-jet in wedge resection in the pig model.

The use of Hydro-jet dissection in LPN in humans has not been formally reported. Basting et al.[60] report the use of Hydro-jet in a series of 24 renal sparing surgeries performed for benign and neoplastic disease. Dissection took between 14 and 35 minutes and the average blood loss was 60mL with no significant complications. Shekarriz[61] describes unpublished data that hydro-dissection was successfully used in 6 open partial nephrectomies for RCC without hilar control. Dissection time was 20-30 minutes, blood loss ranged from 150-500 mL (mean 265 mL) and there were no complications.

4.1.5 Microwave coagulation

Microwave tissue coagulation (MTC) with the Microtaze device (Azwell, Osaka, Japan) utilizes a needle-type monopolar electrode which is inserted into the kidney repeatedly prior to renal incision. 2450 MHz of microwave energy is applied to tissue surrounding the electrode forming a conical-shaped wedge of coagulated tissue extending up to 10mm. Partial nephrectomy is then performed in the plane of coagulated tissue resulting in a relatively blood-free field. MTC necessitates mobilization of the entire kidney for appropriate probe insertion and has the potential for serious complications, as subsequently described.

Terai et al [62] have used MTC to perform LPN in 18 patients with peripheral tumors. They report a mean operative time of 240 minutes (range 131-390 minutes). Minimal blood loss occurred in 14 patients and 100-400mL blood loss occurred in the remaining. Postoperative complications which were managed conservatively included a hematoma in an anticoagualated patient and a 14-day urinary leak. A renal arteriovenous fistula that required embolization occurred in one patient. Finally, pelvicalyceal stenosis resulting in a nonfunctional kidney occurred in another patient. Similar complications have also been reported in OPN [63, 64]. Yoshimura et al [65], Satoh et al [66] and Itoh et al [67] have reported smaller MTC LPN series without such complications.

4.1.6 Radiofrequency ablation

Radiofrequency ablation (RFA) involves the delivery of energy via a needle causing coagulation around the inserted probe. Investigators have successfully used interstitial ablative technologies (like radiofrequency ablation and cryotherapy) as definitive in situ management of select renal lesions. Ablated tumors are left in situ, necessitating concerns about the oncologic effectiveness of ablation in the target lesion and the cost of radiographic follow-up. In RFA-assisted LPN, radiofrequency coagulation can be used prior to partial nephrectomy to achieve energy-based tissue destruction followed by resection of the ablated tissue. Resection of ablated tissue is relatively bloodless obviating the need for hilar clamping.

Wu et al [68] have recently published a series comparing 36 patients undergoing LPN with hilar clamping to 42 patients undergoing RFA-assisted robotic clampless partial nephrectomy. Tumors were larger in the RFA group (2.8 vs. 2.0cm), more often endophytic (52.6% vs. 16.1%) and collecting system reconstruction occurred more often (78.6% vs. 30.6%). Although operative time was longer in the RFA group (373 vs. 250 minutes), blood loss, transfusion rates, renal function and complication rates did not differ between groups. Zeltser et al [69] have also published a series of 32 tumors treated with RFA-assisted LPN.

Mean blood loss was 80 mL and there were no recurrences at a mean follow-up of 31 months. Other authors have also published series on this technique[70-72].

4.1.7 TissueLink

Another option that may be used for dissection and hemostasis is the TissueLink Floating Ball (TissueLink Medical, Inc., Dover, NH). This is a monopolar device that employs radiofrequency current for dissection and uses saline as a cooling medium. A total of 34 patients in several series were identified by us [73-76] which all had appropriate operative time, oncologic control, complications and blood loss when compared to other hemostatic devices.

4.2 Hemostatic materials

Hemostatic materials involve the application of a substance to the resection bed to effect hemostasis. Classes of hemostatic materials include fibrin sealants, gelatin matrix sealants, hydrogel based sealants and oxidized cellulose. The use of multiple hemostatic materials is routine in centers performing LPN [77].

These materials differ in their mechanism, cost, application conditions, uses, and tissue reaction. A rigorous comparison of these materials is beyond the scope of this chapter due to the number of products and absence of appropriate comparative studies. Concerns that arise when using these products include cost, risk allergic reaction, potential transmission of prion and other infectious diseases, and the need to mix two components and/or sequentially apply them.

Fibrin products include Tisseel (Baxter), Beriplast (CSL BehringGmbH), Hemaseel (HMN), Costasis (Cohesion Technologies), Vivostat (Vivostat A/S), and Evicel (Ethicon, Johnson & Johnson). Fibrin products must be applied to a dry surface and may offer both hemostasis and sealing of the collecting system [78]. Generally, these products include a concentrated solution of human fibrinogen which is mixed with thrombin and calcium chloride. The addition of aprotinin helps to slow the natural fibrinolysis occurring at the resection site. Natural bioabsorption eventually occurs from plasma-mediated lysis [79]. Fibrin sealants may also come in sprays [80]. Autologous fibrin sealants, such as Vivostat, have been developed in attempts to minimize this risk of infectious and allergic complications. Authors have demonstrated that fibrin sealants may be effective as the sole hemostatic technique or used in conjunction with other methods [79, 81, 82].

Gelatin matrix products provide thrombin, calcium, and bovine-derived gelatin granules. These agents include FloSeal (Baxter), which is our preferred hemostatic flowable agent to use during LPN. FloSeal may be applied to a wet surface and function only in parenchymal hemostasis. Unlike fibrin sealants, thrombin in these products converts fibrinogen from the patient's blood into a fibrin clot. The gelatin granules swell on contact with blood, creating a composite hemostatic plug with physical bulk that mechanically controls hemorrhage [83]. Gill et al [83] have reported a series of 131 patients, in which they compared their conventional technique of sutured renorraphy over a Surgicel bolster to the same technique with the addition of Floseal. FloSeal significantly reduced overall complications (37% vs. 16%) and had a trend towards lower rates of hemorrhagic complications (12% vs. 3%). Wille et al [84], Richter et al [85] and Bak et al [86] have also described positive series.

Bovine serum albumin and glutaraldehyde tissue adhesive (BioGlue, Cryolife, Kennesaw, GA) is another sealant that is applied to a dry surface and controls both the renal parenchyma and collecting system. Glutaraldehyde exposure causes the lysine molecules of the bovine serum albumin, extracellular matrix proteins, and cell surfaces to bind to each other, creating a strong covalent bond. The reaction is spontaneous without needing the patient's coagulation factors. The glue begins to polymerize within 20 to 30 seconds and reaches maximal strength in approximately 2 minutes, resulting in a strong implant. The degradation process takes approximately 2 years, and it is then replaced with fibrotic granulation tissue. Several series support the use of BioGlue [87, 88] .

Oxidized cellulose products include Surgicel (Johnson & Johnson, Somerville, NJ), Gelfoam (Pfizer, Inc., New York, NY) and Surgifoam (Johnson & Johnson). These products have hemostatic properties and can also be left as a bolster within the kidney to tamponade bleeding. Authors report the use of the bulk of these products to close fill parenchymal defects [89] although it is associated with a foreign-body reaction [90].

While numerous other hemostatic agents exist, these products represent the most frequently used materials. Newer products are currently being developed using various in vivo and in vitro models [91-93].

5. Morbidity

LPN improves upon the morbidity of open PN. Investigators from Cleveland Clinic analyzed the complications of their initial 200 cases treated with LPN for a suspected renal tumor [94] and reported that 66 (33%) patients had a complication: 36 (18%) patients had urologic complications, the majority of which was bleeding, and 30 (15%) patients had non-urologic complications. This experienced team also reported a decreased complication rate (16%) since they began using a biologic hemostatic agent as an adjunctive measure. Gill et al[19] compared 100 patients who underwent LPN with 100 patients who underwent OPN. The median surgical time was 3 hours vs 3.9 hours (p < 0.001), estimated blood loss was 125 ml vs 250 ml (p < 0.001), and mean WIT was 28 minutes vs 18 minutes (p < 0.001). The laparoscopic group required less postoperative analgesia, a shorter hospital stay, and a shorter convalescence. Intraoperative complications were higher in the laparoscopic group (5% vs 0%; p = 0.02), and postoperative complications were similar (9% vs 14%; p = 0.27). Functional outcomes were similar in the two groups: median preoperative serum creatinine (1.0 vs 1.0 mg/dl, p < 0.52) and postoperative serum creatinine (1.1 vs 1.2 mg/dl, p < 0.65).

Similarly, Beasley et al[95] retrospectively compared the result of laparoscopic PN to OPN using a tumor size-matched cohort of patients. Although the mean operative time was longer in the laparoscopic group (210 ± 76 minutes versus 144 ± 24 minutes; p < 0.001), the blood loss was comparable between the two groups (250 ± 250 ml vs 334 ± 343 ml; p = not statistically significant). No blood transfusions were performed in either group. The hospital stay was significantly reduced after LPN compared with the open group (2.9 ± 1.5 days vs 6.4 ± 1.8 days; p < 0.0002), and the postoperative parenteral narcotic requirements were lower in the LPN group (mean morphine equivalent 43 ± 62 mg vs 187 ± 71 mg; p < 0.02).

These initial results have been reproduced in recent studies. In an analysis of 1800 OPN and LPN cases for single renal T1 tumours, LPN was associated with shorter operative time, decreased operative blood loss, and shorter hospital stay (p<0.01) [27]. Another multicentre study of 10 years' worth of data demonstrated decreased transfusion incidence and estimated blood loss less (293 vs 418 cc) in LPN compared to OPN [96].

Interestingly, published studies have not demonstrated increased morbidity for LPN for T1b tumors. A retrospective study at a single centre compared operative and post-operative complications in patients who underwent LPN for tumors > 4cm to those who underwent LPN for tumors ≤ 4cm. The authors concluded that there were no significant differences observed with respect to operating time, transfusion requirements, post-operative complications, or hospital stay, suggesting that LPN, from a morbidity standpoint, is feasible for tumors > 4 cm in carefully selected patients [97].

Despite the absence of a prospective randomized controlled trials, these congruent series suggest improved morbidity from LPN relative to open PN.

6. Oncologic results

Longitudinal studies for LPN for tumors ≤ 4 cm and > 4 cm have demonstrated the efficacy and safety of this approach comparable to OPN and other laparoscopic techniques. The 3 year cancer-specific survival for patients with a single cT1N0M0 RCC has been reported similar for OPN and LPN (99.3% LPN and 99.2% OPN) [27]. In a 5 year, intermediate-term study, comparing laparoscopic radical nephrectomy (LRN) and LPN (n=35) for T1b-T3N0M0 RCC, overall mortality (11% in each group), cancer-specific mortality (3% in each group) and recurrence (3% vs 6%) rates (p=0.4) were equivalent [9]. Recurrence-free survival in each group was 96%. The longest follow-up study to date is a retrospective 7-year follow-up study comparing oncologic outcomes of LPN and OPN for a single cT1 cortical tumor 7cm or less. Metastases free survival with a minimum of 7 years follow-up was equivalent in both groups (97.5% LPN vs. 97.3% OPN, p=0.47.) After multivariable analysis that accounted for the propensity to undergo LPN, surgical approach was not associated with a significant difference in the odds of metastases (OR 2.18, 95% CI 0.85-5.89) [98].

Promising oncologic outcomes have also been reported for LPN with respect to more complex tumors. Porpilgia et al published a retrospective case series of 100 consecutive patients LPN for tumors ≤ 4 cm and tumors greater than 4 cm, demonstrating that in spite of statistically significant differences in tumor size and location (p=0.002), the incidence of positive surgical margins was equivalent and acceptable pathologic results were achieved in both groups [11]. Similarly, a study comparing bilateral OPN to bilateral LPN for bilateral kidney tumors demonstrated equivalent cancer-specific and recurrence-free survival rates in both groups over a mean follow-up of 5.5 years [13].

7. Emerging techniques: Robot-assisted LPN and Laproendoscopic Single-Site (LESS) surgery

Robot-assisted LPN (RPN) has recently been introduced at several centres around the world. In general, its indications are the same as for OPN and LPN[99], and the transperitoneal approach is used most often[18]. Preliminary data suggests that RPN is equivalent to LPN in terms of WIT, perioperative status, and functional outcomes, but the main drawbacks of RPN remain cost and need for trained personnel.

Studies comparing RPN to OPN, comparing RPN to LPN, and investigating the outcomes of RPN for hilar and more complex tumours suggest that RPN is safe, feasible, and provides equivalent functional outcomes to the existing standard procedures [100-103]. In some instances, it also results in a shorter hospital stay [100, 102]. A small study involving 11 patients examined the intra-operative use of indocyanine green to facilitate near infrared fluorescent imaging during RPN. The imaging was used to successfully delineate the renal vasculature in all cases. Interestingly, of the 10 patients with malignancies that were eventually confirmed via histopathology, 7 of these tumors were hyper-fluorescent compared to the surrounding renal parenchyma during the intra-operative imaging [104]. Similarly, Laparoendoscopic Single-Site (LESS) partial nephrectomy is an emerging technique that has been proven feasible for small, exophytic, easily approachable tumors [18]. Further data, prospective studies, and greater surgical experience are needed to truly realize the potential of these emerging technologies.

8. Cost effectiveness

Emerging data suggests that LPN is the most cost-effective procedure for small renal masses. A simulation analysis for cost-effectiveness– based on the case of a healthy 65-year old patient with an asymptomatic, unilateral small renal mass, and using quality adjusted life-years as a measure of benefit– concluded that immediate LPN was the most cost-effective nephron-sparing strategy [105]. In this model, LPN was favorable to OPN, laparoscopic or percutaneous ablation, active surveillance, and nonsurgical management with observation. A direct financial analysis conducted in a retrospective Canadian study demonstrated a lower total hospital cost after LPN (4839 dollars ± 1551 dollars vs. 6297 dollars ± 2972 dollars; $p < 0.05$) when compared to OPN [95]. Similarly, a retrospective meta-analysis of 2745 procedures (OPN, LPN, and RPN) confirmed that despite similar OR times, LPN was more cost effective than OPN because of a shorter length of hospital stay. Additionally, despite a longer length of stay compared to RPN, LPN was more cost effective due to lower instrumentation costs [106]. These analyses suggest that LPN currently represents the most economical option with regard to nephron-sparing procedures.

9. Summary

Partial nephrectomy is a standard of care for the surgical management small renal masses. In the past decade, laparoscopic partial nephrectomy has advanced to offer equivalent functional and oncologic outcomes, when compared to open partial nephrectomy and laparoscopic radical nephrectomy, at lower cost. Although the appropriate amount of WIT remains controversial, emerging technology (including hemostatic devices and robotic systems) will continue to facilitate improvement in the surgical management of renal masses.

10. References

[1] Clayman, R.V., et al., *Laparoscopic nephrectomy: initial case report.* J Urol, 1991. 146(2): p. 278-82.

[2] McDougall, E.M., et al., *Laparoscopic partial nephrectomy in the pig model.* J Urol, 1993. 149(6): p. 1633-6.

[3] Winfield, H.N., et al., *Laparoscopic partial nephrectomy: initial case report for benign disease.* J Endourol, 1993. 7(6): p. 521-6.

[4] Finelli, A. and I.S. Gill, *Laparoscopic partial nephrectomy: contemporary technique and results.* Urol Oncol, 2004. 22(2): p. 139-44.

[5] Pouliot, F., et al., *Multivariate analysis of the factors involved in loss of renal differential function after laparoscopic partial nephrectomy: a role for warm ischemia time.* Can Urol Assoc J, 2011. 5(2): p. 89-95.

[6] Campbell, S.C., et al., *Guideline for management of the clinical T1 renal mass.* J Urol, 2009. 182(4): p. 1271-9.

[7] Ljungberg, B., et al., *Renal cell carcinoma guideline.* Eur Urol, 2007. 51(6): p. 1502-10.

[8] Herr, H.W., *Partial nephrectomy for unilateral renal carcinoma and a normal contralateral kidney: 10-year followup.* J Urol, 1999. 161(1): p. 33-4; discussion 34-5.

[9] Simmons, M.N., C.J. Weight, and I.S. Gill, *Laparoscopic radical versus partial nephrectomy for tumors >4 cm: intermediate-term oncologic and functional outcomes.* Urology, 2009. 73(5): p. 1077-82.

[10] Kim, J.M., et al., *Comparison of Partial and Radical Nephrectomy for pT1b Renal Cell Carcinoma.* Korean J Urol, 2010. 51(9): p. 596-600.

[11] Porpiglia, F., et al., *Does tumour size really affect the safety of laparoscopic partial nephrectomy?* BJU Int, 2011. 108(2): p. 268-73.

[12] Shikanov, S., et al., *Laparoscopic partial nephrectomy for technically challenging tumours.* BJU Int, 2010. 106(1): p. 91-4.

[13] Ching, C.B., et al., *Functional and oncologic outcomes of bilateral open partial nephrectomy versus bilateral laparoscopic partial nephrectomy.* J Endourol, 2011. 25(7): p. 1193-7.

[14] Tsivian, A., et al., *Laparoscopic partial nephrectomy for multiple tumours: feasibility and analysis of peri-operative outcomes.* BJU Int, 2010.

[15] Deklaj, T., et al., *Localized T1a renal lesions in the elderly: outcomes of laparoscopic renal surgery.* J Endourol, 2010. 24(3): p. 397-401.

[16] Marszalek, M., et al., *Laparoscopic partial nephrectomy: a matched-pair comparison of the transperitoneal versus the retroperitoneal approach.* Urology, 2011. 77(1): p. 109-13.

[17] Wright, J.L. and J.R. Porter, *Laparoscopic partial nephrectomy: comparison of transperitoneal and retroperitoneal approaches.* J Urol, 2005. 174(3): p. 841-5.

[18] Lee, S.Y., J.D. Choi, and S.I. Seo, *Current status of partial nephrectomy for renal mass.* Korean J Urol, 2011. 52(5): p. 301-9.

[19] Gill, I.S., et al., *Comparative analysis of laparoscopic versus open partial nephrectomy for renal tumors in 200 patients.* J Urol, 2003. 170(1): p. 64-8.

[20] Winfield, H.N., et al., *Laparoscopic partial nephrectomy: initial experience and comparison to the open surgical approach.* J Urol, 1995. 153(5): p. 1409-14.

[21] Wolf, J.S., Jr., B.D. Seifman, and J.E. Montie, *Nephron sparing surgery for suspected malignancy: open surgery compared to laparoscopy with selective use of hand assistance.* J Urol, 2000. 163(6): p. 1659-64.

[22] Gill, I.S., et al., *Laparoscopic partial nephrectomy for renal tumor: duplicating open surgical techniques.* J Urol, 2002. 167(2 Pt 1): p. 469-7; discussion 475-6.

[23] Janetschek, G., et al., *Laparoscopic nephron sparing surgery for small renal cell carcinoma.* J Urol, 1998. 159(4): p. 1152-5.

[24] Ward, J.P., *Determination of the Optimum temperature for regional renal hypothermia during temporary renal ischaemia.* Br J Urol, 1975. 47(1): p. 17-24.

[25] Novick, A.C., *Renal hypothermia: in vivo and ex vivo.* Urol Clin North Am, 1983. 10(4): p. 637-44.

[26] McLoughlin, G.A., M.R. Heal, and I.M. Tyrell, *An evaluation of techniques used for the production of temporary renal ischaemia.* Br J Urol, 1978. 50(6): p. 371-5.

[27] Gill, I.S., et al., *Comparison of 1,800 laparoscopic and open partial nephrectomies for single renal tumors.* J Urol, 2007. 178(1): p. 41-6.

[28] Tatsugami, K., et al., *Impact of cold and warm ischemia on postoperative recovery of affected renal function after partial nephrectomy.* J Endourol, 2011. 25(5): p. 869-73; discussion 873-4.

[29] Thompson, R.H., et al., *Comparison of warm ischemia versus no ischemia during partial nephrectomy on a solitary kidney.* Eur Urol, 2010. 58(3): p. 331-6.

[30] Becker, F., et al., *Assessing the impact of ischaemia time during partial nephrectomy.* Eur Urol, 2009. 56(4): p. 625-34.

[31] McDougall, E.M., A.M. Elbahnasy, and R.V. Clayman, *Laparoscopic wedge resection and partial nephrectomy--the Washington University experience and review of the literature.* JSLS, 1998. 2(1): p. 15-23.

[32] Harmon, W.J., L.R. Kavoussi, and J.T. Bishoff, *Laparoscopic nephron-sparing surgery for solid renal masses using the ultrasonic shears.* Urology, 2000. 56(5): p. 754-9.

[33] Koo, H.J., D.H. Lee, and I.Y. Kim, *Renal hilar control during laparoscopic partial nephrectomy: to clamp or not to clamp.* J Endourol, 2010. 24(8): p. 1283-7.

[34] Gerber, G.S. and B.R. Stockton, *Laparoscopic partial nephrectomy.* J Endourol, 2005. 19(1): p. 21-4.

[35] Shao, P., et al., *Laparoscopic partial nephrectomy with segmental renal artery clamping: technique and clinical outcomes.* Eur Urol, 2011. 59(5): p. 849-55.

[36] Novick, A.C., et al., *Operative urology at the Cleveland Clinic.* 2006, Humana Press: Totowa, N.J. p. xiv, 552 p.

[37] Simon, J., et al., *Optimizing selective renal clamping in nephron-sparing surgery using the Nussbaum clamp.* Urology, 2008. 71(6): p. 1196-8.

[38] Huyghe, E., et al., *Open partial nephrectomy with selective renal parenchymal control: a new reliable clamp.* Urology, 2006. 68(3): p. 658-60.

[39] Mejean, A., et al., *Nephron sparing surgery for renal cell carcinoma using selective renal parenchymal clamping.* J Urol, 2002. 167(1): p. 234-5.

[40] Denardi, F., et al., *Nephron-sparing surgery for renal tumours using selective renal parenchymal clamping.* BJU Int, 2005. 96(7): p. 1036-9.

[41] Rodriguez-Covarrubias, F., et al., *Partial nephrectomy for renal tumors using selective parenchymal clamping.* Int Urol Nephrol, 2007. 39(1): p. 43-6.

[42] Verhoest, G., et al., *Laparoscopic partial nephrectomy with clamping of the renal parenchyma: initial experience.* Eur Urol, 2007. 52(5): p. 1340-6.

[43] Simon, J., et al., *Laparoscopic partial nephrectomy with selective control of the renal parenchyma: initial experience with a novel laparoscopic clamp.* BJU Int, 2009. 103(6): p. 805-8.

[44] Toren, P., et al., *Use of a novel parenchymal clamp for laparoscopic and open partial nephrectomy.* Can Urol Assoc J, 2010. 4(5): p. E133-6.

[45] Gill, I.S., et al., *A new renal tourniquet for open and laparoscopic partial nephrectomy.* J Urol, 1995. 154(3): p. 1113-6.

[46] Cadeddu, J.A., et al., *Hemostatic laparoscopic partial nephrectomy: cable-tie compression.* Urology, 2001. 57(3): p. 562-6.

[47] Wilhelm, D.M., et al., *Feasibility of laparoscopic partial nephrectomy using pledgeted compression sutures for hemostasis.* J Endourol, 2003. 17(4): p. 223-7.

[48] Beck, S.D., et al., *Endoloop-assisted laparoscopic partial nephrectomy.* J Endourol, 2002. 16(3): p. 175-7.

[49] Shanberg, A.M., M. Zagnoev, and T.P. Clougherty, *Tension pneumothorax caused by the argon beam coagulator during laparoscopic partial nephrectomy.* J Urol, 2002. 168(5): p. 2162.

[50] Min, S.K., J.H. Kim, and S.Y. Lee, *Carbon dioxide and argon gas embolism during laparoscopic hepatic resection.* Acta Anaesthesiol Scand, 2007. 51(7): p. 949-53.

[51] *Fatal gas embolism caused by overpressurization during laparoscopic use of argon enhanced coagulation.* Health Devices, 1994. 23(6): p. 257-9.

[52] Hernandez, A.D., et al., *A controlled study of the argon beam coagulator for partial nephrectomy.* J Urol, 1990. 143(5): p. 1062-5.

[53] Lucioni, A., et al., *Efficacy of the argon beam coagulator alone in obtaining hemostasis after laparoscopic porcine heminephrectomy: a pilot study.* Can J Urol, 2008. 15(3): p. 4091-6.

[54] Jackman, S.V., et al., *Utility of the harmonic scalpel for laparoscopic partial nephrectomy.* J Endourol, 1998. 12(5): p. 441-4.

[55] Tomita, Y., et al., *Use of the harmonic scalpel for nephron sparing surgery in renal cell carcinoma.* J Urol, 1998. 159(6): p. 2063-4.

[56] Guillonneau, B., et al., *Laparoscopic partial nephrectomy for renal tumor: single center experience comparing clamping and no clamping techniques of the renal vasculature.* J Urol, 2003. 169(2): p. 483-6.

[57] Moinzadeh, A., et al., *Water jet assisted laparoscopic partial nephrectomy without hilar clamping in the calf model.* J Urol, 2005. 174(1): p. 317-21.

[58] Shekarriz, H., et al., *Hydro-jet assisted laparoscopic partial nephrectomy: initial experience in a porcine model.* J Urol, 2000. 163(3): p. 1005-8.

[59] Corvin, S., et al., *Use of hydro-jet cutting for laparoscopic partial nephrectomy in a porcine model.* Urology, 2001. 58(6): p. 1070-3.

[60] Basting, R.F., N. Djakovic, and P. Widmann, *Use of water jet resection in organ-sparing kidney surgery.* J Endourol, 2000. 14(6): p. 501-5.

[61] Shekarriz, B., *Hydro-Jet technology in urologic surgery.* Expert Rev Med Devices, 2005. 2(3): p. 287-91.

[62] Terai, A., et al., *Laparoscopic partial nephrectomy using microwave tissue coagulator for small renal tumors: usefulness and complications.* Eur Urol, 2004. 45(6): p. 744-8.

[63] Murota, T., et al., *Retroperitoneoscopic partial nephrectomy using microwave coagulation for small renal tumors.* Eur Urol, 2002. 41(5): p. 540-5; discussion 545.

[64] Akiyama, T., et al., *Renal arteriovenous fistula developing after tumor enucleation using a microwave tissue coagulator.* Int J Urol, 2001. 8(10): p. 568-71.

[65] Yoshimura, K., et al., *Laparoscopic partial nephrectomy with a microwave tissue coagulator for small renal tumor.* J Urol, 2001. 165(6 Pt 1): p. 1893-6.

[66] Satoh, Y., et al., *Renal-tissue damage induced by laparoscopic partial nephrectomy using microwave tissue coagulator.* J Endourol, 2005. 19(7): p. 818-22.

[67] Itoh, K., et al., *Posterior retroperitoneoscopic partial nephrectomy using microwave tissue coagulator for small renal tumors.* J Endourol, 2002. 16(6): p. 367-71.

[68] Wu, S.D., et al., *Radiofrequency ablation-assisted robotic laparoscopic partial nephrectomy without renal hilar vessel clamping versus laparoscopic partial nephrectomy: a comparison of perioperative outcomes.* J Endourol, 2010. 24(3): p. 385-91.

[69] Zeltser, I.S., et al., *Intermediate-term prospective results of radiofrequency-assisted laparoscopic partial nephrectomy: a non-ischaemic coagulative technique.* BJU Int, 2008. 101(1): p. 36-8.

[70] Gettman, M.T., et al., *Hemostatic laparoscopic partial nephrectomy: initial experience with the radiofrequency coagulation-assisted technique.* Urology, 2001. 58(1): p. 8-11.

[71] Jacomides, L., et al., *Laparoscopic application of radio frequency energy enables in situ renal tumor ablation and partial nephrectomy.* J Urol, 2003. 169(1): p. 49-53; discussion 53.

[72] Oefelein, M.G., *Delayed presentation of urinoma after radiofrequency ablation-assisted laparoscopic partial nephrectomy.* J Endourol, 2006. 20(1): p. 27-30.

[73] Sundaram, C.P., et al., *Hemostatic laparoscopic partial nephrectomy assisted by a water-cooled, high-density, monopolar device without renal vascular control.* Urology, 2003. 61(5): p. 906-9.

[74] Stern, J.A., et al., *TissueLink device for laparoscopic nephron-sparing surgery.* J Endourol, 2004. 18(5): p. 455-6.

[75] Tan, Y.H., et al., *Hand-assisted laparoscopic partial nephrectomy without hilar vascular clamping using a saline-cooled, high-density monopolar radiofrequency device.* J Endourol, 2004. 18(9): p. 883-7.

[76] Coleman, J., et al., *Radiofrequency-assisted laparoscopic partial nephrectomy: clinical and histologic results.* J Endourol, 2007. 21(6): p. 600-5.

[77] Breda, A., et al., *Use of haemostatic agents and glues during laparoscopic partial nephrectomy: a multi-institutional survey from the United States and Europe of 1347 cases.* Eur Urol, 2007. 52(3): p. 798-803.

[78] Msezane, L.P., et al., *Hemostatic agents and instruments in laparoscopic renal surgery.* J Endourol, 2008. 22(3): p. 403-8.

[79] Pruthi, R.S., J. Chun, and M. Richman, *The use of a fibrin tissue sealant during laparoscopic partial nephrectomy.* BJU Int, 2004. 93(6): p. 813-7.

[80] Pick, D.L., et al., *Sprayed fibrin sealant as the sole hemostatic agent for porcine laparoscopic partial nephrectomy.* J Urol, 2011. 185(1): p. 291-7.

[81] Schips, L., et al., *Autologous fibrin glue using the Vivostat system for hemostasis in laparoscopic partial nephrectomy.* Eur Urol, 2006. 50(4): p. 801-5.

[82] Gidaro, S., et al., *Efficacy and safety of the haemostasis achieved by Vivostat system during laparoscopic partial nephrectomy.* Arch Ital Urol Androl, 2009. 81(4): p. 223-7.

[83] Gill, I.S., et al., *Improved hemostasis during laparoscopic partial nephrectomy using gelatin matrix thrombin sealant.* Urology, 2005. 65(3): p. 463-6.

[84] Wille, A.H., et al., *Laparoscopic partial nephrectomy using FloSeal for hemostasis: technique and experiences in 102 patients.* Surg Innov, 2009. 16(4): p. 306-12.

[85] Richter, F., et al., *Improvement of hemostasis in open and laparoscopically performed partial nephrectomy using a gelatin matrix-thrombin tissue sealant (FloSeal).* Urology, 2003. 61(1): p. 73-7.

[86] Bak, J.B., A. Singh, and B. Shekarriz, *Use of gelatin matrix thrombin tissue sealant as an effective hemostatic agent during laparoscopic partial nephrectomy.* J Urol, 2004. 171(2 Pt 1): p. 780-2.

[87] Hidas, G., et al., *Sutureless nephron-sparing surgery: use of albumin glutaraldehyde tissue adhesive (BioGlue).* Urology, 2006. 67(4): p. 697-700; discussion 700.

[88] Nadler, R.B., et al., *Use of BioGlue in laparoscopic partial nephrectomy.* Urology, 2006. 68(2): p. 416-8.

[89] Abou-Elela, A., et al., *Use of oxidized cellulose hemostats (surgicel) to support parenchymal closure and achieve hemostasis following partial nephrectomy.* Surg Technol Int, 2009. 18: p. 75-9.

[90] Sabino, L., et al., *Evaluation of renal defect healing, hemostasis, and urinary fistula after laparoscopic partial nephrectomy with oxidized cellulose.* J Endourol, 2007. 21(5): p. 551-6.

[91] Rane, A., et al., *Evaluation of a hemostatic sponge (TachoSil) for sealing of the renal collecting system in a porcine laparoscopic partial nephrectomy survival model.* J Endourol, 2010. 24(4): p. 599-603.

[92] Bernie, J.E., et al., *Evaluation of hydrogel tissue sealant in porcine laparoscopic partial-nephrectomy model.* J Endourol, 2005. 19(9): p. 1122-6.

[93] Murat, F.J., et al., *Evaluation of microporous polysaccharide hemospheres for parenchymal hemostasis during laparoscopic partial nephrectomy in the porcine model.* JSLS, 2006. 10(3): p. 302-6.

[94] Ramani, A.P., et al., *Complications of laparoscopic partial nephrectomy in 200 cases.* J Urol, 2005. 173(1): p. 42-7.

[95] Beasley, K.A., et al., *Laparoscopic versus open partial nephrectomy.* Urology, 2004. 64(3): p. 458-61.

[96] Park, H., et al., *Comparison of laparoscopic and open partial nephrectomies in t1a renal cell carcinoma: a korean multicenter experience.* Korean J Urol, 2010. 51(7): p. 467-71.

[97] Nouralizadeh, A., et al., *Laparoscopic partial nephrectomy for tumours >4 cm compared with smaller tumours: perioperative results.* Int Urol Nephrol, 2011. 43(2): p. 371-6.

[98] Lane, B.R. and I.S. Gill, *7-year oncological outcomes after laparoscopic and open partial nephrectomy.* J Urol, 2010. 183(2): p. 473-9.

[99] Van Haute, W., A. Gavazzi, and P. Dasgupta, *Current status of robotic partial nephrectomy.* Curr Opin Urol, 2010. 20(5): p. 371-4.

[100] Cho, C.L., et al., *Robot-assisted versus standard laparoscopic partial nephrectomy: comparison of perioperative outcomes from a single institution.* Hong Kong Med J, 2011. 17(1): p. 33-8.

[101] Dulabon, L.M., et al., *Multi-institutional analysis of robotic partial nephrectomy for hilar versus nonhilar lesions in 446 consecutive cases.* Eur Urol, 2011. 59(3): p. 325-30.

[102] Lee, S., et al., *Open versus robot-assisted partial nephrectomy: effect on clinical outcome.* J Endourol, 2011. 25(7): p. 1181-5.

[103] Rogers, C.G., et al., *Robotic partial nephrectomy for renal hilar tumors: a multi-institutional analysis.* J Urol, 2008. 180(6): p. 2353-6; discussion 2356.

[104] Tobis, S., et al., *Near infrared fluorescence imaging with robotic assisted laparoscopic partial nephrectomy: initial clinical experience for renal cortical tumors.* J Urol, 2011. 186(1): p. 47-52.

[105] Chang, S.L., et al., *Cost-effectiveness analysis of nephron sparing options for the management of small renal masses.* J Urol, 2011. 185(5): p. 1591-7.

[106] Mir, S.A., et al., *Cost comparison of robotic, laparoscopic, and open partial nephrectomy.* J Endourol, 2011. 25(3): p. 447-53.

4

Health-Related Quality of Life After Radical Nephrectomy and Kidney Donation

Archil Chkhotua, Tinatin Pantsulaia and Laurent Managadze
National Center of Urology
Georgia

1. Introduction

Radical nephrectomy (RN) is a treatment of choice for the patients with renal cell carcinoma (RCC) achieving excellent results, especially in local stages of the disease. Oncological results of RN are well evaluated on a large number of patients. However, studies on a postoperative health-related quality of life (HRQol) of these patients are very limited (Novara G et al., 2010; Poulakis V et al., 2003; Clark PE et al., 2001). There are no publications available comparing the HRQoL of patients after RN with that of healthy individuals and other forms of nephrectomy.

Living kidney transplantation provides excellent results with the lowest complication and the highest graft and patient survival rates (Hariharan et al., 2000). However, it should not be forgotten that donors are healthy persons voluntarily donating an organ and their postoperative health and HRQol should be a matter of utmost importance. It has been shown that kidney donation does not cause serious medical problems like: deterioration of kidney function, arterial hypertension or proteinuria (El-Agroudy et al., 2007). Although advocated in the literature, psychosocial assessment and monitoring of living kidney donors is not yet routinely performed. There are only limited reports in the literature examining HRQol issues in the donors.

The HRQol concept is well-known in clinical medicine and is frequently applied for the assessment of surgical or other treatment modalities to determine their therapeutic success. HRQol has become a leading criteria in many outcome studies alongside with somatic and economic factors and is frequently listed as outcome parameter in many medical societies' guidelines. Despite methodological difficulties in making HRQol measurable, there are numerous surveys and questionnaires used for this purpose. The Short Form-36 (SF-36), Giessen Subjective Complaints List-24 (GBB-24) and Zerssen's Mood-Scale (Bf-S) are internationally validated and frequently used questionnaires for this purpose (Ware & Sherbourne CD, 1992; Giessing et al., 2004; Zerssen D, 1976).

The importance of this topic is underlined by the fact, that available data on psychological well-being and HRQol of the patients after RN and kidney donors are limited and somewhat controversial. It would be very interesting to know as to whether there are differences between countries, races, or social groups, with regard to HRQol of the patients and donors. While some of these studies are providing evidences that the donor HRQol is at least comparable or even better than that of the general population (Giessing et al., 2004;

Ibrahim et al, 2009; Feltrin et al, 2008; Johnson et al, 1999; Smith et al, 2003; Isotani et al, 2002; Fehrman-Ekholm et al, 2000; Tanriverdi et al, 2004; Lima et al, 2006), others are showing the negative impact of the donation on donors' HRQol (Giessing et al., 2004; Johnson et al, 1999; Smith et al, 2003; Jackobs et al., 200; Reimer et al., 2006; Schover et al., 1997; Zargooshi, 2001; Tellioglu et al., 2008). There are no studies comparing the HRQol of kidney donors with the patients who underwent neprectomy due to the urological diseases.

The aim of the current study was to assess the HRQol of the patients who underwent RN due to the RCC and compare it with age- and sex-matched healthy persons and our kidney donors.

2. Subjects and methods

The study population consisted of:

Group I: 52 patients who underwent nephrectomy due to the RCC

Group II: 120 age- and sex matched healthy individuals

Group III: The kidney donors operated at our institution from January 2005 to December 2008 (n=57).

The patients (Group I) and the kidney donors (Group III) have been followed-up prospectively. The questionnaires have been sent to them after a follow-up of at least 3 months.

The Group I consisted of the 98 consecutive patients operated at our institution for RCC. Three questionnaires (SF-36, GBB-24 and Bf-S) have been mailed to all the patients. 7 (7%) patients have been reported as dead at the time of evaluation, 10 (10%) were lost of follow-up and 29 (30%) didn't respond. We've received the completed questionnaires from 52 patients (53%). The mean follow-up was 28 months (range: 4-35 months). None of the patients had clinical signs of renal insufficiency or other substantial co-morbidities (diabetes etc). Radical or partial nephrectomy without adjuvant immunotherapy was performed in all patients. The pathological stage distribution of the tumors was the following: T1 – 21 (40%); T2 – 13 (25%); T3 – 18 (35%) patients. 14 (27%) cancers were G1, 20 (38%) - G2 and 18 (35%) - G3. Morphological evaluation revealed clear cell RCC in all 52 patients. 2 patients had lymph node and 1 patient had distant metastases at the time of surgery. 18 (34.6%) tumors were discovered incidentally, 29 (55.8%) were locally symptomatic and 5 patients (9.6%) had a systemic disease symptoms. All patients were operated on in one department.

The control group has been generated by using probability-based methods to ensure representativeness of the general population of the Country. The subjects from other psychological surveys have been provided by the national psychological association for this purpose. The control group consisted of 120 healthy volunteers with the mean age of 51±9 years (18-70 years). They were matched with the donors and patients on the basis of: age, sex, race and ethnicity. Exclusion criteria were chronic diseases, with the exception of controlled systemic hypertension and previous non-major surgical interventions.

61 living kidney transplants have been performed at our institution since January 2005 to December 2008. The mean follow-up of the donors was 32 months (range: 4-57 months). All the transplants were performed from genetically related donors. 19 donors (31%) were male and 42 (69%) were female. The mean donor age was 49±9 years. The most frequent form of donation was parent to child (86.5%). In 2.7% of cases organ was offered by sibling and in 5.4% - by cousin and uncle each.

All transplant operations were approved by the ethical committee of the Ministry of Health of Georgia. All the patients and donors were studied according to protocols accepted at our centre. Donor nephrectomy was done by open extraperitoneal approach. All transplants have been performed according to ABO compatibility and negative direct cross-match.

All the donors are alive. They have been followed either by our nephrology department or by associated institutions, with which our center cooperates closely. Three questionnaires (SF-36, GBB-24 and Bf-S) have been mailed, e-mailed, or handed out to all the donors who could be contacted, with a follow-up of at least 3 months. If no answer was returned, we called the donor, motivated him or her for participation, and sent the questionnaires again. If the donor could not be contacted, we talked to the recipient and asked for assistance. Thus, we have received answers from 57 (93%) donors who could be contacted.

The evaluation procedure was completely anonymous and all the respondents were free of any charges related to filling or sending the questionnaires.

2.1 Short form-36 questionnaire

The SF-36 questionnaire was developed in the United States (Ware & Sherbourne CD, 1992). It is a standardized instrument for measuring HRQol on eight different scales: physical function (PF), physical role (PR), social function (SF), general health perception (GH), vitality (V), bodily pain (BP), mental health (MH), and emotional role (ER). Thirty-six questions have to be answered, and a score is computed for each scale, ranging from 0 (least well-being) to 100 (greatest well-being). This form has been adapted by psychologists for use in Georgia with adequate translation and minor changes to the content of the form.

2.2 Giessen subjective complaints list-24 questionnaire

Giessen Subjective Complaints List-24 questionnaire (GBB-24) assesses physical complaints attributable to psychosomatic reasons (Giessing et al., 2004). The questionnaire has six questions, each referring to four items (cardiac complaints, gastric complaints, limb pain and fatigue tendency) for which participants are asked to rate their complaints (0-no complaints, 4-strong complaints). The sum of these four items reflects the fifth item, "overall subjective complaints" (0–96 points).

2.3 Bf-S questionnaire

Bf-S questionnaire is a self-rating scale developed by Zerssen in 1975 (Zerssen D, 1976). It is a 28 question scale designed to assess the person's mood. The questionnaire has been used for the analysis of patient's self-feeling pre- and/or post event (operation, donation etc.).

The study design was approved by the internal review board of the institution as conforming to the provisions of the Declaration of Helsinki. All participants provided written informed consent.

2.4 Statistical analysis

Statistical analysis was performed using computer software (SPSS 12.0 for Windows, Lead Technologies Inc. 2003. Chicago, IL.). Normality of data distribution was examined with

Kolmogorov-Smirnov test. The different scores in the groups were compared with ANOVA, Mann Whitney and Kruskal Wallis tests. Age-dependency of the scores was analysed by the Pearson correlation and linear regression. A p value of less than 0.05 was considered significant.

3. Results

The age, sex distribution and mean follow-up was not different between the groups. At the time of the study, 97.8% of the recipients were alive and 89% of these had a functioning graft. Overall, 12 minor complications occurred in 9 donors (15%) (table 1).

Complication	N	%
Pneumonia	1	1.7
Pneumothorax	2	3.5
UTI	3	5.2
Postoperative hernia	3	5.2
Impaired wound healing	3	5.2

Table 1. Postoperative donor complications

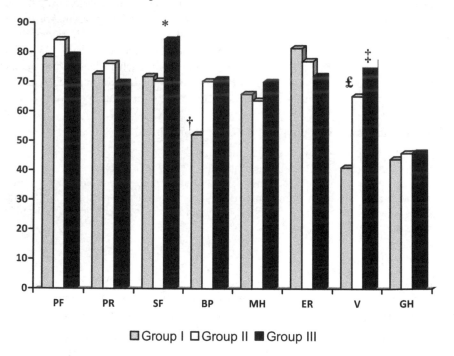

□ Group I □ Group II ■ Group III

* p=0.0001vs.Group II and p=0.0209 vs. Group I
† p=0.0357 vs. Group III and p=0.0375 vs. Group II
‡ p=0.0478 vs. Group II and p=0.0006 vs. Group I
£ p=0.0128 vs. Group I

Fig. 1. Comparison of the mean (±SE) SF-36 scores between the groups

For the SF-36 items: "Social function", "Bodily pain" and "Vitality", donors scored significantly better than controls and patients. "Bodily pain" and "Vitality" indexes of the controls were significantly higher than that of the patients (Fig. 1). The SF-36 scores were not different between males and females.

We analyzed the age dependency of the SF-36 scores in all three groups. The correlation coefficients, corresponding p values and 95% CIs of the eight different SF-36 scores against age are shown in table 1. The correlation coefficients of "Social function" in Group III; "Social function", "Mental health" and "Vitality" in Group II were moderately high (-541, -0.341, -292 and -0.292, respectively); their 95% CIs were narrow (-0.768- -0.195, -0.568- -0.067, -0.530- -0.012 and -0.529- -0.011, respectively) and their p values were significant (0.0037, 0.0158, 0.0413 and 0.0416, respectively), showing a negative correlation with age. Low correlation coefficients of other SF-36 scores, especially in Group I, together with a wide range of 95% CIs including 0, indicated that these scores were not age-related (table 2).

SF-36 score	Correlation Coefficient	P value	95% Lower CI	95% Upper CI
Group I				
PF	-0.235	0.7345	-0.925	0.817
PR	-0.792	0.1282	-0.986	0.310
SF	0.334	0.6238	-0.778	0.939
BP	-0.703	0.2167	-0.978	0.472
MH	-0.326	0.6323	-0.938	0.781
ER	0.212	0.7610	-0.825	0.922
V	-0.670	0.2521	-0.976	0.520
GH	-0.312	0.6479	-0.937	0.787
Group II				
PF	-0.219	0.1307	-0.471	-0.066
PR	-0.243	0.0924	-0.491	0.041
SF	-0.341	0.0158	-0.568	-0.067
BP	-0.212	0.1439	-0.466	0.073
MH	-0.292	0.0413	-0.530	-0.012
ER	-0.017	0.4236	-0.386	0.0169
V	-0.292	0.0416	-0.529	-0.011
GH	-0.116	0.4313	-0.384	0.171
Group III				
PF	-0.045	0.8724	-0.529	0.461
PR	-0.140	0.6106	-0.595	0.382
SF	-0.541	0.0037	-0.768	-0.195
BP	-0.058	0.8340	-0.538	0.451
MH	0.008	0.9784	-0.490	0.501
ER	-0.304	0.2573	-0.695	0.226
V	0.284	0.2923	-0.246	0.684
GH	-0.068	0.8069	-0.545	0.443

Table 2. Pearson correlation analysis of the age dependency of SF-36 scores in different groups

The four scores which showed significant correlations with age ("Social function" in Group III; "Social function", "Mental health" and "Vitality" in Group II) were evaluated further with a linear regression model. Figs. 2 and 3 show the regression plots of the three scores ("Social function" in Group III; "Social function" and "Vitality" in Group II) against age. Regression analyses confirmed the results of the Pearson correlation regarding the linearity of their relationship with age. As to "Mental health" in Group II, regression analyses didn't verify linearity of the relationship.

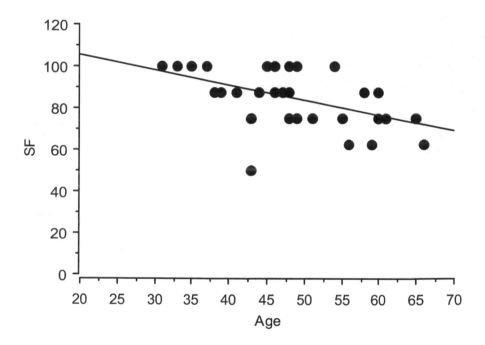

$Y = 120,103 - 0,728 * X; R^2 = 0,245, p=0.0040$

Fig. 2. Regression plot of SF-36 score for "social function" against age in the donors

In all five GBB-24 items the donors scored higher than the controls and patients. For the "gastric complaints" the difference was statistically significant. In this item the patients scored significantly worse than controls and donors (Fig. 4). The GBB-24 scores were not correlated with age. Comparison of the scores between males and females showed that in the Group II, in four out of five items ("Overall complaints", "Fatigue tendency", "Limb pain" and "Cardiac complaints") males scored significantly higher than females (Fig. 5). The differences in other groups were not significant (data not shown).

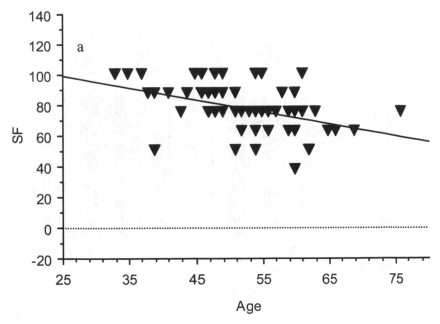

Y = 118,649 - 0,781 * X; R^2 = 0,190; p=0.0003

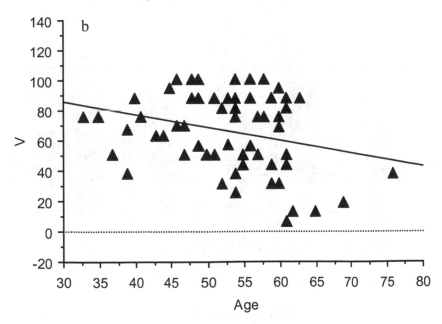

Y = 111,364 - 0,848 * X; R^2 = 0,073 ; p=0.0290

Fig. 3. Regression plots of the SF-36 scores for "social function" (a) and "vitality" (b) against age in the control group

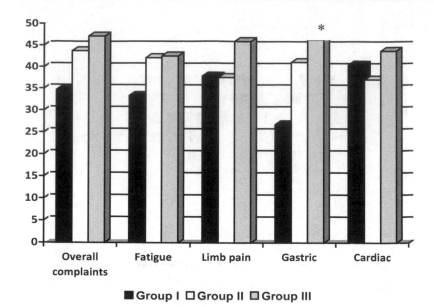

* p=0.0080 vs. Group I and p=0.0293 vs. Group II

Fig. 4. Comparison of the GBB-24 scores between the groups

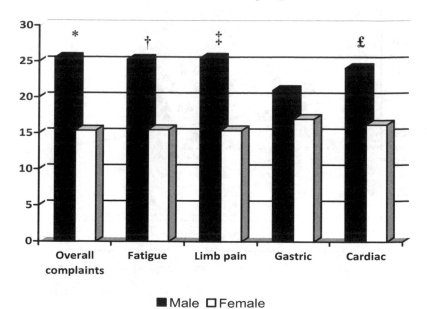

* p=0.0067, † p=0.0433, ‡ p=0.0088, £ p=0.0326.

Fig. 5. Comparison of the GBB-24 scores between males and females in the control group

The mood analyses have shown that Bf-S scores of the donors were significantly higher than that of the controls and patients. The controls scored better than the patients (Fig. 6). The Bf-S scores were not age-related and didn't differ between males and females (data not shown).

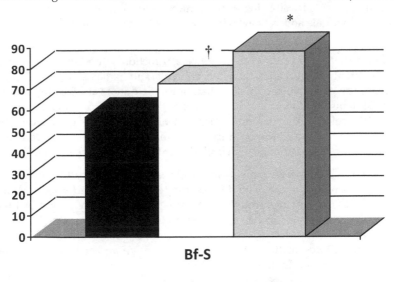

Bf-S

■ Group I □ Group II ▨ Group III

* p=0.0007 vs. Group II and p<0.0001 vs. Group I
† p=0.0183 vs. Group I

Fig. 6. Comparison of the Bf-S scores between the groups

4. Discussion

RN and nephron sparing surgery are the treatments of choice for the patients with RCC. Oncological results and complications of these forms of treatment are extensively evaluated showing excellent outcomes in the patients with local disease stages. However, information on the HRQol of these patients is scarce. There are very few publications assessing and comparing the HRQol of the patients after different forms of surgical treatment of RCC.

The studies on the donors' psychological well-being and HRQol have been conducted since the early years of kidney transplantation. Yet, this topic remains largely under-evaluated and unknown. Most of the existing studies have limitations such as: retrospective design; lack of matching the groups for age or gender; use of non-standardized and validated questionnaires; comparison of the results with references validated for another cultural background; too few participants or low response rates. Nonetheless, these studies suggest hypotheses that require evaluation in a well-designed prospective manner. It should be considered that disparities among the countries in terms of religion, culture, customs, environment, and other factors can influence the HRQol.

In this study we assessed postoperative HRQol of the patients who underwent RN in comparison with our living kidney donors and age and sex matched healthy individuals.

Three different questionnaires have been used to complexly evaluate their: postoperative HRQol (SF-36), subjective complaints (GBB-24) and mood (Bf-S). This type of design is original in existing literature and gives an opportunity to deeper analyse physical, psychosocial and spiritual well-being of the patients after RN in comparison with healthy, non-operated individuals and persons who underwent the same operation for non-medical indications.

We have shown that in three SF-36 items: "Social function", "Bodily pain" and "Vitality" donors scored significantly better than the controls and patients. In "Bodily pain" and "Vitality" items the patients scored worse than both, the donors and healthy individuals. In all five GBB-24 items the donors had higher scores than the controls and patients, but only for the "Gastric complaints" the difference reached statistical significance. Incomplete sample number may be the reason of it. In mood analyses the patients scored significantly worse than the controls and donors, with both these differences being substantial.

The reason of worse scores of the patients in comparison with the healthy subjects should be physical complains related to the main disease and/or operation performed. Also, it should be considered that after passing through the treatment process they do not feel themselves completely healthy. The better scores of the donors in somatic parameters can be explained by the fact that they are selected group of individuals, well-evaluated and with better general health than representatives of the common population. The better scores in psychosocial parameters is caused by the fact that donating an organ is associated with giving a second life to the family member and/or close relative, psycho-social mobilization of the donor and consequently, the better mood.

The new findings of this study are: negative correlation of HRQol scores with age; and gender differences in subjective complaints. We have shown that "Social function", "Mental health" and "Vitality" indexes of the healthy individuals are decreasing with age. The same was true only for the "Social function" of the donors. Significant postoperative improvement in some of the HRQol parameters could be the reason why these differences have not been detected in the donors. As to the "Social function", this domain is much more dependent on time and external factors than "Mental health" or "Vitality" and kept negative correlation with age.

Four out of five GBB-24 scores were found to be significantly higher in males as compared with females. Again, this difference was evident in the control group and disappeared in the donors and patients. This result corresponds with the outcomes of early studies showing that: a) females tend to have more health complaints than their male counterparts; b) they do receive more diagnostic workups; and c) they receive prescriptions more often during office visits than men do (Verbrugge & Steiner, 1985). Significant postoperative HRQol worsening in the patients and HRQol improvement in the donors was probably the reason why the difference was not evident in these groups. Both of these concepts need further evaluation with higher sample numbers in order to assess importance of the findings.

This study has some limitations. The most important is a lack of an ideal control group. We've used the healthy individuals from general population as controls. As far as the donors are, on the whole, healthier than representatives of the general population, it would be even more informative to compare their results with the persons who were evaluated and accepted as donors, but finally didn't donate a kidney. However, this kind of analyses would be impossible to perform with relatively small number of transplants performed in our country. An ongoing multicenter study from the US is addressing this issue and will probably come up with the results in the next few years (http://www.clinicaltrials.gov/ct2/results?term=NCT00608283). Relatively small sample number, especially in Group III, can be considered as another shortcoming of this study. Nevertheless, taking into consideration that they comprise 85% of transplants performed in Georgia, and a very high response rate, this group is representative for the Country.

Prospective design and high response rate are the most important advantages of this study. The response rate of 94% is the highest reported in the literature using these questionnaires. It was caused by the fact that the questionnaires have been handed out personally to almost all the donors by nephrologists. On the contrary, the questionnaires have been mailed to the patients (Group I) and only half of them responded. Another advantage of this study is a comparison of pairs of subjects and controls matched for gender and age. Only few studies have evaluated the matched pairs (Fehrman-Ekholm et al, 2000) whereas others have compared their findings with the scores of general population (Johnson et al, 1999; Karrfelt et al, 1998). The present study is also the first to include post-nephrectomy patients, and apply the Bf-S questionnaire to the study groups.

5. Conclusion

In conclusion, the HRQol of living kidney donors and healthy individuals is similar and better than HRQol of the patients operated due to the medical indications. The future prospective studies with higher number of participants will enhance our knowledge of factors influencing HRQol of the living kidney donors and patients after nephrectomy.

6. References

Clark, PE., et al. (2001). Quality of life and psychological adaptation after surgical treatment for localized renal cell carcinoma: impact of the amount of remaining renal tissue. *Urology*, Vol. 57, No. 2, (February 2001), pp. 252-256.

El-Agroudy, AE.; et al. (2007). Long-term follow-up of living kidney donors: a longitudinal study, *British Journal of Urology International*, Vol. 100, No. 6, (December 2007), pp. 1351-1355.

Feltrin, A.; et al. (2008). Experience of donation and quality of life in living kidney and liver donors, *Transplant International*, Vol. 21, No. 5, (may 2008), pp. 466-472.

Fehrman-Ekholm, I.; et al. (2000). Kidney donors don't regret: follow-up of 370 donors in Stockholm since 1964. *Clinical Transplantation*, Vol. 69, No. 10, (May 2000), pp. 2067-2071.

Giessing, M.; et al. (2004). Quality of Life of Living Kidney Donors in Germany: A Survey with the Validated Short Form-36 and Giessen Subjective Complaints List-24 Questionnaires. *Transplantation*; Vol. 78, No. 6, (September 2004), pp. 864-872.

Hariharan, S.; et al. (2000). Improved graft survival after renal transplantation in the United States, 1988 to 1996. *New England Journal of Medicine*, Vol. 342, No.9, (March 2000), pp. 605-612.

Ibrahim, HN.; et al. (2009). Long-Term consequences of kidney donation. *New England Journal of Medicine*, Vol. 360, No. 5, (January 2009), pp. 459-469.

Isotani, S. ; et al. (2002). Quality of life of living kidney donors: the short-form 36-item health questionnaire survey. *Urology*, Vol. 60, No. 4, (October 2002), pp. 588-592.

Jackobs, S.; et al. (2005). Quality of life following living donor nephrectomy comparing classical flank incision and anterior vertical mini-incision. *World Journal of Urology*, Vol. 23, No. 5, (November 2005), pp. 343-348.

Johnson, EM.; et al. (1999). Long-term follow-up of living kidney donors: quality of life after donation. *Transplantation*, Vol. 67, No. 5, (March 1999), pp. 717-721.

Karrfelt, HME.; et al. (1998). To be or not to be a living donor: questionnaire to parents of children who have undergone renal transplantation. *Transplantation*, Vol. 65, No. 7, (April 1998), pp. 915-918.

Lima, DX.; Petroianu A. & Hauter HL. (2006). Quality of life and surgical complications of kidney donors in the late post-operative period in Brazil. *Nephrol Dialusis and Transplantation*, Vol. 21, No. 11, (November 2006), pp. 323823-42.

Novara, G., et al. (2010). Factors predicting health-related quality of life recovery in patients undergoing surgical treatment for renal tumors: prospective evaluation using the RAND SF-36 Health Survey. *European Urology,*Vol 57, No. 1, (January 2010), pp. 112-120.

Poulakis, V., et al. (2003). Quality of life after surgery for localized renal cell carcinoma: comparison between radical nephrectomy and nephron-sparing surgery. *Urology*, Vol. 62, No. 5, (November 2003), pp. 814-820.

Reimer, J.; et al. (2006). The impact of living-related kidney transplantation on the donor's life. *Transplantation*, Vol. 81, No. 9, (May 2006), pp. 1268-1273.

Schover, LR.; et al. (1997). The psychosocial impact of donating a kidney: long-term follow-up from a urology based center. *Journal of Urology*, Vol. 157, No. 5, (May 1997), pp. 1596-1601.

Smith, GC.; et al. (2003). Prospective psychosocial monitoring of living kidney donors using the SF-36 health survey. *Transplantation*, (September 2003), Vol. 76, No. 5, pp. 807-809.

Smith, GC.; et al. (2004). Prospective psychosocial monitoring of living kidney donors using the Short Form-36 health survey: results at 12 months. *Transplantation*, Vol. 78, No. 9, (November 2004), pp. 1384-1389.

Tanriverdi, N. ; et al. (2004). Quality of life and mood in renal transplantation recipients, donors, and controls: preliminary report. *Transplant Proceedings*, Vol. 36, No. 1, (January-February 2004), pp. 117-119.

Tellioglu, G.; et al. (2008). Quality of life analysis of renal donors. *Transplant Proceedings* , Vol. 40, No. 1, (January-February 2008), pp. 50-52.

Verbrugge, LM. & Steiner, RP. (1985). Prescribing drugs to men and women. *Health Psychology*. Vol. 4, No. 1, pp. 79-98.

Ware, JE Jr. & Sherbourne, CD. (1992). The MOS 36-item short-form health survey (SF-36). I. Conceptual framework and item selection. *Medical Care*, Vol. 30, No. 6, (June 1992), pp. 473-483.

Zargooshi, J. (2001). Quality of life of Iranian kidney donors. *Journal of Urology*, Vol. 166, No. 5, (November 2001), pp. 1790-1799.

Zerssen, D. (1976). Die Befindlichkeitsskala. - Manual. Weinheim: Beltz Test. Beltz-Test GmbH.

5

Clinical Spectrum of Patients with Renal Cell Carcinoma

Mehrnaz Asadi Gharabaghi
Tehran University of Medical Sciences
Iran

1. Introduction

The classic triad of flank pain, palpable mass and hematuria exists in less than 20 percent of patients with renal cell carcinoma, and the tumor may become large in its origin before any local sign or symptom arises. Therefore, it is common to detect the tumor only after the metastasis develops.

Renal cell carcinoma (RCC) may present with diverse range of clinical manifestations. Many cases of renal cell carcinoma are unsuspected initially. The same is true for tumor recurrence even several years after primary tumor resection. For instance, it is not uncommon for a thyroid nodule to be the presenting feature of metastatic RCC. Renal cell carcinoma may masquerade any other illness so it is named tumor of internal medicine. Here the clinical presentations of the tumor within different body organs are discussed. In the followings, the clinical spectrum is arranged by each system in the body. The symptoms and signs of tumor in the urinary system are discussed separately. The systemic manifestations of cancer-related treatment are not discussed here.

2. Skin manifestations

Dermatological manifestations of renal cell carcinoma are not common. However, there are reports of coetaneous metastases as the primary clue to the tumor diagnosis (Mueller et al., 2004; Srinivasan, 2010). Skin nodules are more common. Scalp is the most prevalent site followed by chest and abdomen (Arrabal-Polo et al, 2009; Dorairajan et al., 1999).

Small vessel vasculitis limited to skin has been noted in renal cell carcinoma. It causes papules, nodules and even skin ulceration. Maynard et al reported a case of an adult male with renal cell carcinoma that initially presented with leukocytoclastic vasculitis involving skin, joints and gastrointestinal tracts (Maynard, 2010).

Palmar fibromatosis,acanthosis nigricans,hypertrichosis lanuginose,paraneoplastic erythroderma, bullous pemphigoid, and acquired ichthyosis are rare coetaneous manifestations of internal malignancies that are rarely reported in cases of renal cell carcinoma (Klein et al., 2009; Tebbe et al.,1991).

Hence, it cannot be over emphasized that an occult cancer such as renal cell carcinoma needs to be considered in evaluation of an elderly patient presenting with systemic vasculitis or certain dermatologic disorders.

3. Musculoskeletal manifestations

Renal cell carcinoma avidly involves the skeleton .After lung; the skeleton is the second most common site for metastases (Fottner et al., 2010). It ranks as the sixth solid tumor responsible for bone metastases that cause severe bone pain or debilitating skeletal complications such as pathologic fractures and spinal cord compression. Pelvis, ribs and vertebrae are the most prevalent sites for bone metastases. Patients with bone involvement portend a grave prognosis and most of them die within a year. Various therapeutic modalities such as chemo radiotherapy, surgery and bisphosphonates have been introduced with variable success (Lipton et al., 2004).

A 54 year-old man presented with multiple pathologic fractures of thoracic vertebrae to my department. He was finally diagnosed to suffer from advanced renal cell carcinoma. He was a truck driver and noticed the severe back pain while fixing his truck. The fractures occurred when he was tightening the screws forcefully. Therefore, it seems prudent to look for a kidney cancer while confronting bone metastasis with unknown origin.

Cancer and autoimmunity is a well-known inter-disciplinary entity .Tumor products behave as haptens triggering an overwhelming autoimmune response within the body. The autoimmune disorder may herald the presence of an occult cancer.

Inflammatory myopathies, myositis and inclusion body myositis are reported as paraneoplastic syndromes associated with renal cell carcinoma. Klausner et al reported a case of 45- year -old man presented with polymyosistis that finally diagnosed to have renal cell carcinoma (Klausner et al, 2002). Similarly, Respicio et al reported a case of concurrent renal cell carcinoma, interstitial lung disease and polymyositis in a 58 year-old man (Respicio et al., 2007).It is not exactly known whether it is possible to predict the type of solid tumor at the time of inflammatory mysoitis by means of tumor biologic markers. Amoura et al reported that markers as CA-125 and CA19-9 may predict developing the offending tumor in advance and need to be included in evaluation of patients with inflammatory myopathic syndromes(Amoura et al.,2005).

A syndrome resembling to polymyalgia rheumatica (PMR) has been described as a paraneoplastic manifestation of solid tumors. The syndrome is not steroid responsive. Yet, it is not clear whether it will be improved after nephrectomy (Sidhom et al., 1993). Hence, it is reasonable to look for an occult solid tumor such as renal cell carcinoma in a patient with PMR refractory to steroids. Niccoli et al reported three patients presenting with PMR mimicking syndrome heralding renal cell carcinoma. They suggested that besides inefficacy of steroids, absence of morning stiffness and characteristic sonographic findings of shoulder are features of PMR mimicking syndrome associated with RCC (Niccoli et al., 2002).

RS3PE (remitting symmetric sero negative synovitis with pitting edema) is a syndrome with symptoms similar to PMR; it occurs in patients older than 50 and may be associated with solid tumors or hematologic malignancies. It is mandatory to rule out an occult malignancy in the setting of RS3PE syndrome. Lung, breast, prostate and rarely kidney cancers have been reported as the underlying solid tumors in patients with this syndrome (Juncadella et al., 2003; Marto et al., 2010; Russel, 2005).

Other rare rheumatic manifestations of renal cell carcinoma include metastatic monoarthritis and multi centric reticulo histiocytosis (MR). The latter is a syndrome presenting with coetaneous nodules and severe destructive arthritis .It may be associated with an internal malignancy. Tan et al reported two cases of MR associated with urologic malignancies (Placed et al, 2010; Tan et al.2011).

4. Nervous system manifestations

Paraneoplastic neuropathy is a well-known autoimmune neuropathy associated with anti neuronal nuclear antibody. Roy et al (Roy et al., 2002) reported chronic sensory motor polyneuropathy in a 65-year-old man several months before the diagnosis of RCC. Allen et al also reported a case of acute demyelinating neuropathy in a case of papillary renal cell carcinoma that resolved following nephrectomy (Allen et al., 2011). Torvik et al reported three cases with necrotizing vasculitic involvement of peripheral nerves that were diagnosed to have renal cell carcinoma through postmortem follow up (Torvik & Berntzen, 1968).

Numb chin syndrome is numbness of lower lip, chine and gingiva of anterior lower teeth. It may be associated with a visceral malignancy such as lung, breast cancer or leukemia; however, it has been reported in renal cell carcinoma. Inferior alveolar/mental nerve is involved due to metastasis to mandible or nerve sheath infiltration by tumor (Divya et al., 2010; Lata & Kumar, 2010).

Opsoclonus is an ocular dyskinesia characterized by involuntary, repetitive, rapid conjugate saccades. It is most commonly seen in children. In an adult, it may herald an internal malignancy. Koukoulis A et al reported a case of paraneoplastic opsoclonus in a 64 year- old man. The patient was diagnosed to have papillary renal cell carcinoma 6 months after the diagnosis of opsoclonus (Koukoulis et al., 1998).

Antinueronal nuclear antibody type 1 (classically known as anti –Hu) is detected in cancer associated autoimmune neurologic disorders (lucchinetti et al., 1998) .Patients develop various forms of neurologic disease including Lambert-Eaton myasthenic syndrome, encephalitis, cerebellar ataxia and so forth. For instance, Ammar et al reported a case of 64-year- old woman who presented with acute cerebellar ataxia as the initial manifestation of renal cell carcinoma (Ammar et al., 2008). There is also a report of bilateral diaphragmatic paralysis as a paraneoplastic neurologic disease secondary to RCC that ameliorated after nephrectomy (Rijnders & Decramer, 2000).Therefore, it is appropriate to investigate for an occult cancer when confronting an idiopathic bilateral diaphragmatic paralysis.

Brain and spinal metastases are common in advanced stages of RCC. However, solitary brain metastasis and relevant clinical findings such as headache and focal neurologic deficit may be the presenting signs of the cancer (Candiano et al., 2010). Spinal metastases are usually extra dural but intradural involvement with resulting neurologic deficits, especially cauda equina syndrome were reported (Lin et al., 2011). Back pain and sciatica due to metastatic nerve root infiltration of lumbo sacral nerves have been reported in RCC patients (Shakeel et al., 2009). Intramedullary spinal metastasis that are the rarest type of spinal involvement have also been reported as the presenting sign in RCC (Asadi et al., 2009; Donovan& Freeman, 2006; Gómez de la Riva et al., 2005; Schijns et al., 2000). Although uncommon, an occult cancer such as renal cell carcinoma needs to be considered in differential diagnosis of the above-mentioned syndromes.

5. Vascular system manifestations

Renal vein and caval thromboses are among the well- known thrombotic events associated with renal cell carcinoma. Left-sided varicocele that does not decompress after taking the recumbent position is a well -known complication of the locally advanced RCC. It is due to tumor thrombus extending along the renal vein that blocks drainage of left spermatic vein into inferior vena cava (IVC).It is not just left spermatic vein that may become clogged .Right spermatic vein is at risk too. Shinsaka et al reported a case of right varicocele as a result of RCC thrombus in right spermatic vein without simultaneous caval thrombosis (Al-Taan et al., 2007;Shinsaka et al., 2006).Furthermore, prothrombotic state as a paraneoplastic feature of RCC may cause thrombosis in unusual sites such as subclavian veins(Hameed et al.,2011). Hence, it is worthwhile to consider RCC in evaluating patients with idiopathic venous thrombosis, especially in an unusual site.

6. Hematologic manifestations

Cytopenia, especially anemia is a common feature of the tumor. Polycythemia may also be seen, although less frequently (Mohammed Ilyas et al., 2008). Although, micro angiopathic hemolytic anemia, hemolytic uremic syndrome and disseminated intravascular coagulopathy may occur because of cancer chemotherapy in RCC, the tumor rarely presents with such a hematologic manifestation as thrombocytopenia .Yet, there are reports of metastatic RCC presenting with thrombocytopenia due to bone marrow carcinomatosis (Florcken et al., 2009).

Disturbation in fibrinolysis system is a well –known feature of hematologic and non-hematologic tumors such as prostate cancer. Plasminogen is converted to plasmin; tissue plasminogen activator (t PA) or urokinase- type plasminogen activator (uPA) promotes the conversion. Some tumors express high level of tPA activity. This feature not only brings some sort of bleeding diathesis but also seems to be vital for tumor survival. In fact, the variable expression of fibrinolysis system components in a given cancer may affect the prognosis. For instance, patients with greater expression of u-PA on breast cancer cells have shorter survival and increased chance of relapse (Bell, 1996).In renal cell carcinoma, it has been demonstrated that expression of plasminogen inhibitor-1 is an independent poor prognostic factor as it promotes tumor angiogenesis and metastasis (Choi et al.,2011;Zubcaet al.,2010). Therefore, changes in hematologic parameters are not only paraneoplstic features of RCC but also of prognostic value.

7. Pulmonary manifestations

Lung metastases are common in natural history of RCC. Single or multiple variable –sized pulmonary nodules are usually detected in patients with advanced RCC. Regarding large reserve volume of lung, tumor burden may become so huge before any respiratory symptom such as dyspnea or cough develops. Besides this common mode of presentation, lymphangitic carcinomatosis may develop in setting of metastatic RCC. It is an interstitial lung disorder caused by lymphangitic spread of tumors such as breast, lung and rarely kidney cancer. It usually manifests with obstinate cough and progressive dyspnea. Wallach et al reported a case of 68 year -old man who presented with respiratory symptoms 20 months after nephrectomy for stage III RCC. He had lymphangitic carcinomatosis.

According to their review of literature, there are less than 10 reports of such patients (Wallach et al., 2011).

RCC metastases are not confined to lung parenchyma. There are reports of endobronchial metastases from RCC .Therefore hemoptysis or a pulmonary atelectasis may result from endobronchial spread of RCC.As the tumor is a hyper vascular one, it is mandatory to take precaution while planning local therapeutic modalities for symptomatic metastases (Mathai et al., 2007; Suyama et al., 2011).

Malignant pleural effusion secondary to RCC is rare and usually seen with papillary and clear cell histological types. There are reports of special cases of malignant effusion secondary to RCC.As an example; Chetcuti K et al reported a case of massive spontaneous hemothorax in a 78 year- old man with a history of RCC. The culprit was a chest wall metastasis of RCC (Chetcuti et al., 2010; Teresa et al., 2011).

Mediastinal lymph adenopathy and masses are seen in advanced stages of renal cell carcinoma or as presenting features of primary tumor or tumor recurrence. They are closely correlated with poor prognosis (Mattana et al., 1996; Winter et al., 2010). Niikura S et al reported a case of 62 year- old man presented with mediastinal lymph node enlargements 19 years after nephrectomy for RCC (Niikura et al., 1999).

Pulmonary infarction due to tumor emboli within pulmonary circulation is an unusual manifestation of renal cell carcinoma .The tumor emboli originates from thrombus extending along vena cava, right sided heart or proximal part of pulmonary artery (Shiono et al.,2001;Wieder et al.,2003). The disease presents with acute or sub acute cor pulmonale and cytological study of pulmonary artery sample helps diagnosis.

Despite the grave prognosis associated with pulmonary involvement in patients with RCC, there is a report by Okubo Y et al who described a patient with an obstinate cough as the sole manifestation of non- metastatic RCC .Cough disappeared after nephrectomy and recurred with tumor relapse (Okubo et al., 2007).

8. Cardiac manifestations

Heart may be involved in different manners by a non-cardiac tumor. For example, certain chemotherapeutic drugs and radiotherapy have deleterious effects on heart. Opportunistic infection of cardiac chambers has been demonstrated because of immune suppression in cancer patients. The tumor may involve the pericardium and less frequently, myoendocardium.So malignant pericardial effusion is a common finding in advanced cancer patients (Kim et al., 2010). Although uncommon, there are reports of malignant pericardial effusion secondary to RCC (Zustovich et al., 2008).

In RCC, vena cava thrombosis can extend beyond the hepatic veins into the right atrium (Kalkat et al., 2008) .However; there are reports of cardiac metastasis mimicking primary cardiac tumors without concurrent cava involvement (Aburto et al., 2009; Talukder et al., 2010). For instance, Lee HJ et al demonstrated a case of 77- year- old man with 2- month history of RCC in whom cardiac metastasis caused left ventricular outflow tract obstruction (Lee et al., 2010). Miyamoto MI et al reported a case of metastatic renal carcinoma with a left atrial mass mimicking myxoma. They demonstrated that the mass was RCC metastasis derived from pulmonary vein tumor extension. The pulmonary vein itself had been involved from adjacent mediastinal lymph nodes (Miyamoto& Picard, 2002). Cardiac metastasis in a patient with known history of primary cancer is not challenging to diagnosis. Yet it is not uncommon for a RCC to present initially with a cardiac mass (Crouch & Tak,2002).Therefore, it needs to be vigilant to the presence of an occult cancer when evaluating a cardiac mass even if it resembles a primary cardiac tumor and there is no extra cardio respratory symptom.

Not only myopericardium is involved in RCC but also the endocardium may become diseased in RCC. Non-bacterial endocarditis is a well –known disease entity in various diseases such as HIV infection, connective tissue disorders and cancers. The exact mechanism is not yet defined but thrombophilic state associated with malignancy may be responsible. The most primary cancer site is pancreas (Johnson et al., 2010). In literature review, there is few report of RCC associated with non-bacterial thrombotic endocarditis.

9. Gastrointestinal manifestations

Gastrointestinal (GI) tract is involved by RCC in different ways. Stauffer's syndrome constitutes reversible abnormalities in liver function tests including enzymes and pro thrombin time. It may present as hepatocellular or cholestatic liver disease. It is not due to liver metastasis and actually caused by humoral effects of inflammatory cytokines produced by the tumor. Therefore, the abnormalities disappear after tumor resection by nephrectomy (Kranidiotis et al., 2009). However, there are reports of renal cell carcinoma metastases to various organs of gastrointestinal tracts.

Oral cavity metastases from RCC have been demonstrated. In fact, intraoral soft tissue metastases are not common. They usually originate from lung and breast cancers. Metastatic oral cavity lesions rarely present as the initial feature of an occult cancer. For instance, Maestre-Rodríguez O reported a case of 55- year-old man who underwent resection of a gingival tumor that finally diagnosed to be metastatic RCC (Will et al., 2008; Maestre-Rodríguez et al., 2009). Esophageal metastasis producing local symptoms such as dysphagia is not surprising in a case of an advanced RCC (de los Monteros-Sanchez et al., 2004). Hematogenous spread of RCC to stomach is seen, albeit with concomitant metastases in other organs, especially lungs (Pollheimer et al., 2008).Although uncommon, gastric metastasis and upper gastrointestinal bleeding may be the initial feature of RCC. Tiwari P et al reported a 58- year-old woman with a 2-week history of melena. The source of bleeding was a 3cm×5cm vascular polypoid antral mass .She was finally diagnosed to have metastatic RCC (Tiwari et al., 2010).

Intraluminal metastases from RCC may be the source of intestinal bleeding or less commonly intussusceptions. They may behave as the leading point for an intestinal obstruction and intussusceptions. Periampullary region, duodenum and jejunum rank the most common sites .Yet, other sites as large bowel may be involved too (Eo et al., 2008; Loualidi et al., 2004; Nozawa et al., 2003; Papachristodoulou et al., 2004; Roviello et al., 2006; Sadler et al., 2007 Takeda et al., 2011). The above cases highlight the importance of considering RCC metastasis as a source of intestinal bleeding and/or obstruction, especially in patients with a known cancer history.

Liver is the organ that is frequently involved in advanced RCC (Staehler et al., 2010). Yet it is not the only solid organ within GI tract involved by RCC. Pancreatic metastasis may occur due to a close proximity to the left kidney. However, the pancreas may be involved as a nest for metastatic deposits even years after nephrectomy. Yokonishi T et al reported pancreatic metastasis in a 74 year -old man who had history of nephrectomy due to RCC 25 years before (Yokonishi et al., 2010). The physicians must be alert to pancreatic metastasis from renal cell carcinoma and differentiate it from primary tumors of the gland because the prognosis differs in each case. Ghavamian R et al reviewed 23 patients with metastatic RCC to the pancreas .They found that imaging features of metastatic RCC resembled the primary RCC and differed from pancreatic tumours such as adenocarcinoma. RCC is a hyper vascular tumour, hence the metastasis enhances in early phase of contrasted abdominal computed tomography. They also noticed that the mean interval for pancreatic metastases to develop after nephrectomy was 9.8 years (Ghavamian et al., 2000).

Budd-Chiari syndrome defined by presence of abdominal pain, hepatomegaly and ascites has also been reported as a manifestation of renal cell carcinoma. The syndrome caused by tumor thrombus extending along vena cava. As a result, hepatic venous drainage system will be blocked .It may become fulminate if not treated on time (Moragnoni et al., 2010; Shih et al., 2009).

Bowel ischemia may be seen in RCC not only as a complication of immunotherapy but also as a consequence of embolic infarcts from tumor thrombus in left heart (Low et al.,1989;Sparano etal.,1991).

Sinistral portal hypertension refers to gastric variceal hemorrhage secondary to splenic vein thrombosis. It is most common in the setting of pancreatic pathologies such as pancreatitis, pseudocysts and cancer. There is no concurrent liver dysfunction (Singhal et al., 2006). Joya Seijo MD et al reported a case of sinistral portal hypertension and gastric bleeding as the initial manifestation of left sided RCC infiltrating the pancreas (Joya Seijo et al., 2004). RCC may rarely present with variceal bleeding. A 51- year- old man presented to our hospital with an episode of upper gastrointestinal bleeding twelve years after nephrectomy for a clear cell RCC. He was diagnosed to have downhill esophageal varices. They were formed by compressing effects of enlarged mediastinal lymph nodes upon the azygous vein .Pathologic review of the lymph nodes revealed recurrence of clear cell carcinoma.

10. Endocrinologic system

Like any other organ, endocrine system is not safe from RCC. Metastatic RCC may invade pituitary gland and mimics a nonfunctional pituitary adenoma (Kramer et al., 2010). Panhypopituitarism, suprasellar extension, headache, hemianopia, galactorrhea and diabetes insipidus are reported because of RCC metastasis to pituitary gland (Gopan et al., 2007). Although uncommon, thyroid metastasis in RCC has been demonstrated that can be of diagnostic challenge to be differentiated from primary thyroid tumors (Cimino-Mathews et al,2011).Adrenal, testicular and ovarian metastases have been reported in the course of disease even years after primary nephrectomy (Guney et al.,2010;Wu et al.,2010). Toquero L et al reported a case of 54- year old woman with a pelvic mass as an initial presentation of RCC. The mass was actually ovarian metastasis from RCC (Toquero et al., 2009).Ovarian metastases usually originate from stomach, colon, breast cancers and lymphoma. However,

RCC needs to be considered in differential diagnosis. The patients with this sort of metastasis in either testis or ovary usually seek medical care because of localized symptoms rather than a symptom relevant to hypogonadism.It is may be due to age of patients who are usually in 50s-70s.

11. Paraneoplastic syndromes

There are constellation of signs, symptoms and laboratory data abnormalities not related to tumor local effect or its metastases. Some of them such as Stauffer's syndrome have been mentioned above. Most of them are cytokine mediated such as neoplastic fever (Alsirafy et al., 2011) .The remaining may be due to tumor products. Humoral hypercalcemia of malignancy is a paraneoplastic feature of various tumors. In RCC, it is multi factorial. Widespread bone metastases, parathormone-related peptide and increased production of 1, 25 hydroxyvitamin D are responsible. Therefore, hypercalcaemia in patients with RCC may respond to administration of steroids (Shivnani et al., 2009).

Glucose metabolism abnormalities have been demonstrated in association with RCC. The tumor can produce insulin like growth factor II resulting in hypoglycemia (Berman & Harland, 2001).On the other hand, hyper glycemia is reported as a paraneoplastic endocrinopathy in patients with RCC(Jobe et al.,1993).For instance, Yumura Y et al reported 2 patients whose diabetes was controlled after nephrectomy for RCC (Yumura et al.,2007).

Although hypertension is a complication of targeted therapy in RCC patients, it may develop as a paraneoplastic feature of kidney cancer not related to treatment (kirkali,2011).Some of the patients show increased blood level of renin and plasma renin activity as a possible cause of their increased blood pressure(Steffens et al.,1992).

Gynecomastia attributable to human chorionic gonadotropin overproduction has been reported as another paraneoplastic endocrinopathy in RCC (Mohammed Ilyas et al., 2008).It has also been demonstrated that expression of beta subunit of human chorionic gonadotropin is associated with adverse prognosis in RCC (Hotakainen et al., 2002, 2006).

Cancerous erythrocytosis is another rare para neoplastic disorder associated with RCC caused by over expression of erythropoietin and hypoxemia induced factor. However, only a small percentage of patients with over expression of erythropoietin develop paraneoplastic erythrocytosis (Wiesener et al., 2007).Although uncommon, paraneoplastic erythrocytosis of RCC may have grave sequels; Kruyt ND et al reported a case of 65- year - old man who presented with neurologic deficits due to multiple cerebral infarctions as the initial presentation of RCC. His erythrocytosis and cognitive dysfunction relieved after nephrectomy for newly diagnosed RCC (Kruyt & Wessels, 2006).

Although above-mentioned paraneoplastic syndromes are not common in RCC, they are of value for both diagnosis and estimating the prognosis of the primary tumor.

12. Miscellaneous abnormalities

RCC behaves unpredictably so it is common to confront its metastasis in unusual sites. The followings are some examples. It has been reported that renal cell carcinoma may initially present as an orbital mass, a mass within paranasal sinuses, gallbladder metastasis, cerebellopontine angle or superior vena cava syndrome due to supraclavicular lymph nodes involvement (Cobo-Dolset al., 2006; Fang et al., 2010; Panarese et al., 2002; sakura et al., 2007; Mudiayanselage et al., 2008).

13. Conclusion

The classic triad of flank pain, hematuria and palpable abdominal mass occurs in a small fraction of patients with renal cell carcinoma, so it is wise to be aware of various clinical presentations of the disease. The above-mentioned clinical features are summarized in Table-1.

Skin
coetaneous metastases, Skin nodules, Small vessel vasculitis, Palmar fibromatosis,Acanthosis nigricans, Hypertrichosis lanuginose,Paraneoplastic erythroderma, Bullous pemphigoid,Acquired ichthyosis
Musculoskeletal system
Bone metastases, Inflammatory myopathies, Myositis , Inclusion body myositis, Polymyalgia rheumatica- like syndrome, RS3PE (remitting symmetric sero negative synovitis with pitting edema), Metastatic monoarthritis and multi centric reticulo histiocytosis (MR)
Nervous system
Paraneoplastic neuropathy, Numb chin syndrome, Opsoclonus, Lambert-Eaton myasthenic syndrome, Encephalitis, Cerebellar ataxia, Bilateral diaphragmatic paralysis, Brain and spinal metastases
Vascular system
Renal vein and caval thromboses, Left sided varicocele, Prothrombotic state and thrombosis in unusual sites
Hematologic system
Cytopenia,Polycythemia, Micro angiopathic hemolytic anemia, Hemolytic uremic syndrome, Disseminated intravascular coagulopathy, Disturbation in fibrinolysis system
Pulmonary system
Single or multiple variable –sized pulmonary nodules, Lymphangitic carcinomatosis, Malignant pleural effusion, Mediastinal lymph adenopathy, Pulmonary infarction due to tumor emboli
Heart
Malignant pericardial effusion, Cardiac metastasis mimicking primary cardiac tumors, Non-bacterial endocarditis
Gastrointestinal tract
Stauffer's syndrome, Oral cavity metastases, Esophageal metastasis, Gastric metastasis and upper gastrointestinal bleeding, Intraluminal metastases, Hepatic and pancreatic metastases, Budd-Chiari syndrome, Bowel ischemia due to tumor emboli, Sinistral portal hypertension, Gastric variceal bleeding
Endocrinologic system
Panhypopituitarism ,Metastasis to thyroid, adrenal, ovaries and testes
Paraneoplastic syndromes
Hypercalcaemia, Hypoglycemia, Hyperglycemia, Polycythemia, Gynecomastia, Hypertension

Table 1. Clinical spectrum of patients with renal cell carcinoma

14. References

Aburto, J., Bruckner, BA. Blackmon, SH., Beyer, EA. &Reardon, MJ. (2009). Renal cell carcinoma, metastatic to the left ventricle. *Tex Heart Inst J.*, 36(1):48-9, 19436786.

Allen, JA., Yang, XJ. & Sufit, RL. (2011).Reversible demyelinating neuropathy associated with renal cell carcinoma. *Neuromuscular Disord*, 21(3):227-31, 21195618.

Alsirafy, SA., El Mesidy, SM., Abou-Elela, EN. & Elfaramawy, YI. (2011). Naproxen test for neoplastic fever may reduce suffering.*J Palliat Med.*, 14(5):665-7, 21291328.

Al-Taan, OS. Featherstone, JM., Rees, AM., Young, WT. & Stephenson TP. (2007).Renal cell carcinoma in a horseshoe kidney presenting as an acute, left sided varicocele.*Int Urol Nephrol.*, 39(2):369-71, 16835726.

Ammar, H., Brown, SH., Malani, A., Sheth, HK., Sollars, EG., Zhou, SX., Gupta ,C. &Mughal ,S. (2008 May). A case of paraneoplastic cerebellar ataxia secondary to renal cell carcinoma.*South Med J.*, 101(5):556-7, 18414160.

Amoura, Z., Duhaut ,P., Huong, DL., Wechsler, B., Costedoat-Chalumeau, N., Francès, C., Cacoub ,P., Papo ,T, Cormont ,S., Touitou, Y., Grenier, P., Valeyre, D.& Piette, JC.(2005). Tumor antigen markers for the detection of solid cancers in inflammatory myopathies.*Cancer Epidemiol Biomarkers Prev.*, 14(5):1279-82, 15894686.

Arrabal-Polo, MA. Arias-Santiago, SA. Aneiros-Fernandez, J., Burkhardt-Perez, P., Arrabal-Martin, M., &Naranjo-Sintes, R. (2009). Cutaneous metastases in renal cell carcinoma: a case report. report. *Cases J.*, 25; 2:7948-51, 19918439.

Asadi, M., Rokni-Yazdi, H., Salehinia, F. & Allameh, FS. (2009). Metastatic renal cell carcinoma initially presented with an intramedullary spinal cord lesion: a case report.*Cases J.*, 2:7805-8, 19918485.

Bell, WR. (1996). The fibrinolytic system in neoplasia.*Semin Thromb Hemost.* , 22(6):459-78, 9122711.

Berman, J. &Harland, S. (2001).Hypoglycaemia caused by secretion of insulin-like growth factor 2 in a primary renal cell carcinoma.*Clin Oncol (R Coll Radiol).* , 13(5):367-9, 11716231.

Candiano, G., Pepe, P., Grasso, G. &Aragona, F. (2010).Headache: a unique clinical presentation for renal cell carcinoma (RCC).*Arch Ital Urol Androl.* , 82(4):184-6, 21341558.

Chetcuti, K., Barnard, J., Loggos, S., Hassan, M., Srivastava, V., Mourad, F., Makhzoum, Z. & Bittar, MN. (2010). Massive hemothorax secondary to metastatic renal carcinoma.*Ann Thorac Surg.*, 89(6):2014-6, 20494072.

Choi, JW., Lee, JH., Park, HS. & Kim, YS. (2011).PAI-1 expression and its regulation by promoter 4G/5G polymorphism in clear cell renal cell carcinoma.*J Clin Pathol.*, July1, (Epub head of print), 21725041.

Cimino-Mathews, A., Sharma, R., &Netto, GJ. (2011). Diagnostic use of PAX8, CAIX, TTF-1, and TGB in metastatic renal cell carcinoma of the thyroid.*Am J Surg Pathol.* , 35(5):757-61.21451364.

Cobo-Dols, M., Alés-Díaz, I., Villar-Chamorro, E., Gil-Calle, S., Alcaide-García, J., Montesa-Pino, A., Gutiérrez-Calderón, V. & Benavides-Orgaz, M. (2006).Solitary metastasis in a nasal fossa as the first manifestation of a renal carcinoma.*Clin Transl Oncol.* , 8(4):298-300, 16648109.

Crouch, ED. & Tak, T. (2002).Renal cell carcinoma presenting as right atrial mass.*Echocardiography*, 19(2):149-51, 11926979 de los Monteros-Sanchez, AE., Medina-Franco, H., Arista-Nasr, J. & Cortes-Gonzalez ,R. (2004). Resection of an esophageal metastasis from a renal cell carcinoma.*Hepatogastroenterology,* 51(55):163-4, 15011855.

Divya, KS., Moran, NA. & Atkin, PA. (2010). Numb chin syndrome: a case series and discussion. *Br Dent J.,* 208(4):157-60, 20186196.

Donovan, DJ. &Freeman, JH. (2006). Solitary intramedullary spinal cord tumor presenting as the initial manifestation of metastatic renal cell carcinoma: case report.*Spine (Phila Pa 1976).* , 15; 31(14):E460-3., 16778676.

Dorairajan ,LN., Hemal ,AK., Aron, M., Rajeev, TP., Nair, M., Seth, A., Dogra, PN.&Gupta, NP.(1999). Cutaneous metastases in renal cell carcinoma.*Urol Int.* , 63(3):164-7, 10738187.

EO, WK., Kim, GY. & Choi, SI. (2008). A case of multiple intussusceptions in the small intestine caused by metastatic renal cell carcinoma.*Cancer Res Treat.* , 40(2):97-9, 19688056.

Fang, X., Gupta, N., Shen, SS., Tamboli, P., Charnsangavej, C., Rashid, A. & Wang, H. (2010).Intraluminal polypoid metastasis of renal cell carcinoma in gallbladder mimicking gallbladder polyp.*Arch Pathol Lab Med.,* 134(7):1003-9, 20586628.

Florcken ,A., Loew, A., Koch, M., Gebauer, B., Dorken, B. & Riess, H. (2009).Severe thrombocytopenia in a patient with metastatic renal cell carcinoma.*Onkologie.* , 32(11):670-2, 19887872.

Fottner, A., Szalantzy, M., Wirthmann, L., Stähler, M., Baur-Melnyk, A., Jansson, V. &Dürr, HR. (2010).Bone metastases from renal cell carcinoma: patient survival after surgical treatment.*BMC Musculoskelet Disord.* , 3; 11:145-50, 20598157.

Ghavamian, R., Klein, KA., Stephens, DH., Welch, TJ., LeRoy, AJ., Richardson, RL., Burch, PA. &Zincke H. (2000).Renal cell carcinoma metastatic to the pancreas: clinical and radiological features.*Mayo Clin Proc.,* 75(6) :581-5, 10852418.

Gómez de la Riva, A., Isla ,A., Pérez-López, C., Budke, M., Gutiérrez, M. & Frutos, R. (2005). [Intramedullary spinal cord metastasis as the first manifestation of a renal carcinoma].*Neurocirugia (Astur).* , 16(4):359-64, 16143809.

Gopan, T., Toms, SA., Prayson ,RA., Suh, JH., Hamrahian, AH. & Weil, RJ. (2007). Symptomatic pituitary metastases from renal cell carcinoma.*Pituitary,* 10(3):251-9, 17541748.

Guney, S., Guney, N., Ozcan, D., Sayilgan, T. & Ozakin, E. (2010).Ovarian metastasis of a primary renal cell carcinoma: case report and review of literature.*Eur J Gynaecol Oncol.* , 31(3):339-41, 21077484.

Hameed, A., Pahuja, A., Thwaini, A. &Nambirajan, T. (2011).Subclavian vein thrombosis: an unusual presentation of renal cell carcinoma. *Can Urol Assoc J.,* 5(2):E27-8, 21470547.

Hotakainen, K., Lintula, S., Ljungberg, B., Finne, P., Paju, A., Stenman, UH. &Stenman ,J. (2006).Expression of human chorionic gonadotropin beta-subunit type I genes predicts adverse outcome in renal cell carcinoma.*J Mol Diagn.* , 8(5):598-603, 17065429.

Hotakainen, K., Ljungberg, B., Paju, A., Rasmuson, T., Alfthan, H. & Stenman, UH. (2002). The free beta-subunit of human chorionic gonadotropin as a prognostic factor in renal cell carcinoma.*Br J Cancer.* , 86(2):185-9, 11870503.

Jobe ,BA., Bierman, MH. & Mezzacappa, FJ. (1993). Hyperglycemia as a paraneoplastic endocrinopathy in renal cell carcinoma: a case report and review of the literature.*Nebr Med J.,* 78 (11):349-51, 8309485.

Johnson, J.A., Everett, B.M., Katz, J.T. & Loscalzo, J. (2010).Clinical Problem-Solving Painful Purple Toes. *N Engl J Med.*, 362:67 – 73, 0807291.

Joya Seijo, MD., del Valle Loarte, P., Marco Martínez, J., Herrera Merino, N.& Agud Aparicio, JL.(2004). carcinoma. An *Med Interna.*, 21(6):283-4, 15283642.

Juncadella, E., Ramentol, M., Rozadilla, A., &Ferre, J . (2003). RS3PE syndrome and renal cancer. *Med Clin (Barc).*, 8;121(16):638-9, 14636547.

Kalkat, MS., Abedin, A., Rooney, S., Doherty, A., Faroqui, M., Wallace, M. & Graham, TR. (2008).Renal tumours with cavo-atrial extension: surgical management and outcome.*Interact Cardiovasc Thorac Surg.*, 7(6):981-5, 18550606.

Kim, SH., Kwak, MH., Park, S., Kim, HJ., Lee, HS., Kim, MS., Lee, JM., Zo, JI., Ro, JS. & Lee, JS. (2005). Clinical characteristics of malignant pericardial effusion associated with recurrence and survival. *Cancer Res Treat.* , 42(4):210-6, 21253323.

Kirkali, Z. (2011).Adverse events from targeted therapies in advanced renal cell carcinoma: the impact on long-term use.*BJU Int.*, 107(11):1722-32, 21251188.

Klausner, AP., Ost, MC., Waterhouse RL ,Jr. &Savage SJ. (2002). Occult renal cell carcinoma in a patient with polymyositis.*Urology.* , 59(5):773-6, 11992921.

Klein, T., Rotterdam, S., Noldus, J. &Hinkel, A. (2009). Bullous pemphigoid is a rare paraneoplastic syndrome in patients with renal cell carcinoma. *Scand J Urol Nephrol.* , 43(4):334-6, 19308806.

Koukoulis ,A., Cimas, I. &Gómara, S. (1998).Paraneoplastic opsoclonus associated with papillary renal cell carcinoma. J *Neurol Neurosurg Psychiatry.*, 64(1):137-8, 9436748.

Kramer, CK., Ferreira, N., Silveiro, SP., Gross, JL., Dora, JM. &Azevedo, MJ. (2010).Pituitary gland metastasis from renal cell carcinoma presented as a non-functioning macroadenoma.*Arq Bras Endocrinol Metabol.* , 54(5) :498-501,20694412.

Kranidiotis, GP., Voidonikola, PT., Dimopoulos, MK. & Anastasiou-Nana, MI. (2009). Stauffer's syndrome as a prominent manifestation of renal cancer: a case report. Cases J., 2(1):49-52, 19144140.

Kruyt ND& Wessels PH. (2006).Cerebral infarction due to polycythaemia as the initial manifestation of renal cell carcinoma.*Ned Tijdschr Geneeskd.* , 150(17):969-72, 17225738.

Lata, J& Kumar, P. (2010). Numb chin syndrome: a case report and review of the literature. *Indian J Dent Res.* , 21(1):135-7, 20427925.

Lee, HJ., Park, JI., Lim, BH., Seo, JW., Kang, EM., Lee, BU. & Kim, YJ. (2010). Left ventricular metastasis from renal cell carcinoma causing left ventricular outflow tract obstruction. *Korean Circ J.*, 40(8):410-3, 20830256.

Lin, TK., Chen, SM. & Jung, SM. (2011).Solitary intradural extramedullary metastasis of renal cell carcinoma to the conus medullaris.*Kaohsiung J Med Sci.*, 27(1):45-8, 21329893.

Lipton, A., Colombo-Berra, A., Bukowski, RM., Rosen, L., Zheng, M. &Urbanowitz, G. (2004).Skeletal complications in patients with bone metastases from renal cell carcinoma and therapeutic benefits of zoledronic acid.*Clin Cancer Res.*, 15; 10(18 Pt 2):6397S-403S, 15448038.

Loualidi, A., Spooren, PF., Grubben, MJ., Blomjous, CE. & Goey, SH. (2004).Duodenal metastasis: an uncommon cause of occult small intestinal bleeding.*Neth J Med.*, 62(6):201-5, 15460501.

Low, DE. Frenkel, VJ., Manley, PN., Ford, SN. & Kerr, JW. (1989). Embolic mesenteric infarction: a unique initial manifestation of renal cell carcinoma. *Surgery*, 106(5):925-8, 2683176.

Lucchinetti, CF., Kimmel, DW. &Lennon, VA. (1998). Paraneoplastic and oncologic profiles of patients seropositive for type 1 antineuronal nuclear autoantibodies. *Neurology.* , 50(3):652-7, 9521251.

Marangoni, G., O'Sullivan, A., Ali, A., Faraj, W. & Heaton, N. (2010).Budd-Chiari syndrome secondary to caval recurrence of renal cell carcinoma.*Hepatobiliary Pancreat Dis Int.*, 9(3):321-4, 20525562.

Marto, G., Klitna, Z., Biléu, MC. & Barcelos, A. (2010). Remitting seronegative symmetric synovitis with pitting oedema syndrome, associated with prostate adenocarcinoma: a cse report.*Acta Reumatol Port.* , 35(3) :358-60, 20975640.

Mathai, AM., Rau, AR., Shetty, AB., Kamath, MP. & Prasad, SC. (2007). Endobronchial metastasis from renal cell carcinoma: a case report. Indian *J Pathol Microbiol.* , 50(2):379-81, 17883082.

Mattana, J., Kurtz, B., Miah, A. & Singhal, PC. (1996). Renal cell carcinoma presenting as a solitary anterior superior mediastinal mass.*J Med.*, 27(3-4):205-10, 8289968.

Maynard, JW., Christopher-Stine, L. & Gelber, AC. (2010). Testicular pain followed by microscopic hematuria, a renal mass, palpable purpura, polyarthritis, and hematochezia.*J Clin Rheumatol.*, 16 (8):388-91, 21085014.

Miyamoto, MI. & Picard, MH. (2002). Left atrial mass caused by metastatic renal cell carcinoma: an unusual site of tumor involvement mimicking myxoma.*J Am Soc Echocardiogr.* , 15(8):847-8, 12174358.

Mohammed Ilyas, MI., Turner, GD. & Cranston, D. (2008). Human chorionic gonadotropin-secreting clear cell renal cell carcinoma with paraneoplastic gynaecomastia.*Scand J Urol Nephrol.* , 42(6):555-7, 19031270.

Mueller, TJ., Wu, H., Greenberg, RE., Hudes, G., Topham, N., Lessin, SR. &Uzzo RG. (2004). Cutaneous metastases from genitourinary malignancies.*Urology*, 63 (6):1021-6, 15183939.

Niccoli, L., Salvarani, C., Baroncelli, G., Padula, A., Olivieri, I. &Cantini F. (2002).Renal cell carcinoma mimicking polymyalgia rheumatica. Clues for a correct diagnosis.*Scand J Rheumatol.* , 31(2):103-6, 12109644.

Niikura, S., Hirata, A., Kunimi, K., Yokoyama, O., Koshida, K., Uchibayashi, T., Namiki, M., Nishino, A. & Kameda, K. (1999). Renal cell carcinoma recurrence in the mediastinum lymph node 19 years after nephrectomy: a case report.*Hinyokika Kiyo.* , 45(6):419-21, 10442285.

Nozawa, H., Tsuchiya, M., Kobayashi, T., Morita, H., Kobayashi, I., Sakaguchi, M., Mizutani, T., Tajima, A., Kishida, Y., Yakumaru, K., Kagami, H. & Sekikawa, T. (2003).Small intestinal metastasis from renal cell carcinoma exhibiting rare findings.*Int J Clin Pract.* , 57(4):329-31, 12800466.

Okubo, Y., Yonese, J., Kawakami, S., Yamamoto, S., Komai, Y., Takeshita, H., Ishikawa, Y. & Fukui, I. (2007).Obstinate cough as a sole presenting symptom of non-metastatic renal cell carcinoma.*Int J Urol.*, 14(9):854-5, 17760755.

Panarese, A., Turner, J. & Fagan, PA. (2002). Renal carcinoma metastasis: an unusual cerebellopontine angle tumor.*Otolaryngol Head Neck Surg.*, 127(3):245-7, 12297820.

Papachristodoulou, A., Mantas, D., Kouskos, E., Hatzianastassiou, D. & Karatzas, G. (2004).Unusual presentation of renal cell carcinoma metastasis.*Acta Chir Belg.*, 104(2):229-30, 15154588.

Placed, IG., Alvarez-Rodriguez, R., Pombo-Otero, J., Vázquez-Bartolomé, P., Hermida-Romero, T.& Pombo-Felipe, F.(2010). Metastatic renal cell carcinoma presenting as shoulder monoarthritis: diagnosis based on synovial fluid cytology and immunocytochemistry.*Acta Cytol.* , 54(5) :730-3, 20968165.

Pollheimer, MJ., Hinterleitner, TA., Pollheimer, VS., Schlemmer, A. &Langner, C. (2008). Renal cell carcinoma metastatic to the stomach: single-centre experience and literature review. *BJU Int.* , 102 (3):315-9, 18336607.

Respicio, G., Shwaiki, W. & Abeles, M. (2007).A 58-year-old man with anti-Jo-1 syndrome and renal cell carcinoma: a case report and discussion.*Conn Med.*, 71(3):151-3, 17405398.

Rijnders, B. & Decramer, M. (2000). Reversibility of paraneoplastic bilateral diaphragmatic paralysis after nephrectomy for renal cell carcinoma. *Ann Oncol.* , 11(2):221-5, 10761760.

Roviello, F., Caruso, S., Moscovita Falzarano, S., Marrelli, D., Neri, A., Rampone, B., De Marco, G., Perrotta, ME. & Mariani, F. (2006).Small bowel metastases from renal cell carcinoma: a rare cause of intestinal intussusception.*J Nephrol.* 19(2):234-8, 16736429.

Roy, MJ., May, EF. & Jabbari B. (2002). Life-threatening polyneuropathy heralding renal cell carcinoma.*Mil Med.*, 167(12):986-9, 12502172

Russell EB. (2005). Remitting seronegative symmetrical synovitis with pitting edema syndrome: followup for neoplasia.*J Rheumatol.* , 32(9):1760-1, 16142875.

Sadler, GJ., Anderson, MR., Mos, MS. & Wilson, PG. (2007).Metastases from renal cell carcinoma presenting as gastrointestinal bleeding: two case reports and a review of the literature.*BMC Gastroenterol.* , 7:4-7, 17766757.

Sakura, M., Tsujii, T., Yamauchi, A., Tadokoro, M., Tsukamoto, T., Kawakami, S., Yonese, J. & Fukui, I. (2007). Superior vena cava syndrome caused by supraclavicular lymph node metastasis of renal cell carcinoma.*Int J Clin Oncol.* , 12(5):382-4, 17729122.

Schijns, OE., Kurt, E., Wessels, P., Luijckx, GJ. & Beuls, EA. (2000). Intramedullary spinal cord metastasis as a first manifestation of a renal cell carcinoma: report of a case and review of the literature.*Clin Neurol Neurosurg.* , 102(4):249-254, 11154816.

Shakeel, M., Kumaravel, M., Mackenzie, JM. &Knight, DJ. (2009). An uncommon cause of sciatica.*J Coll Physicians Surg Pak.*, 19(2):127-9, 19208321.

Shih, KL., Yen ,HH., Su ,WW., Soon ,MS., Hsia, CH.& Lin ,YM.(2009). Fulminant Budd-Chiari syndrome caused by renal cell carcinoma with hepatic vein invasion: report of a case.*Eur J Gastroenterol Hepatol.* , 21(2):222-4, 19212212.

Shinsaka, H., Fujimoto, N. & Matsumoto, T. (2006).A rare case of right varicocele testis caused by a renal cell carcinoma thrombus in the spermatic vein.*Int J Urol.*, 13 (6):844-5, 16834679.

Shiono, Y., Kishimoto, K., Furuta, N., Igarashi, H., Hatano, T., Miki, K., Oishi, Y.& Kiyota, H. (2001). Pulmonary infarction caused by the spontaneous migration of the vena caval tumor thrombus of right renal cell carcinoma: a case report.*Hinyokika Kiyo .Acta urologica japoniva.* , 47(11):781-4, 11771170.

Shivnani, SB., Shelton, JM., Richardson, JA. & Maalouf, NM. (2009). Hypercalcemia of malignancy with simultaneous elevation in serum parathyroid hormone--related peptide and 1, 25-dihydroxyvitamin D in a patient with metastatic renal cell carcinoma.*Endocr Pract.* , 15(3):234-9, 19364692.

Sidhom, OA., Basalaev, M. & Sigal LH. (1993). Renal cell carcinoma presenting as polymyalgia rheumatica. Resolution after nephrectomy. *Arch Intern Med.*, 13; 153(17):2043-5, 8357289.

Singhal, D., Kakodkar, R., Soin, AS., Gupta, S. & Nundy, S. (2006). Sinistral portal hypertension .a case report. *JOP.* , 10; 7(6):670-3, 17095850.

Sparano, JA., Dutcher, JP., Kaleya, R., Caliendo, G., Fiorito, J., Mitsudo, S., Shechner, R., Boley, SJ., Gucalp, R. & Ciobanu, N. (1991). Colonic ischemia complicating immunotherapy with interleukin-2 and interferon-alpha. *Cancer*, 68(7):1538-44, 1893354.

Srinivasan, N., Pakala, A., Al-Kali, A., Rathi, S. & Ahmad, W. (2010). Papillary renal cell carcinoma with cutaneous metastases. *Am J Med Sci.*, 339(5):458-61, 20234300.

Staehler, MD., Kruse, J., Haseke, N., Stadler, T., Roosen, A., Karl, A., Stief, CG., Jauch, KW. &Bruns, CJ. (2010). Liver resection for metastatic disease prolongs survival in renal cell carcinoma: 12-year results from a retrospective comparative analysis. *World J Urol.*, 28(4):543-7, 20440505.

Steffens, J., Bock, R., Braedel, HU., Isenberg, E., Bührle, CP. & Ziegler, M. (1992). Renin-producing renal cell carcinomas--clinical and experimental investigations on a special form of renal hypertension.*Urol Res.*, 20(2):111-5, 1553788.

Suyama, H., Igishi, T., Makino, H., Kaminou, T., Hashimoto, M., Sumikawa, T., Tatsukawa, T. &Shimizu, E. (2011). Bronchial artery embolization before interventional bronchoscopy to avoid uncontrollable bleeding: a case report of endobronchial metastasis of renal cell carcinoma. *Intern Med.*, 50(2):135-9, 21245638.

Takeda, T., Shibuya, T., Osada, T., Izumi, H., Mitomi, H., Nomura, O., Suzuki, S., Mori, H., Matsumoto, K., Kon, K., Abe, W., Beppu, K., Sakamoto, N., Nagahara, A., Otaka, M., Ogihara, T., Yao, T. &Watanabe S. (2011). Metastatic renal cell carcinoma diagnosed by capsule endoscopy and double balloon endoscopy. *Med Sci Monit.* , 17(2):CS15-7, 21278196.

Talukder, MQ., Deo, SV., Maleszewski ,JJ. & Park SJ. (2010). Late isolated metastasis of renal cell carcinoma in the left ventricular myocardium.*Interact Cardiovasc Thorac Surg.*, 11(6):814-6, 20847070.

Tan, BH., Barry, CI., Wick, MR., White, KP., Brown, JG., Lee, A., Litchfield, AH., Lener, EV.&Shitabata, PK.(2011). Multicentric reticulohistiocytosis and urologic carcinomas: a possible paraneoplastic association. *J Cutan Pathol.* , 38(1):43-8, 20726933.

Tebbe, B., Schlippert, U., Garbe, C. & Orfanos, CE. (1991). Erythroderma "en nappes claires" as a marker of metastatic kidney cancer. Lasting, successful treatment with rIFN-alpha-2a.*Hautarzt.* , 42(5):324-7, 1831444.

Teresa, P., Maria Grazia, Z., Doriana, M., Irene, P. & Michele, S. (2011).Malignant effusion of chromophobe renal-cell carcinoma: Cytological and immunohistochemical findings.*Diagn Cytopathol.* , Jan 6. [Epub ahead of print], 21213172.

Tiwari, P., Tiwari, A., Vijay, M., Kumar, S. & Kundu, AK. (2010). Upper gastro-intestinal bleeding - Rare presentation of renal cell carcinoma.*Urol Ann.*, 2(3):127-9, 20981203.

Toquero, L., Aboumarzouk, OM. & Abbasi, Z. (2009). Renal cell carcinoma metastasis to the ovary: a case report. *Cases J.*, 2:7472-5, 19829972.

Torvik, A. & Berntzen, AE. (1968). Necrotizing vasculitis without visceral involvement. Postmortem examination of three cases with affection of skeletal muscles and peripheral nerves.*Acta Med Scand.*, 184(1-2):69-77, 4387508.

Wallach, JB., McGarry, T. & Torres, J.(2011).Lymphangitic metastasis of recurrent renal cell carcinoma to the contralateral lung causing lymphangitic carcinomatosis and respiratory symptoms.*Curr Oncol.*, 18(1):e35-7, 21311270.

Wieder, JA., Laks, H., Freitas, D., Marmureanu, A. & Belldegrun, A. (2003). Renal cell carcinoma with tumor thrombus extension into the proximal pulmonary artery.*J Urol.*, 169(6):2296-7, 12771776.

Wiesener, MS., Münchenhagen, P., Gläser, M., Sobottka, BA., Knaup, KX., Jozefowski, K., Jürgensen, JS., Roigas, J., Warnecke, C., Gröne, HJ., Maxwell, PH., Willam, C.& Eckardt, KU. (2007). Erythropoietin gene expression in renal carcinoma is considerably more frequent than paraneoplastic polycythemia.*Int J Cancer.*, 121(11):2434-42, 17640059.

Will, TA., Agarwal, N. & Petruzzelli,GJ. (2008). Oral cavity metastasis of renal cell carcinoma: a case report.*J Med Case Reports.*, 2:313-6, 18823541.

Winter, H., Meimarakis, G., Angele, MK., Hummel, M., Staehler, M., Hoffmann, RT., Hatz, RA. &Löhe, F. (2010).Tumor infiltrated hilar and mediastinal lymph nodes are an independent prognostic factor for decreased survival after pulmonary metastasectomy in patients with renal cell carcinoma.*J Urol.*, 184(5):1888-94, 20846691.

Wu, HY., Xu, LW., Zhang, YY., Yu, YL., Li, XD. & Li, GH. (2011). Metachronous contralateral testicular and bilateral adrenal metastasis of chromophobe renal cell carcinoma: a case report and review of the literature.*J Zhejiang Univ Sci B.*, 11(5):386-9, 20443217.

Yokonishi ,T., Ito, Y., Osaka, K., Komiya, A., Kobayashi, K., Sakai, N., Noguchi, S., Kishi, H., Satomi, Y., Mogaki, M., Tsuura, Y., Mizuno, N. &Ikeda, I. (2010).Pancreatic metastasis from renal cell carcinoma 25 years after radical nephrectomy.*Hinyokika Kiyo.*, 56(11):629-33, 21187708.

Yumura, Y., Yamashita, Y., Senga, Y., Jinza, S. &Goro, A. (2007). Two cases of renal cell carcinoma with diabetes mellitus that was healed after nephrectomy.*Hinyokika Kiyo.*, 53(5):301-5, 17571714.

Zubac, DP., Wentzel-Larsen, T., Seidal, T. & Bostad, L. (2010).Type 1 plasminogen activator inhibitor (PAI-1) in clear cell renal cell carcinoma (CCRCC) and its impact on angiogenesis, progression and patient survival after radical nephrectomy.*BMC Urol.*, 10:20-4, 21129210.

Zustovich, F., Gottardo, F., De Zorzi, L., Cecchetto, A., Dal Bianco, M., Mauro, E. &Cartei, G. (2008).Cardiac metastasis from renal cell carcinoma without inferior vena involvement: a review of the literature based on a case report. Two different patterns of spread?*Int J Clin Oncol.*, 13(3):271-4, 18553240.

Maestre-Rodríguez ,O., González-García, R., Mateo-Arias, J., Moreno-García, C., Serrano-Gil, H., Villanueva-Alcojol, L., Campos-de-Orellana, AM. & Monje-Gil, F. (2009). Metastasis of renal clear-cell carcinoma to the oral mucosa, an atypical location.*Med Oral Patol Oral Cir Bucal.*, 14(11):e601-4, 19680203.

Mudiyanselage, SY., Prabhakaran, VC., Davis, GJ. & Selva, D. (2008).Metastatic renal cell carcinoma presenting as a circumscribed orbital mass.*Eur J Ophthalmol.*, 18(3):483-5, 18465741.

6

Management of Renal Cell Carcinoma Metastasis of the Spine

Alessandro Gasbarrini[1], Christiano Esteves Simões[2],
Michele Cappuccio[3] and Stefano Boriani[1]
[1]Department of Oncologic and Degenerative Spine Surgery, Rizzoli Institute
[2]Department of Orthopedics and Traumatology – Spine Unit, Felício Rocho Hospital
[3]Department of Orthopedics and Traumatology – Spine Surgery, Maggiore Hospital
[1,3]Italy
[2]Brazil

1. Introduction

Renal cell carcinoma (RCC) is the most frequent malignant neoplasm of the kidneys, accounting for 85% of all renal cancers, and 2% of all adult malignancies. Forty-five percent of these tumors have been diagnosed as locally advanced or metastatic disease (Stage IV, according to the American Joint Committee on Cancer staging system), and the five-year survival rate varies between 0 to 8% according to the United States National Cancer Data Base (American Cancer Society, 2011). Bones metastases from renal cell carcinoma occur in up to 50% of patients (Swanson et al., 1981), and from this group approximately one half is located in the spine. RCC is the fourth most common metastatic tumor of the spine and the most common cancer to present as a neurologic deficit secondary to an undetected primary malignancy. According to Les et al, the prognosis is generally worse when metastases occur in the axial skeleton rather than in the extremities. In general, the average survival of all patients diagnosed with metastatic RCC is about four months and only 10% of these survive for one year (Thyavihally et al., 2005).

The RCC has a well know angiotropism associated to the anatomical and hemodynamic characteristics of the blood supply of the spine, and to the persistence of hematopoietic tissue inside the vertebral body, making this region the most susceptible localization for the metastases in the spine.

Vertebral lesions determine a severe compromise of the quality of life, with pain that can become intractable and a high risk of vertebral fracture and/or paralysis. The substitution of the healthy bone with the metastatic tissue cause a weakening of the vertebra, and sometimes an acute fracture with spinal canal invasion, that can be the most dramatic result from the clinical point of view.

Kidneys cancer cells are not usually susceptible to chemotherapy agents and traditional radiation therapy. Only a small number of patients have been shown good responses to these drugs vinblastine, floxuridine, 5-fluorouracil (5-FU), capecitabine, and gemcitabine, and therefore it should be reserved for cases in which target drugs and/or immunotherapy are not effective. Radiation therapy can be used for patients that the general health is too poor to have surgery, however it is not routinely recommended because there is no evidence that it can improve survival.

The management of bone metastasis from RCC is often a difficult task. The progressive improvement in the survival rate of the patients due to new forms of treatment, and the radiation therapy, and chemotherapy resistance associated to this tumor, imposes a great challenge to its proper treatment. The role of the spine surgeon in these cases, is to choose the best treatment considering not only the factors associated with the primary tumor, but specially the individual characteristics of every patient.

New therapies, known as "target therapies", directed to specific molecular targets implicated in angiogenesis and tumor proliferation have presented encouraging results. Even though these results coupled with a fuller understanding of molecular pathways in RCC have paved the way for new targets in the treatment of kidney cancer. These drugs are often used as the first line of treatment against advanced kidney cancers. While they may shrink or slow the growth of the cancer, it does not seem that any of these drugs can actually cure RCC (American Cancer Society, 2011). Immunotherapy associated to surgery should also be considered the first treatment of choice in selected cases or in cases of failure of previous treatment with target therapies. In the authors' experience, this treatment has been the one to show the best results so far. The surgical treatment of the spine metastasis varies from local decompression to en bloc resection of the lesion. Although the en bloc resection does not have the objective to cure the patient from the disease, it should be considered to minimize the risk of local disease progression (Les et al., 2001). However, many patients treated with en bloc resection can still develop local recurrence.

2. Metastatic pathways to the spine

The tumor dissemination to the bone can come from three pathways: direct extension, the lymphatic vessels and, the most frequent, the hematogenous pathway. The most frequent site in the vertebrae is the vertebral body, because of its abundant vascularization and the presence of bone marrow inside.

In 1928, Ewing suggested that the metastatic diffusion was influenced only by mechanical factors. The abundant tortuous vessels inside the vertebral body contribute to the metastatic embolus deposit locally and the localization of the blood vessels near the vertebral end plate can explain the normal localization of the metastases in the spine. Batson showed in 1940 the role of the paravertebral venous plexus in the metastatic dissemination of pelvic and abdominal tumors to the spine. This valveless plexus allows a retrograde blood flow from the inferior vena cava to the paravertebral venous plexus any time that the intra-abdominal or intra-thoracic pressure rises, even if temporally. This retrograde flow can deliver metastatic embolus direct to the spine, escaping from the natural filters of the organism, as the liver and lungs.

Renal cell carcinoma presents a peculiar venotropism, which is the capacity of its cells to reach the venous circulation. The diffusion can occur through an anterograde flow in the renal vein to the inferior cave vein reaching the right atrium, or through a retrograde diffusion. Moreover, the anatomical connections between the renal venous circulation and the paravertebral venous plexus through the azygos and hemiazygous systems can also favor a metastatic implantation at the spine.

The associations of the well-known angiotropism of the renal cell tumors, the anatomical and the hemodynamic characteristics of the spinal circulation, and the persistence of the hematopoietic tissue inside the vertebral spongeous bone matter are the responsible for the high frequency of metastasis of RCC.

3. Diagnosis

3.1 Clinical diagnosis

The early diagnosis of metastatic spinal disease is important because functional outcomes depend on neurologic condition at the time of presentation. The presentation of spinal metastases can vary widely from back pain to different degrees of neurologic deficit including complete paralysis at the lesion level. Pathologic fracture and a complete spinal cord lesion are the worse conditions associated to the spinal disease and, in most of the cases, can and should be avoided. Clinically, the symptoms associated to RCC spinal metastases do not differ from most of the other metastatic primary tumors. The past history of renal cell carcinoma is usually the most important clue to localize the primary site. Often, spinal metastases can occur in patients submitted in the past to nephrectomy to treat RCC, and that have been considered as "no evidence of disease" for several years.

Back pain is the most common symptom caused by spinal metastases, and often precedes the neurologic symptoms by weeks, sometimes even months. In some cases, back pain can be the first symptom related to the original cancer disease, and the primary site diagnosis is reached through a biopsy of the spinal lesion. There are mainly three different sources of back pain: mechanical, radicular and local pain. The mechanical pain is caused by the spinal instability secondary to the structural abnormality of the spine, and is also known as axial back pain (Gokaslan and York, 1998). The instability can be diagnosed because of its clinical symptoms or with obvious alterations such as pathologic fractures. This pain is movement-related and exacerbate by sitting or standing which increases the axial load on the spine. Patients presenting with pathological fractures of the spine may also present pain in recumbence and often give a history of sleeping upright in a chair for several weeks. The presumed mechanism is extension of the unstable kyphosis. At the beginning, mechanical pain maybe relieved with narcotics or an external orthosis, however it does not respond to steroids. The source of local pain can also be increased by the muscle, tendon, ligament and/or joint capsule strain that secondarily occurs from the vertebral body damage. Radicular pain may occur when spinal metastases compress or irritate an exiting nerve root, yielding pain in the dermatomal distribution of the involved nerve root. This type of pain is often described as "sharp," "shooting," or "stabbing" (Perrin et al., 1982). The periosteal stretching and/or a local inflammatory process stimulate the pain fibers within the periosteum causing local pain. It is predominantly nocturnal or early morning pain and generally improves with activity during the day, and it is usually described as a persistent "gnawing" or "aching" pain originated from the affected spinal segment. Inflammatory pain usually responds to administration of low dose steroids.

The second most common presenting complaint is motor dysfunction. Myelopathic abnormalities begins with hyperreflexia, clonus, Babisnki reflex and can progress to weakness, proprioceptive sensory loss, and loss of pain and temperature below the level of spinal cord compression. Autonomic dysfunction can occur secondarily to spinal cord compression or cauda equina compression. Bladder dysfunction is the most common autonomic finding and often correlates with the degree of motor dysfunction (Schiff 2004). The proper identification of neurologic deficit is of paramount importance, considering the motor function at the time of diagnosis correlates with the prognosis (Arguello et al., 1990). Unfortunately, the presence of back pain is extremely common in the general population, and it is likely that delay diagnoses of vertebral metastases occur in the presence of only back or neck pain. For these reasons, in every patient with a past history of RCC, the hypothesis of vertebral metastasis must be considered until proven otherwise.

Generally, the motor dysfunction is associated with sensory dysfunctions, such as anesthesia, hyperesthesia, hypoesthesia and/or paraesthesia. Complains of sensory abnormalities can occur in the dermatomal distribution of the radicular pain or weakness, while the patients with myelopathy may elicit a sensory level across the chest or abdomen.

The clinical evaluation of spinal patients should include general performance status, a pain assessment and a quantitative neurologic score. The most common method of pain assessment is the visual analog scale. The performance status reflects ambulation, medical comorbidities and extent of the disease. A patient may have normal motor strength, but be unable to walk from loss of proprioception, fracture of lower limbs or from a variety of other reasons.

The neurologic status is assessed using the modified Frankel grading system (McGuire et al., 1998) and/or the American Spinal Injury Association (ASIA) score (Table 1). Both systems assess the motor function with a score of "E" being normal and "A" being a complete paralysis.

Grade	Description
A	Complete: No motor or sensory function is preserved in the sacral segments S4-S5.
B	Incomplete: Sensory but not motor function is preserved below the neurological level and extends through the sacral segments S4-S5.
C	Incomplete: Motor function is preserved below the neurological level, and the majority of the key muscles below the neurological level have a muscle grade less than 3.
D	Incomplete: Motor function is preserved below the neurological level, and the majority of the key muscles below the neurological level have a muscle grade greater than 3.
E	Normal: Motor and sensory function is normal.

Table 1. ASIA impairment scale.

The modified Frankel score system divides the clinical-neurologic status in seven stages:

- A: Complete loss of the motor and sensitive functions.
- B: Presence of sensory but absence of voluntary motor functions.
- C: Motor deficit that allows the deambulation, but only with antibrachial support and lower limbs bracing.

- D1: High degree of motor deficit that allows deambulation using only an antibrachial support, and/or bladder or bowel paralysis.
- D2: Moderate degree of motor deficit that allows the deambulation without support or bracing, and/or bladder or bowel neurologic dysfunction.
- D3: Mild motor deficit with a normal bladder and bowel functions.
- E: Complete motor and sensitive function (osteotendinous reflexes can be abnormal)

3.2 Diagnostic imaging

Plain radiography (with or without myologram), myelography, computed tomography (CT) (with or without myelogram), magnetic resonace imaging (MRI), and positron emission tomography (PET) all play important roles in the imaging assessment of spinal cancer and metastatic lesions from RCC.

3.2.1 Plain films

Plain radiographs are readily available, easy to perform, relatively low cost, and provides a detailed assessment of osseous structures. Lytic or sclerotic areas of bone, pathologic compression fractures, deformity, and paraspinal masses can be seen, however, according to Gabriel et al., up to 50% of the bone must be eroded before there is a noticeable change on plain radiographs.

3.2.2 Computed tomography (CT)

CT provides a detailed assessment of osseous structures and the extent of tumor involvement within the bone. It is indispensible for pre-operative staging according to the Weinstein-Boriani-Biagini and surgical planning (Boriani et al., 1997). When associated to myelography, it demonstrates any suspected compression of the neural elements caused by tumor extension to the canal or osseous fragments from a pathologic fracture.

The CT is very important also to evaluate the risk of pathologic fracture based on the tumor's extension in the vertebrae.

3.2.3 Nuclear scintigraphy

Nuclear scintigraphy or bone scan demonstrates areas of active bone metabolism. A major advantage of bone scans is its cost-effective ability to scan the entire axial and appendicular skeleton at the same time and its capacity of revealing lesions at an earlier stage when compared to plain films. Its disadvantage is the low specificity, as increased metabolic activity in the presence of inflammation or infection. The image correlation with CT and MRI is necessary due to its low imaging resolution. The PET scanning with ^{18}F-fluorodeoxygucose is more sensitive and specific for whole body metastatic evaluations, but as with bone scans, it also necessitates concomitant use of CT or MRI. Koga et al, assessed the diagnostic value of bone scan in 205 patients with confirmed renal cell carcinoma, and concluded that bone scan may be omitted in patients with stages T1-3aN0M0 tumors and no bone pain because of the low proportion of missed cases with bone metastasis (Koga et al., 2001).

3.2.4 Magnetic Resonance Imaging (MRI)

MRI is currently the gold standard imaging technique for assessing the spinal metastasis. It combines excellent spatial and contrast resolution. MRI is also more sensitive than CT, and bone scans, and does not exposes patients to ionizing radiation. It provides superior resolution of soft-tissue structures such as paraspinal muscles, intervertebral disc, spinal cord and nerve roots. Standard MRI protocols include T1-weighted images (T1 WIs) without and with intravenous contrast, T2-weighted images (T2WIs) in axial, coronal and sagittal reconstructions. Fat suppression techniques are useful in evaluating osseous lesions that enhance with contrast. Disadvantages include relatively long acquisition times, insurmountable safety contra-indications in some patients, and lower sensitivity to osseous structural abnormalities.

3.2.5 Angiography

Metastasis from hypervascular tumors as RCC may have diagnostic and therapeutic benefits from angiography. Pre operative angiography can provides the knowledge about the tumors vascular supply and allows preoperative embolization, decreasing the blood loss during the intralesional excision.

3.3 Anatomopathologic diagnosis

Percutaneous biopsy to confirm the diagnosis is paramount. Although imaging modalities can provide a great definition of the anatomical aspects of the lesions the correct diagnosis is mandatory prior to the treatment planning. Patients with well-known primary cancer can present with a spinal lesion from another hidden metastatic tumor or a primary bone tumor associated. CT guided percutaneous trocar biopsies provide relatively easy access to most lesions with success rates approaching 90%. Traspedicular biopsy is the most adequate technique because of the smaller contamination of the adjacent tissues, facilitating its removal during the resection.

4. Management of spinal metastasis

When dealing with spinal metastasis factors need to be taken into consideration by the oncologist, spine surgeon, anesthesiologist and the entire multidisciplinary group involved in the caring of these patients. Considering that metastatic disease to the spine a systemic disease, at first, the curative excision of the entire secondary lesion does not seems necessary, particularly in the spine because of its anatomical characteristics and morbidity. The palliative treatment frequently applied has the primary objective to decrease the pain, stabilize the spine and, whenever is necessary, decompress the adjacent neural structures. The intralesional excision of the tumor (inadequate oncological margins) can be complete or incomplete, allowing a circumferential decompression of the spinal cord and a better local control of the disease.

RCC is well known as radiation therapy and chemotherapy resistant, and immunotherapies with cytokines based on interferon alpha and interleukin-2 (IL2) have shown poor results with significant toxicities. New therapies directed to molecular targets implicated in angiogenesis and tumor proliferation are being developed. Sunitinib is considered one of the new reference first-line treatment for RCC metastasis, however despite all the progress in recent years, complete responses are still very rare, and many important issues regarding the use of these agents in the management of metastatic renal cell cancer still need to be properly addressed.

Surgical treatment has been the only recognized therapy to improve the quality of life in the patients with RCC metastatic disease in the spine. In most of the cases the surgery does not improve the survival prognosis of these patients but it can dramatically improve the their life quality. Moreover, in a small group of patients with solitary spinal RCC metastases the en bloc resection has shown to substantially improve the overall survival time. In their retrospective work, Thyavihally et al. demonstrated the complete resection of either synchronous or metachronous solitary metastases from RCC is justified and can contribute to a long-term survival in a selective group of patients. They also concluded that patients with long interval between diagnosis and development of metastasis and early stage of the primary tumor have a better prognosis after en bloc resection of the metastases.

The treatment goals of spinal metastasis is different than the primary bone tumors, the first one aims the patient's quality of life while the main target of primary bone tumor is to preserve life. The best treatment" should include local control of the disease and restoration of the spinal function.

4.1 Treatment planning

Surgical indications for spinal metastasis in general, have been subject of controversy because the ideal moment, patient and surgical technique are still trying to be defined in the literature. Many strategies have been proposed trying to appropriately direct the best surgical treatment. In 1987 Tokuhashi et al. published a point-addition-type scoring system for the preoperative prediction of the survival period to select treatment options. This score system was later on revised and magnified its the application to the group with conservative treatment. The general condition (Karnofsky performance status), the number of extraspinal bone metastases, the number of metastases in the vertebral column, the presence of metastases to major internal organs (lungs, liver, kidneys, and brain), the primary site of cancer, and the severity of spinal cord palsy were the items evaluated. Each parameter ranged from 0 to 5 points, and the total score was 15 points. RCC was considered as moderate prognosis receiving three points in the item "primary site of cancer". Tomita et al, also have described a scoring system based on the primary tumor, the presence of metastases to the vital organs and number of bone metastases. These systems have been used among the spine surgeons with reasonable results, unfortunately the scores systems are too simple, based in numbers that allocates extremely different types of patient in the same group, and also they do not consider the clinical status and other physicians opinions involved in the patient's care before deciding the best treatment option.

In 2008, the authors published their own treatment algorithm to guide the decision planning when dealing with spine metastasis, based on a retrospective study of 43 patients (Cappuccio et al., 2008). According to Cappucio et al., multidisciplinary treatment could be beneficial, and a failure to do so, is very like to end in a suboptimum prognosis and could even lead to sever impairment. The treatment planning, including the surgical planning should involve not only the spine surgeon, but also the nonsurgical physicians (anesthetist, oncologist, radiotherapist), and it should be chosen on each individual patient. Gasbarrini et al., conducted a semi-prospective clinical study in 2010 with 202 patients to evaluate the efficacy of this algorithm which furthermore evolved to a flow chart (Figure 1).

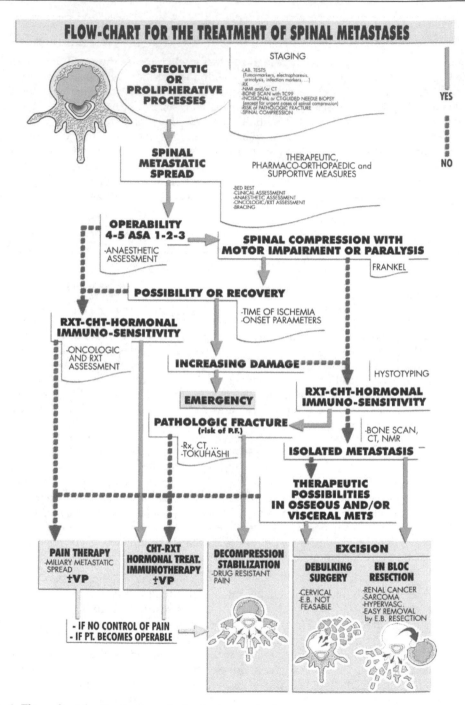

Fig. 1. Flow chart for the treatment of spinal metastasis.

According to this flow-chart, all spinal tumors must be staged, and the first question when planning the treatment is to discuss with the oncologist about the life expectancy of the patient and to reach a consensus with the anesthesiologist if the patient is operable or not (based on the ASA score). Other important items to consider is the neurological status and its capacity to deteriorate or to improve, the presence of pathologic fracture, the sensitivity of the primary tumor to non surgical therapies, and the number of spinal, bone or visceral metastasis. Following the flow chart the best therapeutic option can be achieved, ranging from only pain therapy to surgical procedures as en bloc resections.

Considering the RCC metastases, the surgical treatment is the only method that can improve the patient's quality of life, and in some well selected cases of single spinal metastases, a cure of these patients have been well documented after en bloc resections (Li et al., 2009). Patients with disseminated RCC metastasis, or clinically incapable to be submitted to surgical procedures, pain therapy is indicated.

4.2 Surgical planning

In order to apply the surgical indication determined by the oncological staging and the Gasbarrini's flow chart, it is necessary a complete work-up to evaluate the vertebral tumor that will be treated. The histological diagnosis, preferably obtained by CT-guided biopsy, is fundamental. Magnetic resonance imaging, CT-scan and in some selected cases, angiography, are the imaging techniques indicated to describe the tumor's extension on the transversal and longitudinal planes. The first attempt to determine a surgical staging system to guide the spine surgeons was made by Weistein in 1994. Boriani and Biagini modified this staging system in 1997 (Figure 2).

A. Extraosseous Soft Tissue

B. Intraosseous (Superficial)

C. Intraosseous (Deep)

D. Extraosseous (Extradural)

E. Extraosseous (Intradural)

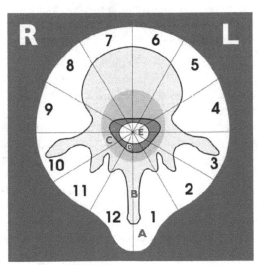

Fig. 2. WBB surgical staging system

4.2.1 Weinstein–Boriani–Biagini (WBB) surgical staging

The WBB surgical staging system is specific for spine tumors and was created to guide the planning of the surgical resection to achieve the appropriate histologic margins. It was first described to treat primary spinal tumors, but its application was later on extended to the treatment of spinal metastasis as well. Pre-operative CT-scan and MRI are required to provide detail of the lesion and the normal tissues surrounding it.

The WBB divides the axial presentation of the vertebrae involved with the tumor into 12 zones similar to a clock face. Zone 1 is located at the left half of the spinous process followed by the others in a counter clockwise sense. Zones 4 and 9 are particularly important to know because they define respectively the left and right pedicles. Vertebrectomy with adequate surgical margins depends upon one of these zones to be free of tumor. The vertebra is further divided into 5 radial zones that define the depth of tumor invasion. These zones are also known as layers, starting from layer A that corresponds to the outside surrounding tissue of the vertebra to layer E that indicates intradural involvement of the tumor. In the cervical spine there is also layer F, which corresponds to the vertebral artery involvement. It is also important to describe the longitudinal extension of the tumor.

4.2.2 Pre-operative Selective Arterial Embolization (SAE)

Vertebral metastases of renal origin are highly vascular and often cause life-threatening intraoperative bleeding. This bleeding may influence the surgeon's ability to have an adequate view of the surgical field, and thus to achieve a complete resection. Preoperative embolization facilitates resection by decreasing intraoperative blood loss, improving visualization of the tumor during surgery, and decreasing tumor size.

Embolization can also be used as a palliative treatment in patients who are poor operative candidates or have recurrent, multiple, or unresectable tumors. It can also be used to treat painful metastatic disease or for patients with neurologic compromise from metastatic lesions by reducing the tumor size, tumor growth, and spinal canal compromise.

In cases of vascular metastatic spinal lesions, as in the RCC metastasis, a preoperative angiography should be performed to demonstrate the hypervascularity of the lesion, to identify the main arterial feeders, and, ultimately, to determine whether the lesion would benefit from the embolization. Angiography of a spinal RCC metastatic lesion typically demonstrates a hyper-dynamic pathologic circulation within the vertebral tumor, enlarged feeding intercostals or lumbar arteries, angiographic blush caused by venous congestion within the tumor nidus, and, possibly, a rapid arteriovenous transit with early filling of draining venous channels (Figure 3A). The enlarged venous pool may contribute to a tumor's mass effect; therefore, embolization may decrease spinal cord compression. Before embolization procedures, it is important to identify the segmental vessels that supply the spinal cord and the radiculomedullary branch of the anterior spinal artery and to determine whether an anterior spinal artery shares the same pedicle as the feeding artery of the tumor. The presence of an anterior spinal artery, also known as artery of Adamkiewicz (Figure 3B), at the same pedicle as the feeding artery at the tumor is considered by many authors a contraindication for embolization due to the risk of spinal cord ischemia, however some authors have demonstrated in animals models that in the presence of more than one artery of Adamkiewicz artery, the embolization of the tumor feeder would not cause damage to the spinal cord. Tomita et al., published in 2009 their techniques on total en bloc spondylectomy and showed that preoperative embolization of bilateral segmental arteries at three levels (at the level of the tumor, and one segment above and another one bellow) should be tried within 48 hours before the operation.

There are many reports of surgeries on metastatic renal cell carcinoma that were aborted because of "uncontrollable bleeding" or excessive blood loss in control groups that did not have preoperative SAE, whereas no case was aborted were complete embolization was done.

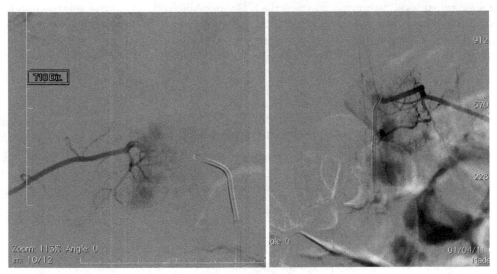

Fig. 3. A. Tumoral "blush" during angiography showing a metastatic RCC lesion in T10; 3B. Artery of Adamkiewicz.

In some cases of neurologic worsening before SAE was done the immediate surgery before the embolization can result into severe complications. Sundaresan et al., had 54% of complications in patients with RCC metastasis that were rushed into surgery without preoperative SAE. Because of this high rate of complications, some authors advocates for a delaying surgery for a few hours to perform preoperative embolization.

The choice of embolic material is based on the territory embolized, the vascular anatomy of the tumor, and the ability of selective delivery of an embolic agent via a catheter. The success of an embolization is judged by reduction in tumor vascularity and lack of tumor blush.

The timing of surgery after preoperative SAE is an important technical consideration. It is recommended that embolization be performed as close as possible to the time of surgery. Minimal blood loss occurs after embolization if surgery is performed within 24 to 48 hours after embolization. Earlier surgeries prevent the development of collateral circulation. The intraoperative blood loss can be reduced from one to two thirds in RCC metastatic lesions (Gottfried et al., 2004).

Complications rates are very low and have been reported to vary from 1% to 2%. Most complications are temporarily and are associated to a post-embolization syndrome that includes malaise, nausea, emesis, low-grade fever, elevated white blood cell count, and local pain usually lasting three to seven days. Permanent paraplegia has been reported in the literature, but fortunately it is very rare.

4.3 Surgical treatment

In the past the patients with spinal metastasis were considered as terminal patients, therefore surgical treatment was reserved for patients with uncontrollable pain with medications, or patients with high risk of pathologic fracture. The surgical approach to the spine is basically anterior or posterior. Both approaches can be also combined in the same surgery or in separated surgical procedures.

The rational behind the adequate surgical option should include:

- The best decompression possible.
- The most efficacious spinal stabilization.
- Removal of the tumor with oncological adequacy.

The correct surgical treatment does not involve simple laminectomy of the spine of any extension. The outcomes of this procedure are comparable to isolated radiation therapy and can result in a severe instability with a high risk of neurological deterioration.

The surgical techniques to be considered are:

1. Spinal decompression and stabilization.
2. Intralesional excision (debulking) and spinal column reconstruction.
3. En bloc resection and spinal column reconstruction.

4.3.1 Decompression and stabilization

This is the fastest and less aggressive surgical procedure aiming to decompress the spinal cord and to stabilize the spine. This procedure does not necessarily include a direct approach to the tumor. It is considered a palliative treatment.

The indications for decompression and stabilization are:

1. Presence, or elevated risk, of pathological fracture in the thoracic and/or lumbar spine.
2. High sensitive tumors to hormonal, chemotherapy or radiotherapy, independently of the neurological status.
3. Patients with extremely poor prognosis aiming only the improvement of the patient's quality of life.

4.3.2 Intralesional excision

Intralesional excision includes a direct approach to the tumoral mass with a partial resection of the tumor in order to reach spinal decompression and tumor mass reduction. This procedure is considered more aggressive than simple decompression and stabilization, especially when dealing with systemic diseases, and it must include a multidisciplinary approach. Selective arterial embolization should be included in the treatment to decrease the hemorrhage, very often life threatening, and also a detailed surgical planning to achieve an adequate excision and to reconstruct the spinal stability. Some times a double approach should be considered.

The indications for intralesional excision are:

1. Tumoral mass compression from radio-resistant metastasis.
2. Pathologic fractures in radio-resistant metastasis.
3. Necessity to reduce the tumoral mass ("debulking") in order to apply adjuvant therapies.

Surgical technique

The surgical technique for intralesional excision depends on the location of the metastases.

In the cervical spine the approach is always anterior, and for the thoracic and lumbar spine, a partial excision can be performed also using a posterior approach.

Cervical Spine: The anterior approach to the cervical spine (from C3 to T1) is well known among the spine surgeons. The approach to C1 and C2 can be transoral or extra-oral. An extension of this approach can be done through a very aggressive trans-mandible technique.

The vertebral arteries are a problem for the circumferential approach. The single anterior approach is indicated in the lower cervical spine for small metastasis (WBB: from sector 4 to 9). Every time that a tumor is located in the posterior elements, invading at least one articular process, a double approach not only is safer, but also indicated for the reconstruction in general.

Thoracic Spine: The metastasis in the thoracic spine can be completely excised through a thoracotomy using the classical anterolateral approach, technically challenging in the cervical-thoracic junction. Using only a posterior approach is also possible to perform a complete curettage of the lesion, legating one nerve root.

Thoracoscopy can also be used for intracapsular excision (McLain 2001).

Lumbar Spine: In the lumbar spine, the anterior approach with decompression, and reconstruction usually is the best option for an anterior lesion. A posterior approach at this level needs to scarify one or more nerve roots. The consequences of such action are persistent pain, loss of mobility and spinal cord ischemia.

4.3.3 En bloc resection

Stener in1989, and Roy-Camille in 1990, described the surgical techniques for en bloc resection in the thoracic and lumbar spine. Later in 1994, Tomita et al., described a similar technique for vertebrectomy using a posterior approach developed specially for spinal metastasis.

The preoperative planning is paramount to choose the best technique for en bloc resection. Each vertebral lesion needs to be evaluated carefully and the resection should be "customized". In order to plan the resection, all tumors should be surgically staged according to the WBB system, previously described.

The resection can be made throughout the external surface of the pseudocapsule (marginal resection), or outside of it, along with a margin of healthy tissue (wide resection).

The well accepted indications for en bloc resections are stage three benign tumors and in stage one, or stage two, primary malignant tumors. The indications for spinal metastasis are still controversial, however it should be considered in cases of a solitary metastases of primary tumors with longer life expectancy, as in the RCC.

Types of en bloc resections:

- Sagittal resection: The criteria to obtain oncologically adequate margins include: No extension to the layer D in the WBB system, or limited extension with dissection plane between the tumor's pseudocapsule and the dural sac.
- Posterior resection: According to the WBB system, the indications for posterior elements resection with oncological margins include sectors four and nine free of tumor e no extension to the layer D, or limited extension with dissection plane between the tumor's pseudocapsule and the dural sac.
- Vertebrectomy: The en bloc resection of the vertebral body is oncologically appropriate by a posterior approach only, in cases of tumors located inside the body (no invasion of layer A in the WBB system). If tumor mass is expanding anteriorly in layer A or when the tumor is located at the cervico-thoracic, thoraco-lumbar, lumbo-sacral junction, the surgical procedure should include an anterior release. In these cases, the posterior approach ends with the blunt dissection of the lateral aspect of the vertebral body not involved by the tumor, if exists. Cervical spine en bloc vertebrectomy is also feasible, however this technique is more difficult and associated to a higher morbidity and mortality because of its elevated risk of vertebral artery and spinal cord injuries.

Surgical technique

Sagittal resection: This technique aims at achieving en bloc resection of a tumor excentrically growing: it consists in the piecemeal removal of the uninvolved posterior elements in order to circumferentially release the dura and finalize the resection by a sagittal osteotomy. An anterior approach is required when the tumor is growing anteriorly and a margin of normal tissue must be left under visual control over the tumor, or vital structures must be protected. One or more neuroforamina are involved by tumor and the corresponding nerve root(s) needs to be sacrificed in order to obtain an appropriate margin. The uninvolved posterior elements are removed piecemeal. A complete release of the dural sac from the tumor should be done. Before the osteotomy, the contralateral pedicle is removed so that the dura is not retracted into its hard surface. First, the vertical cut is performed followed by the superior and inferior horizontal cut. The tumor is finally removed in one piece.

Posterior resection: The posterior resection requires both pedicles free of tumor in order to obtain an oncologically appropriate margin. The posterior arch is removed after both pedicles are transected. This technique is rarely used for RCC metastases because the great majority of spinal metastases are located anteriorly in vertebral body.

Vertebrectomy: Usually the surgical procedure is performed in two steps (first with the patient in prone decubitus position followed by a lateral oblique position at 45°), a posterior and anterior approach. For small lesions, inside the vertebral body the procedure can be done only by a posterior access with oncologically adequate margins, according to the technique described by Tomita et al. Although it is possible to perform an en bloc vertebrectomy using only the posterior approach in the lumbar spine, it should be avoided.

This technique involves a great risk of root damage and unlike the thoracic spine where one or more nerve roots can be sacrificed without causing major problems; in the lumbar spine a motor deficit can deteriorate dramatically the quality of life of these patients.

The advantages of the posterior only approach are less surgical time and blood loss, avoidance of the anterior approach and its morbidity, among others. The most important disadvantage is the high risk of spinal cord lesion and the difficult to obtain adequate cutting surfaces on the spinal column in order to reconstruct the anterior column. Nowadays several devices and techniques have been developed to overcome these problems. The use of a spinal cord protector is important in these cases, and should always be applied. In all en bloc vertebrectomies performed using only a posterior approach, the authors used a special device named PROMID®, to protect the spinal cord and guide the saw path through the vertebral body or intervertebral disc. (Figure 4) The device is positioned underneath the dural sac and secured to a rod. Once the Gigli saw passes through the spinal column, the protector restrains it. The little knots on both sides work as the saw guide, avoiding the use of chisels and scalpels that can cause a massive bone bleeding and also injure the spinal cord.

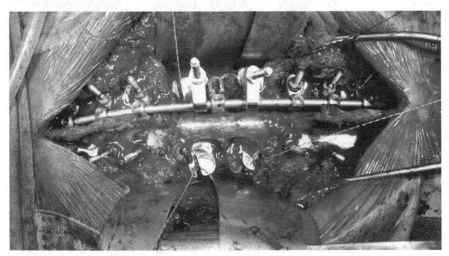

Fig. 4. The spinal cord protector and saw guide device (PROMID®) used during a posterior en bloc vertebrectomy.

The choice of the best surgical treatment is still a matter of debate, however vertebrectomy is becoming more popular among spine surgeons. This technique requires a more experienced surgical team and an adequate clinical support. It is very important to keep in mind that RCC metastases are hypervascular tumors, and intralesional excision can be associated to massive blood loss. On the other hand, en bloc resection is associated to specific techniques, sometimes a combined anterior and posterior approach, and therefore a longer surgical time. It usually requires a prolonged anesthesia, hemodynamic stability, important blood loss compensation and control of body heat loss. To overcome the necessity to complement the surgical procedure with an anterior approach and therefore to deal with its complications, the use of anterior release using thoracoscopy can be done in some selected cases with less morbidity without affecting the oncological management (Cappuccio et al., 2010).

Cappuccio et al., reported a retrospective study comparing the variation of intra-operative hemodynamic parameters (arterial blood pressure, cardiac frequency and hemoglobin levels) between a group of patients submitted to en bloc resection and a group treated by intralesional excision. Surgical timing was significantly higher in the en bloc resection group, however the cardiac frequency, hemoglobin levels and arterial blood pressure were significantly more affected in the patients submitted to intralesional excision. They concluded that constant evolution of the anesthesia techniques allows the execution of surgical treatments that have been forbidden in the past. Hemorrhagic tumors as RCC metastases can be better managed with en bloc resection, even considering that this is a more complex procedure compared to intralesional resection.

Many authors reported the comparison between the different modalities of treatments for RCC spinal metastases. En bloc spondylectomy associated to adjuvant interferon and fractionated radiation presented good results with no recurrence in cases of solitary RCC metastases with epidural extension (Sakaura et al. 2004). In an unpublished series from Boriani, 90 cases of RCC were treated with a variety of techniques, including conventional external beam radiotherapy (4 patients), palliative decompression and instrumentation (19 patients), intralesional gross total resection (42 patients), and en bloc resection (25 patients) with recurrence rates of 100%, 84%, 24%, and 4%, respectively. In the en bloc cohort, 12 patients had no evidence of disease at a median follow-up of 30 months, 5 alive with disease at a median of 28 months, and 8 dead of disease at a median of 8 months. In the en bloc group, 1 patient showed local progression of disease (Bilsky et al., 2009).

4.4 Spinal column reconstruction

The surgical treatment of bone tumors usually results in a bone defect, secondary to curettage or resection that can be reconstructed using different types of implants associated to different methods of osteosynthesis. The complexity of the spinal anatomy requires a more specific and complex technique for resection and reconstruction.

The spinal instability and the criteria for reconstruction of each patient is different case by case, and each type of resection (posterior, corpectomy or vertebrectomy) requires a specific reconstruction technique.

Denis et al., have shown that the stability of the spine is secondary to the integrity of the middle column (posterior longitudinal ligament, posterior portion of the fibrous annulus e the posterior vertebral wall) e the anterior column (anterior longitudinal ligament, anterior portion of the fibrous annulus and the anterior vertebral wall). According to Gurwitz, and Lim et al., in cases where there is a lesion of the anterior column, a posterior stabilization is not sufficiently rigid to resist all weight bearing forces and therefore, needs to be associated to an anterior stabilization. In cases of en bloc vertebrectomy, a circumferential reconstruction is indispensable, in other words, it is necessary to associate a posterior stabilization to the anterior hardware.

The posterior elements resection requires stabilization associated to a lateral arthodesis while corpectomy needs also the substitution of the vertebral body, associated to an anterior stabilization.

4.4.1 Posterior reconstruction

In the majority of the cases an oncological surgical procedure in the spine produces a wide loss of substance associated to a major instability of the spine, thus becoming necessary a rigid stabilization of it. The most indicated system is the utilization of pedicle screws and longitudinal bars above and below the defect. In association for the patients that will not be submitted to radiotherapy, autogenous bone graft should also be used to obtain a permanent postero-lateral arthrodesis.

4.4.2 Anterior reconstruction

The anterior column is responsible for 80% of body weight support in the spine and its reconstruction is mandatory after en bloc vertebrectomies. The maintenance of the biomechanical principles is paramount.

The size of the defect can be measure, and appropriately sized cage can be inserted. The reconstruction can be made using different cages (titanium, carbon fiber, etc.) or a massive allograft bone (femoral shaft). The cages or the bone shafts are filled preferably with autogenous bone. When possible, a connection between the anterior device and the posterior construct should be performed in order to enhance stability of the whole construct.

The number of options for anterior column reconstruction devices is smaller than the posterior reconstruction. They are basically bars, plates and screws or cages that are anchored to the vertebral body. In spinal oncology these implants are frequently used to achieve an anterior stabilization especially at the long term, and also to provide an early rehabilitation.

Orthopedic cement: The use of cement as a spacer, easily adaptable and with a low cost has been abandoned in the past. It has been proven not to be a reliable system at medium and long term (Boriani et al., 1996), being indicated only in selected cases of patients with short life expectancy.

Bone Graft: Bone graft represents the oldest spacer used in the oncological surgery. The bone graft can be used to obtain an interbody fusion or to replace one or more vertebral bodies. The advantage of this kind of graft is its biological integrability. The disadvantages include the necessity of a bank bone (to collect, store, and distribute), risk of infection, the necessity of a long time to consolidate and therefore it needs to be protected (body casts, bed rest, etc.). All bone grafts are somehow damaged in the biological evolution in cases of post-operative radiotherapy (Boriani et al., 1996).

Vertebral prosthesis: There are many options of vertebral body replacement prosthesis. Nowadays the most common used are made of titanium, and recently, made of carbon fibers (Figure 5). The advantages are the immediate stability, they are not damaged by radiotherapy and there is no donor site morbidity. The disadvantages include the higher cost, the necessity to have different sizes available, to be responsible for images artifacts (image distortion in the MRI or CT-s can) and to interfere as an obstacle for post-operative radiotherapy if necessary.

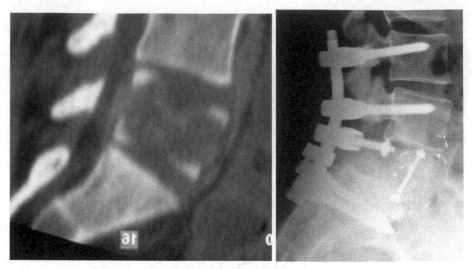

Fig. 5. A Solitary RCC metastasis of L5; 5B. 64 months of follow-up after posterior stabilization and anterior reconstruction with a carbon fiber cage filled with allograft. The bone fusion of the anterior column can be seen thorough the cage.

4.5 Stereotactic radiosurgery

Renal cell carcinoma metastases are well known to be resistant to conventional radiotherapy. In recent years, stereotactic body radiosurgery (SBRS) have allowed the safe delivery of high-dose radiation (image-guided intensity-modulated radiation therapy or spinal radio- surgery) to spinal metastases even in close proximity to the spinal cord and other paraspinal dose-sensitive organs. These treatments are often given in 1 to 5 fractions of high-dose radiation (to ensure safe doses) that are able to limit the dose to the spinal cord (Gerzsten et al., 2009). The aims of SBRS for spinal metastases are to improve on existing rates of clinical response and tumor control, and to reduce the retreatment rate by increasing the biologic equivalent dose (Sahgal et al., 2009).

According to Sahgal et al., the outcomes of spine radiosurgery can be grouped into four categories:

1. Unirradiated patients: spinal metastases in a previously unirradiated volume treated with SBRS.
2. Reirradiated patients: spinal metastases in a previously irradiated volume now containing new, recurrent, or progressive metastatic disease treated with SBRS.
3. Postoperative SBRS patients: spinal metastases treated with SBRS after open surgical intervention, with or without spinal stabilization.
4. Mixed patients: mixed populations involving patients in the previous 3 categories in which outcomes are not separately reported.

Gerzsten et al., reported a durable pain improvement in 94% of patients with RCC metastasis in the spine treated with radiosurgery. In his systematic review of the literature, radiographic control has been reported to be up to 87% in RCC (Gerzsten et al., 2009).

The use of stereotactic radiosurgery as primary option of treatment is indicated in cases of patients undergoing treatment to a symptomatic spine lesion with other significant but asymptomatic spine metastases. These asymptomatic metastases may be treated with radiosurgery to avoid further irradiation to the neural elements as well as to avoid further bone-marrow suppression and permit subsequent systemic therapy. The benefits for this approach include a single treatment that is radiobiologically larger than can be delivered with standard radiotherapy, with a minimal radiation dose to adjacent normal tissue. When used as a primary treatment modality, long- term radiographic tumor control was demonstrated in 90% of cases of isolated RCC metastases.

Stereotactic radiosurgery may be also indicated to treat patients presenting progressive neurologic deficit, where open surgery is contra-indicated, or in cases where the tumor is partially resected (intralesional resection) radiosurgery can be used to treat a residual tumor at a later date. In cases of severe compression of neural elements, the radiosurgery is not indicated and open procedure should be performed. Radiosurgery can also be used after vertebral body cement augmentation, with a local control rate as high as 92% (Gibbs et al., 2009).

Appropriate dose and fractionation schedules have not been determined and differ among institutions. There are institutions where the protocols include single-fraction radiosurgery from eight to 24 Gy or hypofractionated regimens consisting in different doses and number of fractions.

Complications associated to radiosurgery include esophagitis, mucositis, dysphagia, diarrhea, paresthesia, transient laryngitis, and transient radiculitis. Spinal cord injury has been reported, but is considered exceedingly rare.

Although the results so far reported using stereotactic radiosurgery have shown to be satisfying and promising, this technique does not treat spinal instability caused by the majority of the spinal tumors, and is contra-indicated in severe neural compression. Analysis of local tumor control rates after en bloc resection of solitary vertebral RCC metastases and after stereotactic radiosurgery appears to have comparable tumor control rates. The mean follow-up in Gerszten series of 60 patients treated with radiosurgery was 37 months and his final outcomes were comparable to the patients followed by Boriani, which showed 48% of patients with no evidence of disease after 30 months, while 52% presented systemic progression and were dead at eight to 28 months. Long-term prospective randomized studies are still to be done in order to establish to best indications and protocols for the use of stereotactic radiosurgery in RCC metastasis.

Recently, the Spine Oncology Study Group (SOSG) has conducted a systematic review trying to answer the following question "What is the optimal treatment for solitary renal cell metastases without significant epidural disease?". Their conclusion was that there is a very low quality of evidence, however stereotactic radiosurgery should be the first line therapy rather than en bloc resection (Bilsky et al., 2009).

4.6 Other treatment modalities

Radiotherapy is well known to be less effective in RCC metastases. Its use in higher doses to reach a satisfactory response increases the risk of spinal cord lesions, and also the side effects associated to it. The relationship between radiotherapy dose and duration of response has not been well studied, and the results are conflicting in the literature. The palliation of bone pain has been reported to be satisfying by Wilson et.al when compared with the palliation of symptoms at other sites of metastases, but the duration of this effect is still controversial. Higher biological effective dose does not seem to be a predictor of response or of duration of response in the palliative treatment of RCC.

The development of new management techniques of vertebral metastatic lesions has increased. Vertebroplasty, kyphoplasty, and thermablation using radiofrequency techniques have been used. Radiofrequency is fairly used throughout the world, but results evaluating the tumor necrosis have been reported by Gasbarrini et al. in 2009. The purpose of this technique is to selectively destroy the metastatic lesion with local hyperthermia as well as resulting in thrombosis of the local paravertebral veins. In their report, the authors analyzed the tumor necrosis rate under light microscope and also under electronic microscope. They found that good results can be achieved in solid tumors as liver tumors, however the necrosis rate in RCC metastases were different, showing less necrosis rates. Their possible hypothesis for the treatment failure is that in highly vascular tumors is probably difficult to maintain the necessary temperature *in situ* for adequate necrosis. Selective arterial embolization should be considered prior to radiofrequency ablation in RCC metastases.

The use of vertebroplasty, and/or kyphoplasty in spinal metastases has no effect as far as inducing tumor necrosis. Considering the heat generated by the cement and its duration as heat source, these techniques should not be used for that purpose. The use of cement inside the vertebral body is indicated in spinal oncology to increase the vertebrae's resistance and to treat spinal instability secondary to pathologic fractures.

It is very important to always keep in mind that these treatment modalities (vertebroplasty, kyphoplasty, and thermoablation are absolutely palliative and aims only to alleviate the pain.

5. Conclusion

The different therapeutic options and their indications in the treatment of patients with RCC metastatic disease can be distributed as follow:

1. Only radiotherapy:
   - Multiple osseous metastases
   - Untreatable visceral metastases
   - Untreatable primary tumor
   - Patient's poor clinical conditions
2. Decompression, and stabilization associated to radiotherapy:
   - Intractable pain and/or neurological deficit in patients with disseminated disease
   - Untreatable or treatable visceral metastases
3. Intralesional excision and radiotherapy:
   - Solitary bone metastasis (in cases where en bloc resection is contra-indicated)
   - Treatable visceral metastasis
   - En bloc resection not feasible
4. En bloc resection:
   - Solitary bone metastasis
   - Treated primary tumor
   - Absence of visceral metastasis

- Technically feasible
5. Stereotactic radiosurgery:
   - Solitary bone metastasis
   - Absence or with minimal epidural disease
   - Absence of severe spinal instability

Considering all the treatment options, the management of RCC metastases is essentially a surgical treatment. The use of stereotactic radiosurgery has proven to be effective and comparable to en bloc resection for selected cases, however we need to consider that this treatment requires a very specific technology that, so far, is not widely available for the majority of treatment centers and patients throughout the world. This technique also does not provide any kind of mechanical reinforcement to the spinal instability.

The progressive increase of the life expectancy of these patients, associated to the low sensitivity to conventional radiotherapy and the absence of a valid protocol of chemotherapy, makes surgery, associated to immunotherapy, the treatment of election, especially in cases of targeted therapies fail. Furthermore, the vertebral location of the lesion, determines a severe compromise of the quality of life often caused by intractable pain and elevated risk of paralysis and/or pathological fracture. In this last case the surgical treatment is performed in an emergency basis and therefore associated to all the anesthesiology and surgical complication that an urgent procedure can have.

The final results, comparing the en bloc resection to intralesional excision associated to radiotherapy, seems to be similar considering the local control and long term survival. The comparison between the two options as far as morbidity and cost/efficacy favors the en bloc resection.

Isolated surgery is indicated in cases of isolated metastases, and when during the preoperative planning, the procedure is planned to be outside the tumor capsule (extralesional). Selected cases of small tumors in favorable locations, where en bloc spondilectomy is feasible, associated to good prognosis of the primary disease, en bloc resection should be the treatment of choice. This is particularly true in cases of RCC metastases, because of its high risk of local recurrence, after intralesional excision even if combined with radiotherapy. In reality, the worst result after curettage occurs in cases of incomplete excisions (posterior only approach) and the effect of additional radiotherapy is incapable to eradicate the lesion. This findings confirm that the intralesional excision needs to be complete (outside the tumor capsule) in tumors partially or totally radioresitant, like the renal cell carcinoma, becoming necessary a double surgical approach.

Both palliative surgery and intralesional excision may allow, in a good amount of patients, a certain degree of neurological improvement in the short term (improving quality of life), however the survival percentage at mid term is shorter for the patients treated with simple decompression and stabilization of the spine. Although we need to consider that, in general, patients treated with palliative surgery are in worse condition compared to those treated with intralesional excision. In cases of intralesional surgery, the use of adjuvant radiation therapy is indicated even considering the low sensitivity of tumor to this treatment.

Immunotherapy should always be associated to the post-operative radiotherapy, because it has been demonstrated that the association of the adjuvant therapy increases the survival, independently of the surgical technique applied.

The use of isolated radiation therapy is indicated only in the face of multiple RCC metastases in patients with a poor prognosis. Even in those cases, when radiation therapy fails to mitigate pain and/or in the presence of a pathologic fracture with progressive neurological deterioration, a surgical intervention with decompression and stabilization should be performed.

The early diagnosis of the primary tumor, the presence and location of the metastatic disease are paramount. The possibility of detecting the metastatic lesion in an early stage allows the spine surgeon to choose the best treatment for each patient and for each lesion. Unfortunately, the identification of these patients in an advanced stage makes the surgical intervention only a palliative measure used in cases of pathological fractures or severe neurological deficit. On the other hand, the early intervention permits a better local control of the disease, increasing the success possibility as far as improving the neurological status and treating the pain.

6. References

Arguello F, Baggs RB, Duerst RE, Johnstone L, McQueen K, Frantz CN. Pathogenesis of vertebral metastasis and epidural spinal cord compression. *Cancer* 1990;65(1):98–106.

Batson OV. The function of the vertebral veins and their role in the spread of metastases. *Ann Surg* 1940; 112: 138-49.

Batson OV. The vertebral vein system as a mechanism for the spread of metastases. *Am J Roentgenol* 1942; 48: 715-8.

Batson OV. The vertebral vein system. Caldwell lecture. *Am J Roentgenol* 1957; 78:195-212.

Biagini R, Boriani S, Casadei R, Bandiera S, De Iure F, Campanacci L, Demitri S, Orsini U, Di Fiore M.; Resections techniques in the treatment of vertebral neoplasms. *Chir. Org. Mov.* 1997; 82: 341-355.

Bilsky MH, Laufer I., Burch S. Shifting paradigms in the treatment of metastatic spine disease. *Spine* 2009; 34 (22): S101-S107.

Boriani S, Biagini R, De Iure F, Andreoli I, Lari S, Di Fiore M. Lombalgia neoplastica: diagnosi e trattamento. Chir. Organi Mov. 1994; 79: 93-9.

Boriani S, Weinstein JN: Differential diagnosis and surgical treatment of primary benign and malignant Neoplasm. In Frymoyer *The adult spine; Principles and Practice*. 1996; 2nd ed. Lippincott-Raven, Philadelphia.

Boriani S, Weinstein JN, Biagini R: Spine update. Primary bone tumors of the spine. Terminology and surgical staging. 1997; Spine 22: 1036-1044.

Cappuccio M, Gasbarrini A, Van Urk P, et al. Spinal metastasis: a retrospective study validating the treatment algorithm. *Eur Rev Med Pharmaco Sci* 2008; 12:155– 60.

Cappuccio M, Gasbarrini A, Bandello L, Focarazzo E, et al. Il tratamento chirurgico delle metastasi vertebrali da carcinoma renale: problematiche anestesiologiche intraoperatorie. *Clin Ter* 2008; 159 (1): 1-6.

Cappuccio M, Gasbarrini A, Donthineni R, Beisse R, Boriani S. Thoracospcopic assisted en bloc resection of a spine tumor. *Eur Spine J* 2011; 20 (Suppl 2): S202-5.

Crockard A, Quiney R, Taylor B, Lehovsky J: 360 degree surgery for high cervical vertebral tumors. *J.Neurosurg* 1980; 53: 712-21.

Denis F: The three column spine and its significance in the classification of acute thoracolumbar spinal injuries. *Spine* 1983; 8(8): 817-831.

Duensing S, van den Berg-de Ruiter E, Störkel S, Kirchner H, Hänninen EL, Buer J, et al.: Cytogenetic studies in renal cell carcinoma patients receiving low- dose recombinant interleukin-2-based immunotherapy. *Tumour Biol.* 1996; 17: 27-33.

Gabriel K, Schiff D. Metastatic spinal cord compression by solid tumors. *Seminars in Neurology* 2004;24(4):375–83

Gasbarrini A, Cappuccio M, Mirabile L, et al. Spinal metastases: treatment evaluation algorithm. *Eur Rev Med Pharmaco Sci* 2004; 8:265–74.

Gasbarrini A, Cappucio M, Li H, Donthineni R, et al. Treatment of metastases to the vertebrae with radiofrequency ablation: determination of effectiveness by evaluation of tumor necrosis – A preliminary result. *Curr Radiopharm* 2009; 2: 191-194.

Gasbarrini A, Li H, Cappuccio M, Mirabile L, et al. Efficacy evaluation of a new treatment algorithm for spinal metastases. *Spine* 2010; 36 (2): 1466-70.

Gerszten PC, Mendel E, Yamada Y. Radiotherapy and radiosurgery for Metastatic disease: What are the options, indications, and outcomes? *Spine* 2009; 34 (22S): S78-S92.

Gibbs IC, Kamnerdsupaphon P, Ryu MR, et al. Image-guided robotic radiosurgery for spinal metastases. *Radiother Oncol* 2007; 82:185–90.

Gottfried ON, Schloesser PE, Schmidt MH, Stevens EA. Embolization of metastatic tumors. *Neurosurg Clin N Am* 2004; 15:391-99.

Gurwitz GS, Dawson JM, McNamara MJ, Federspiel CF, Spengler DM.: Biomechanical analysis of three surgical approaches for lumbar burst fractures using short-segment instrumentation. *Spine* 1993; 18 (8): 977-982.

Heldwein FL, Escudier B, Smyth G, Souto CAV, Vallancien G. Metastatic renal cell carcinoma management. *Int Braz J Urol* 2009; 35: 256-70.

Jacqmin D, van Poppel H, Kirkali Z, Mickisch G: Renal cancer. *Eur Urol.* 2001; 39: 361-9.

Jemal A, Siegel R, Ward E, Hao Y, Xu J, Murray T, et al. Cancer statistics, 2008. *CA Cancer J Clin.* 2008; 58: 71-96.

Karnofsky DA. Clinical evaluation of anticancer drugs: cancer chemotherapy. *GANN Monogr* 1967; 2: 223–31.

Kawahara N, Tomita K, Murakami H, Demura S. Total en bloc spondilectomy for spinal tumors: surgical techiniques and related basic background. *Othop Clin N Am* 2009; 40: 47-63.

Koga S, Tsuda S, Nishikido M, Ogawa Y, et al. The diagnostic value of bone scan in patients with renal cell carcinoma. *J Urol* 2001; 166(6): 2126-8.

Larkin JM, Eisen T: Kinase inhibitors in the treatment of renal cell carcinoma. *Crit Rev Oncol Hematol.* 2006; 60: 216-26.

Louis R. *Surgery of the spine.* Berlin : Springer – Verlag, 1983.

Manke C, Bretschneider T, Lenhart M, et al. Spinal metastases from renal cell carcinoma: effect of preoperative particle embolization on intraoperative blood loss. *Am J Neuroradiol* 2001; 22: 997-1003.

Marcove RC, Arlen M. *Atlas of Bone Pathology. With Clinical and Radiographic Correlations.* 1st ed. Philadelphia: J.B. Lippincot Co., 1992: 518-34.

McAfee PC, Bohlman HH, Riley LH, et al. Anterior retropharyngeal approach to the upper part of the cervical spine. *J Bone Joint Surg (Am)* 1987; 69: 1371-83.

McLain RF: Spinal cord decompression: an endoscopically assisted approach for metastatic tumors. *Spinal Cord* 2001; 39(9): 482-487.

McGuire RA: Physical examination in spinal trauma. In: Levine AM, Eismont FJ, Garfin SR, Zigler E: *Spine trauma.* W.B. Philadelphia. Saunders Company, 1998: 16-27.

Olerud C, Jonsson H, Lofberg AM, Lorelius LE, Sjostrom L. Embolization of spinal metastases reduces preoperative blood loss. 21 patients operated on for renal cell carcinoma. *Acta Orthop Scand* 1993; 64(1):9–12.

Perrin RG, Livingston KE, Aarabi B. Intradural extramedullary spinal metastasis. A report of 10 cases. *Journal of Neurosurgery* 1982;56(6):835–7.

Roy-Camille R, Mazel Ch, Saillant G, Lapresle Ph: Treatment of malignant tumors of the spine with posterior instrumentation. in: Sundaresan N., Schmidek H.H., Schiller A.L., Rosenthal D.I. (ed.) *Tumors of the Spine. Diagnosis and Clinical Management.* Philadelphia: W.B.Saunders; 1990: 473-492.

Sahgal A, Ames C, Chou D, et al. Stereotactic body radiotherapy is effective salvage therapy for patients with prior radiation of spinal metastases. *Int J Radiat Oncol Biol Phys* 2009; 74:723–31.

Sakaura H, Hosono N, Mukai Y, et al. Outcome of total en bloc spondylectomy for solitary metastasis of the thoracolumbar spine. *J Spinal Disord Tech* 2004; 17:297–300.

Schaberg J, Gainor B.J. A profile of metastatic carcinoma of the spine. *Spine* 1985; 10:19–20.

Stener B.: Complete removal of vertebrae for extirpation of tumors. *Clin Orthop Rel Res* 1989; 245: 72-82.

Sundaresan N, Choi IS, Hughes JE, Sachdev VP, Berenstein A. Treatment of spinal metastases from kidney cancer by presurgical embolization and resection. *J Neurosurg* 1990; 73(4):548–54.

Tae-Hon Lim, An HS, Hong JH, Ahn JY, You JW, Eck J, McGrady LM: Biomechanical evaluation of anterior and posterior fixations in an unstable calf spine model. *Spine* 1997; 22, 3: 261-266.

Thyavihally BY, Mahantshetty U, Chamarajanagar RS, Raibhattanavar SG, Tongaonkar HB. Management of renal cell carcinoma with solitary metastasis. *World J Surg Onc* 2005.Vol 3, No 48.

Tokuhashi Y, Kawano H, Ohsaka S, et al. A scoring system for preoperative evaluation of the prognosis of metastatic spine tumor prognosis. *J Jpn Orthop Assoc* 1989; 63:482–9.

Tokuhashi Y, Matsuzaki H, Toriyama S, et al. Scoring system for the preoperative evaluation of metastatic spine tumor prognosis. *Spine* 1990; 15:1110 –3.

Tokuhashi Y, Matsuzaki H, Sasaki M, et al. Scoring system for the preoperative evaluation of metastatic spine tumor prognosis. *Rinsho Seikei Geka* 1997;32:512–22.

Tokuhashi Y, Matsuzaki H, Okawa A, et al. Indications of operative procedures for metastatic spine tumors: a scoring system for preoperative evaluation of prognosis. *J East Jpn Orthop Traumatol* 1999; 11:31–5.

Tokuhashi Y, Matsuzaki H, Oda H, et al. A revised scoring system for preoperative evaluation of metastatic spine tumors prognosis. *Spine* 2005; 30(19): 2186-91.

Tomita K., Kawahara N., Baba H., Tsuchiya H., Nagata S., Toribatake Y.: Total en bloc spondylectomy for solitary spinal metastases. *International Orthopaedics (SICOT)* 1994; 18: 291-298.

Tomita K, Kawahara N, Baba H,etal.Total enbloc spondylectomy: a new surgical technique for primary malignant vertebral tumors. *Spine* 1997; 22:324 –33.

Tomita K, Kawahara N, Kobayashi T, et al. Surgical strategy for spinal metastases. *Spine* 2001; 26:298–306.

Weinstein JN: Primary Tumors. in: S.Weinstein: *The Pediatric Spine.* New York, Raven Press, 1994.

Wilson D, Hiller L, Gray L, Grainger M, et al. The effect of biological dose on time to symptom progression in metastatic renal cell carcinoma. *Clinical Oncology* 2003; 15: 400-4007.

Part 2

Clinical

7

New Systemic Approaches in the Treatment of Metastatic Renal Cell Carcinoma

Thean Hsiang Tan[1], Judith Lees[1],
Ganesalingam Pranavan[2] and Desmond Yip[2,3]
[1]RAH Cancer Centre, Royal Adelaide Hospital,
[2]Medical Oncology Unit, The Canberra Hospital,
[3]ANU Medical School, Australian National University,
Australia

1. Introduction

Cancer of the kidney comprises approximately 3% of all cancers in males and 2% in females according to Cancer Research UK statistics. (http://info.cancerresearchuk.org) Similar figures are seen globally. The majority (around 90%) of kidney cancers are Renal Cell Carcinomas (RCC), and clear cell carcinomas (adenocarcinomas) are the most common histological subtype. (Cohen & McGovern, 2005) The remaining 20-25% are papillary (Type I and II) (10-15%), chromophobe (4%) and collecting duct (including the rare medullary variant) (<1%) RCCs. (Cohen & McGovern, 2005) Up to a third of patients present at initial diagnosis with evidence of distant metastases, and a third of patients who undergo nephrectomy will have a recurrence within 5 years. These patients are considered candidates for systemic therapy. (Molina & Motzer, 2008)

2. Molecular pathogenesis

2.1 Clear-cell variant renal cell carcinoma

Unravelling of the biology, genetics and intracellular molecular signalling pathways of RCC has greatly improved our understanding of this disease. (Tan et al, 2010) The discovery of von Hippel-Lindau (VHL) tumour suppressor gene as a critical oncogene in the pathogenesis of renal cell carcinoma (clear-cell as well as some of the non-clear-cell variant) has greatly revolutionised the systemic therapy for renal-cell carcinoma where previously treatment had been disheartening. (Choueiri et al, 2008; Cohen & McGovern, 2005) The VHL protein (pVHL) encoded by the VHL tumour suppressor gene serves to regulate the normal cellular response to oxygen deprivation through its interaction with hypoxia-inducible factor (HIF). HIF is a heterodimeric (HIF-α/β) gene transcription factor that consists of an unstable α-subunit and a stable β-subunit. In the presence of normal oxygen tension (or normoxic state), VHL protein is the substrate recognition of an E3 ubiquitin ligase complex that targets HIF-α subunits for destruction by the proteasome as illustrated in Figure 1. (Kamura et al, 2000; Ohh et al, 2000) In the absence of functional VHL proteins, either as a result of mutation or hyper-methylation of the VHL gene as seen in majority of sporadic cases of RCC (equivalent to a physiological hypoxic state), the pVHL-HIF-α interaction is disrupted due to loss of oxygen-dependent hydroxylation of HIF-α subunits leading to their intracellular accumulation. (Maxwell et al, 1999) HIF-α subunits are able to then translocate into the nucleus where they heterodimerize with the HIF-β subunits forming transcriptional factor complexes that induce transcription of various hypoxia-response genes. (Amato, 2011) This in turn leads to the increased production of downstream pro-angiogenic factors such as vascular endothelial growth factor (VEGF), platelet-derived growth factor (PDGF) and transforming growth factor alpha and beta (TGF-α and TGF-β) as illustrated by Figure 1. (Kim & Kaelin, 2004) It is noteworthy that angiogenesis holds the key to tumour survival when the rapidly growing tumour outstrips its own existing blood supply. It utilized the effective HIF mechanism to promote its own survival, growth and progression (metastasis). (Vaupel, 2004)

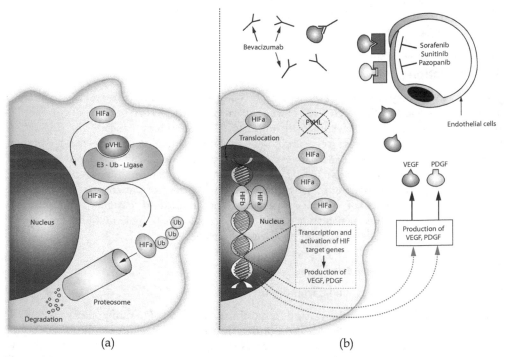

(a)   (b)

Fig. 1. (a) Normoxia/normal VHL gene (b) Hypoxia/inactivated tumour suppressor VHL gene

2.2 Non clear-cell variant renal cell carcinoma

Papillary RCC is the second most common histological subtype of the non-clear cell variant of RCC. (Cohen & McGovern, 2005) It can be further categorized histologically into papillary types I and II with emerging data suggesting an underlying different genetics and molecular pathways. (Furge et al, 2010) Papillary type I RCC is associated with activating mutations of methyl-nitroso-nitroguanidine-induced (MET) oncogene. (Choi et al, 2006; Dharmawardana et al, 2004) These mutations results in ligand-independent activation of intracytoplasmic tyrosine kinase domains which subsequently activate the hepatocyte growth factor/MET pathway. (Choi et al, 2006; Sudarshan & Linehan, 2006) Papillary type II RCC, in contrast is attributed to mutation of the fumarate hydratase (FH) tumour suppressor gene. (Linehan et al, 2007) FH is a tricarboxylic acid (Kreb) cycle enzyme that has a crucial role in aerobic cellular metabolism. (Isaacs et al, 2005) Mutation of FH (inactivation) leads to the generation of a pseudo-hypoxic state with subsequent upregulation of the HIF-α subunits. The mutated FH enzyme allows the accumulation of fumarate which in turn leads to inhibition of HIF-prolyl hydroxylase (HPH), a critical enzymatic regulator of intracellular HIF-α. When HPH is inactivated, the hydroxylation of HIF is disrupted leading to failure of recognition by pVHL; thus preventing the VHL-dependent proteosomal degradation of HIFs. Accumulation of HIF-α leads to downstream transcriptional overexpression of pro-angiogenic factors as described in the previous section. (Isaacs et al, 2005)

Chromophobe RCC accounts for 4% of all RCC. (Cohen & McGovern, 2005) Whilst the exact mechanism underlying its pathogenesis is not well established, the VEGF-angiogenic pathway was again implicated in view of the elevated levels of VEGF and its receptor mRNA in this variant of RCC. The KIT oncogene and the folliculin (FLCN) gene associated with the hereditary form of chromophobe/oncocytic RCC hybrid (Birt-Hogg-Dubé Syndrome) are other molecular targets identified in this variant. (Pavlovich et al, 2002; Yamazaki et al, 2003; Zbar et al, 2002) Due to the rarity of collecting duct RCC (including the virulent medullary variant), the underlying pathogenesis has not been identify. (Oudard et al, 2007a)

3. Prognostic indicators

For patients with recurrent or metastatic disease, a question often faced by the treating physician is their prognosis as treatment is being contemplated. In metastatic RCC, numerous studies have been undertaken to investigate the prognostic markers for metastatic RCC. (Tan et al, 2010) Five prognostic markers linked to the overall survival rate of patients with metastatic RCC have been identified. These include performance status, absence or presence of prior nephrectomy, serum lactate dehydrogenase, corrected serum calcium and haemoglobin level. (Motzer *et al*, 1999) Based on these criteria, patients could be grouped into three prognostic risk categories: favourable (0 risk features), intermediate (1-2 risk features) and poor (≥3 risk features) according to the Memorial Sloan-Kettering Cancer Centre (MSKCC) risk classification. (Motzer *et al*, 1999) Previous radiotherapy, time to systemic therapy, and the presence of hepatic, pulmonary, and retroperitoneal nodal metastasis were found to be independent prognostic factors in later studies. (Mekhail *et al*, 2005) The stratification of the different prognostic factors of renal carcinoma in clinical studies is important to allow comparison of therapies and to gain insight into the cohort of patients that would most benefit from the investigational agent.

When comparing with the clear-cell variant of RCC, localized papillary RCC when resectable, has a more favourable prognosis than conventional clear cell. (Cheville *et al*, 2003; Patard *et al*, 2005) However, metastatic papillary RCC portends a worse prognosis than their clear-cell counterpart. (Margulis *et al*, 2008) The type II papillary variant is thought to be more aggressive than type I with a higher propensity to metastasize early and progress rapidly. (Motzer *et al*, 2004) Chromophobe RCC is considered a good prognostic variant and is associated with earlier stage tumour and longer overall survival compared to clear-cell RCC. In the metastatic setting, the reports from the medical literature are however conflicting. (Beck *et al*, 2004; Cindolo *et al*, 2005; Klatte *et al*, 2008; Motzer *et al*, 2002) Collecting duct RCC is associated with a grave prognosis, with up to one-third of patients presenting with metastatic disease on initial presentation. (Motzer *et al*, 2002)

4. Systemic treatment of metastatic renal cell carcinoma

Metastatic RCC is inherently refractory to chemotherapy and hormonal therapies. (Harris, 1983; Yagoda & Bander, 1989) The response rate of these treatment options are in the order of 10% thereby rendering RCC notoriously difficult to treat. (Yagoda & Bander, 1989) Solitary metastatic lesions may be surgically resected however beyond surgery, the only systemic options available prior to the era of targeted therapy were interferon alpha (IFN-α) and interleukin 2 (IL-2). (Oudard *et al*, 2007b) Allogeneic stem cell transplantation to induce a graft-versus-tumour response has also been examined but at the expense of significant life-threatening toxicities. This is therefore not recommended outside a clinical trial setting. (Barkholt *et al*, 2006; Gommersall *et al*, 2004; Rini *et al*, 2002) Patients with good prognostic features had a response rate of 10-20% to IFN-α and IL-2 and a modest improvement of median survival by ~2.5 months with IFN-α. (1999; Coppin et al, 2005) High dose IL-2 (infusion therapy requiring hospitalization) conferred a durable but small long term disease remission of ~5% in clinical responders. (Fyfe *et al*, 1995; McDermott *et al*, 2005) Both cytokine treatments especially with high dose IL-2 are toxic and difficult to administer. The classical side-effects of flu-like syndrome, depression with suicidal episodes from IFN-α; (Cohen & McGovern, 2005; Motzer *et al*, 1996) hypotension, oliguria, capillary-leak syndrome with secondary multi-organ failure, somnolence and confusion from IL-2 would render both treatments very onerous to patients. (Cohen & McGovern, 2005; Parton *et al*, 2006) Moreover the reported mortality rate of 4% from IL-2 would dilute any modest survival advantage gained. (Fyfe *et al*, 1995) Not surprisingly, the underlying enthusiasm in utilizing these agents as frontline therapy in metastatic RCC has been dampened with the advent of targeted therapies.

4.1 VEGF ligands and receptor inhibitors

Vascular endothelial growth factor (VEGF), platelet-derived growth factor (PDGF) and other angiogenic ligands once produced are able to circulate freely to to interact with cell surface receptors on the endothelial cell. Upon binding of these ligands to their cognate receptors, a cascade of intracellular signalling takes place resulting in downstream activation of Raf and mitogen-activated protein kinase (MAPK) (via phospholipase C-γ). This ultimately leads to the promotion of tumour angiogenesis, endothelial cell survival, proliferation, and migration. (Cebe-Suarez et al, 2006) The discovery of these complex VEGF signalling pathways presented an opportunity as therapeutic targets to treat metastatic RCC. VEGF signaling blockade can be achieved by either the removal of the circulating ligand with monoclonal antibody (bevacizumab) or by inhibiting its receptors with tyrosine kinase inhibitors (TKIs) as illustrated by Figure 1. (Jonasch et al, 2011) The four anti-VEGF therapies approved as of 2011: sunitinib, sorafenib, pazopanib and bevacizumab have revolutionized the treatment of metastatic RCC leading to significant improvement in progression-free survival (PFS) and in some instances overall survival (OS). (Tan et al, 2010)

4.1.1 Sunitinib

Sunitinib is an oral multi-kinase inhibitor that targets several VEGF receptors (VEGF-1, VEGF-2, VEGF-3) and other tyrosine kinase receptors (PDGFR, c-Kit, FLT-3, CSF-1R, and RET). (Abrams et al, 2003; Kim et al, 2006; Mendel et al, 2003; Murray et al, 2003; O'Farrell et al, 2003) Earlier uncontrolled trials showed sunitinib to be active in patients with advanced malignancies including RCC. (Faivre *et al*, 2006)

4.1.1.1 Sunitinib Intermittent Dosing (4 Weeks On / 2 Weeks Off)

The initial phase II study of sunitinib in patients with cytokine-refractory metastatic renal cell cancer assessed the clinical efficacy and safety of sunitinib as second-line therapy. (Motzer et al, 2006) The sixty three patients who failed cytokine-based therapy received 50mg of sunitinib for 4 weeks followed by a 2 week break (4/2), in a 6 week cycle. Forty percent (n=25) of patients had partial response (PR) and 27% (n=17) additional patients demonstrated stable disease (SD) for ≥3 months. The median time to progression and survival were 8.7 months and 16.4 months respectively. (Motzer et al, 2006)

A larger phase II multicentre trial similarly confirmed the anti-cancer efficacy of sunitinib in cytokine refractory patients with metastatic RCC. One hundred and six patients were enrolled and an overall objective response (ORR) of 44% was noted with 1% (n=1) and 43% (n=45) demonstrating a CR and PR respectively. (Motzer et al, 2007b) An additional 22% (n=23) showed SD for ≥ 3 months. The median duration of response for the 46 responding patients was 10 months whilst the median progression free survival (PFS) was 8.3 months. (Motzer et al, 2007b)

As the ORR of sunitinib seen in phase II trials far exceeded the rates previously reported for cytokine therapy as first line treatment of metastatic disease (42% vs. 10–15%), an international landmark phase III trial comparing sunitinib with INF-α for patients with metastatic clear-cell RCC was undertaken. (Costa & Drabkin, 2007; Motzer et al, 2007a) Seven hundred and fifty treatment naïve patients with clear-cell histology and good performance status (ECOG 0 or 1) were randomized in a 1:1 ratio to receive either sunitinib (dose as per earlier studies) or INF-α (9×10^6 units subcutaneously thrice weekly). (Desai *et al*, 2007; Motzer *et al*, 2007a) The median duration of treatment was 6 months (1-15 months) in the sunitinib group and 4 months (1-13 months) in the IFN-α group. The median PFS assessed by an independent third-party review was 11 months in the sunitinib group and 5 months in the IFN-α group, corresponding to a Hazard Ratio (HR) of 0.42 (95% CI 0.32–0.54; p < 0.001). (Motzer et al, 2007a) The investigators' assessment showed similar results, with a PFS of 11 months in the sunitinib and 4 months in the IFN-α group. An updated analysis published in 2009 has shown the ORR of 47% for sunitinib and 12% for IFN-α (p< 0.000001), with a median PFS of 11 months and 5 months, respectively, for sunitinib and IFN-α (p< 0.000001), similar to the original report. (Motzer *et al*, 2009) These results were uniformly seen, regardless of patient's age, gender and prognostic category. (Motzer *et al*, 2009) Patients on sunitinib also experienced a median OS in excess of 2 years. The OS was 26.4 months for sunitinib and 21.8 months for IFN-α (p = 0.051). (Motzer *et al*, 2009) A separate exploratory analysis of patients on both treatment arms who did not receive post-study cancer treatment showed the median OS with sunitinib was twice as long as IFN-α (28.1 months versus 14.1 months respectively, p=0.003). (Motzer *et al*, 2009) Based on these positive results, sunitinib has replaced INF-α in the first line treatment of metastatic RCC.

In addition to the aforesaid clinical trials, sunitinib was also evaluated in an expanded-access programme, designed to allow access to sunitinib in patients with metastatic RCC who would otherwise be excluded from the clinical trials. (Gore et al, 2009) Over 4500 patients, including older patients ($\geq$65 years-old; n=1414), those with poorer performance status (ECOG PS $\geq$2; n=582), non-clear cell histology (n=288) and with brain metastases (n=320) were enrolled in this international, open-label study, thus resembling a more "real-world" setting. (Gore et al, 2009) Patients received a median of five sunitinib treatment cycles, with 56% of patients receiving more than 6 months of sunitinib therapy for a median duration of 15.6 months. In the total evaluable study population (n=4349), the median PFS was 10.9 months and median OS was 18.4 months. (Gore et al, 2009) The median PFS closely resembles the phase III study demonstrating consistent efficacy across patients within and outside clinical trials. No differences were noted in median PFS and OS between patients with or without prior cytokine therapy. Subgroup analysis of elderly patients demonstrated median PFS and OS of 11.3 and 18.2 months respectively. (Gore et al, 2009) In patients with poorer performance status, median PFS and OS were 5.1 months and 6.7 months respectively and lastly in patients with brain metastases with an overall poorer prognosis, a median PFS of 5.6 months and median OS of 9.2 months were observed. (Gore et al, 2009)

4.1.1.2 Sunitinib Continuous Dosing

Sunitinib has also been examined in an open-label multicentre phase II trial using continuous once daily dosing at a dose of 37.5 mg. (Escudier et al, 2009b) One hundred and seven patients were randomised equally to either morning or evening dose for a median 8.3 months. Forty three percent of patients had dose reduction to 25mg due to grade 3-4 adverse effects. (Escudier et al, 2009b) The ORR was 20%, with a median duration of response of 7.2 months, median PFS of 8.2 months and OS of 19.8 months. (Escudier et al, 2009b) The tolerability of the morning and evening dosing as well as the reporting quality of life (QoL) whilst on therapy was similar. Grade 3 diarrhoea, fatigue/asthenia and hand-foot syndrome were however noted more in the evening dosing cohort. This continuous regimen appeared promising and certainly deserves further investigation as this dosing schedule may benefit patients who are not able to tolerate the intermittent sunitinib dosing of 50mg and where one is concerned that the intermittent 37.5mg is suboptimal.

Sunitinib standard dosing schedule (50mg/day; 4 weeks on, 2 weeks off) was compared with continuous dose (37.5 mg/day) in a phase II trial (EFFECT) for patients with locally recurrent clear-cell RCC or metastatic RCC who had received no previous systemic therapy for advanced disease. The intermittent schedule when compared with the continuous schedule showed a trend to improved ORR (32.2% vs. 28.1%; p=0.444) and median PFS (8.5 months vs. 7.0 months; p=0.070). No difference were noted between the median OS (23.1 months vs. 23.5 months, p=0.615). (Motzer et al, 2011b) Interestingly the median OS was lower than the phase III sunitinib vs. INF-α trial which had a median OS of 26 months. The phase III trial had a higher number of patients with better baseline prognostic features (better performance status and more patients had underwent nephrectomy) which may account for better survival results. (Motzer et al, 2011b; Motzer et al, 2007a)

4.1.2 Sorafenib

Sorafenib is an oral multi-kinase inhibitor that inhibits Raf (Raf-1, B-Raf, and mutant *b-raf V600E*), VEGF (VEGF-2, VEGF-3), PDGFR (PDGFR-α, PDGFR-β), c-KIT, FLT3 and RET.

(Carlomango 2006, Wilhelm 2004) A phase II randomized discontinuation trial in 202 patients with metastatic RCC who failed previous systemic treatments were treated with sorafenib at 400 mg BD. (Ratain et al, 2006) Seventy-three patients exhibited tumour shrinkage of more than 25%. Sixty-five patients with stable disease at 12 weeks were randomly assigned to sorafenib (n=32) or placebo (n=33). Patients on sorafenib experienced prolonged median PFS (24 weeks) when compared to placebo (6 weeks) (p = 0.087). (Ratain et al, 2006) A second phase II trial comparing sorafenib with INF-α as first line treatment was undertaken in treatment naïve patients with metastatic RCC. Patients were randomised to receive sorafenib 400mg BD or IFN-α (9 million units thrice weekly). There was an option of dose escalation to sorafenib 600mg BD or crossover from INF-α to sorafenib upon disease progression. There was no significant improvement in PFS of sorafenib vs. placebo, 5.7 months vs. 5.8 months respectively. The ORR was 5% with sorafenib and 9% with IFN-α. (Escudier et al, 2009c)

A subsequent multi-centre placebo controlled phase III trial (TARGET) randomised 903 patients with metastatic clear-cell RCC on 1:1 to receive either placebo or sorafenib 400mg BD. The study cohort consisted of patients who previously received cytokine therapies with IFN-α, IL-2 or a combination of both, or radiotherapy, or had a nephrectomy. After 3 months of therapy, sorafenib resulted in a higher ORR (57% vs. 34%) and statistically significant longer PFS (5.5 months vs. 2.8 months; p< 0.001 with a HR of 0.44) when compared with placebo. (Escudier et al, 2007b) This was consistent with an earlier phase II second line trial that found PFS benefit was independent of age over or under 70 years, prognostic risk, prior cytokine therapy, lung, liver, bone or brain metastases, time from diagnosis, or whether or not the patient had clinical cardiovascular disease. (Beck et al, 2011; Escudier et al, 2007b) The latter included patients with ischemic heart disease, a previous myocardial infarction, left ventricular dysfunction, hypertension, epistaxis or central nervous system ischemia. (Beck et al, 2011) Patients on the placebo arm were permitted to cross over to sorafenib on diagnosis of progressive disease. In the first interim analysis, a trend towards better OS was noted in patients taking sorafenib, and this was unchanged in the final analysis (17.8 vs. 15.2 months, respectively, HR= 0.88; p = 0.146). (Escudier et al, 2007b; Escudier et al, 2009a) However, after placebo patients who crossed over on progression were censored, the difference in OS became significant (17.8 vs. 14.3 months; HR = 0.78; p = 0.029). (Escudier et al, 2007b)

Sorafenib has also been evaluated in two open-label expanded access studies in Europe (The European Advanced Renal Cell Carcinoma Sorafenib (EU-ARCS) and North America ARCCS (NA-ARCCS). The NA-ARCCCS offered insights into sorafenib in the real world setting. (Beck et al, 2008; Beck et al, 2011; Stadler et al, 2010) In Europe, about 1155 patients who failed at least one line of systemic therapy or were unsuitable for cytokine therapy received sorafenib 400mg BD until treatment intolerance or disease progression. Interim analysis revealed a median PFS of 6.9 months (95% CI: 6.2 – 7.5 months). (Beck et al, 2008) The North American access study enrolled 2515 patients in total with 2504 patients having received at least one cycle of sorafenib and therefore evaluable. Patients who had received no prior systemic therapy were allowed enrolment. Except for the difference in the median time from diagnosis (0.6 years vs. 2.2 years), prior nephrectomy rates (77% vs. 89%) and the incidence of >2 sites of metastatic disease prior to study entry (30% vs. 38%), the baseline characteristics were mostly balanced for patients who were treatment-naïve and patients who had at least one prior systemic treatment. The rate of disease progression was similar for fist-line sorafenib patients and patients who had received at least on e prior systemic treatment (16% vs. 17%). Similarly the rates of PFS and disease control (ORR + stable disease) were 83% vs. 84% in the first-line and prior systemic therapy cohorts, respectively. (Eisenhauer *et al*, 2009) These results demonstrate that sorafenib provides similar benefit in first- and second- or later line patient populations in a non-randomised, open access trial. (Stadler *et al*, 2010)

4.1.3 Pazopanib

Pazopanib is an oral multi-targeted receptor tyrosine kinase inhibitor that inhibits VEGF (VEGF-1, VEGF-2, VEGF-3), PDGF (PDGF-α, PDGF-β) and c-KIT. (Hutson *et al*, 2010) Pazopanib showed activity in a phase I trial with 2 partial responders and 4 patients achieving disease stability out of a total 12 patients. (Hurwitz *et al*, 2009) Subsequently, a randomised phase II study to determine the ORR, duration of response and PFS was undertaken on patients with predominantly clear-cell histology who had never been treated or had failed one line of non-multi-kinase therapy. This study was originally designed as a randomized discontinuation study but revised to an open-label study after a planned interim analysis undertaken at 12 weeks showed a response rate of 38%. (Hutson *et al*, 2010) This was confirmed to be similar on an independent review. The final analysis of this trial showed an ORR (CR + PR) of 33.8% with similar response rate between the treatment naïve cohort (34%; 95% CI 26% to 41%) and patients with one previous line of therapy (37%; 95% CI 26% to 49%). The median duration of response was 68 weeks. The estimated median PFS was 11.9 months for pazopanib vs. 6.2 months for placebo. (Rini & Al-Marrawi, 2011)

Pazopanib was subsequently tested in a phase III trial where a total of 233 treatment-naïve and 202 cytokine-pretreated patients with advanced clear-cell RCC were randomized in a 2:1 ratio to pazopanib (n = 290) or placebo (n = 145). (Sternberg *et al*, 2010) Placebo with best supportive care was thought to be an acceptable comparator arm due to the inaccessibility of other tyrosine kinase inhibitors (sunitinib or sorafenib) in some centres at the time of study initiation. Moreover, utilizing placebo control in a randomised double blind design enabled better characterization of the safety and efficacy of the profile of pazopanib. Placebo with best supportive care remained as the comparator arm as cytokines as the standard of care were challenged due to their underlying toxicities. The PFS in the pazopanib arm compared with placebo was significantly prolonged in the overall study population (9.2 months vs. 4.2 months, HR 0.46; p < 0.0001), in treatment naïve patients (11.1 months vs. 2.8 months, HR: 0.40, p < 0.001) and in cytokine-pretreated patients (7.4 months vs. 4.2 months; HR 0.54, p < 0.001). The response rate was 30% with pazopanib versus 3% in the placebo group and the median duration of response was 58.7 weeks. The final OS results were updated at the European Society of Medical Oncology meeting in 2010. A median OS of 22.9 vs. 20.5 months were noted in the pazopanib and placebo arms respectively (p=0.224). The lack of significant benefit was attributed to the early, high rate and prolonged duration of cross-over from placebo to pazopanib. In fact, more placebo than pazopanib patients received subsequent treatment (66% vs. 30% respectively) with 54% of patients on placebo crossing over to the active arm, some occurred as early as week 6 into therapy. (Rini & Al-Marrawi, 2011; Sternberg, 2010) The efficacy of pazopanib as first line therapy is comparable and is an alternative agent in patients who do not tolerate sunitinib. As yet, no head-to-head efficacy data are available to show superiority or non-inferiority between pazopanib and sunitinib and phase III trial (COMPARZ) is currently underway. (NCT00720941, 2011)

4.1.4 Bevacizumab

Bevacizumab is a humanized monoclonal antibody that uniquely targets the VEGF molecule and thus inhibiting this ligand with all of the receptors to which it binds. (Gommersall *et al*, 2004) A randomized phase II trial randomized 116 patients with metastatic clear-cell RCC to either placebo, low-dose (3 mg/kg given fortnightly) or high-dose bevacizumab (10 mg/kg given fortnightly). Accrual was halted when an interim analysis revealed a time to disease progression (TTP) benefit in the (high-dose) bevacizumab arm. A significant prolongation of TTP was observed in the high dose bevacizumab group (p<0.001; HR 2.55) compared to the placebo, and a smaller TTP benefit of borderline significance was reported for those receiving low-dose bevacizumab (p=0.053; HR 1.26). An objective partial response rate of 10.3% in the high-dose bevacizumab arm was noted. (Yang *et al*, 2003) Further data of bevacizumab as monotherapy was derived from a study comparing bevacizumab (10mg/kg; fortnightly) with placebo and bevacizumab with erlotinib (150mg bd), a small-molecule epidermal growth factor receptor (EGFR) inhibitor. Whilst the combination arm was well tolerated, it failed to demonstrate the superiority of this combination over bevacizumab alone. (Bukowski *et al*, 2007b) In both trials, the vast majority of patients treated with bevacizumab demonstrated some degree of tumour shrinkage, although in most instances the extent of tumour shrinkage did not meet the Response Evaluation Criteria in Solid Tumour (RECIST) criteria for PR. Interestingly the efficacy data from these two trials suggest the presence of clinical activity of bevacizumab monotherapy for metastatic RCC. (Elaraj *et al*, 2004) This is in clear contrast with other tumour types (non-small cell lung cancer, metastatic colorectal carcinoma, and metastatic breast carcinoma) where clinical benefit of single-agent bevacizumab without accompanying chemotherapy has been limited. (McDermott & George, 2010)

Two parallel large multicentre randomized international trials both examined the clinical efficacy of bevacizumab and IFN-α versus IFN-α alone, the previous standard of care for systemic treatment of patients with metastatic RCC. (Escudier *et al*, 2007c; Rini *et al*, 2008) Both trial (AVOREN, n=649; CALGB 90206 Intergroup Study, n=732), randomized treatment-naïve patients to IFN-α (9 × 10⁶ units thrice weekly) and bevacizumab (10 mg/kg fortnightly) or placebo and IFN-α. The only difference was that the AVOREN study was placebo-controlled and the CALBG 90206 Intergroup study was an open labelled trial. (McDermott & George, 2010)

In the AVOREN study, the ORR was higher in the bevacizumab arm (31.4% vs. 12,8%, p=0.0001) with 70% of this group of patients demonstrating tumour shrinkage compared to 39% of patients on the IFN- α and placebo arm. The median PFS after a median follow-up of 22 months demonstrated a better median survival in the bevacizumab arm (10.2 months vs. 5.5 months; *p* = 0.0001). The improvement in PFS was evident irrespective of age, tumour subtype (clear cell or mixed), baseline VEGF level, and creatinine clearance. When stratified according to the MSKCC criteria, significant PFS benefits are seen in the low- and intermediate-risk groups but not detected in the poor risk category. As the number of patients enrolled in this poor subgroup were small (<10% of the enrolled patient), it is difficult to undertake any meaningful interpretation. (Escudier *et al*, 2007c)

A subsequent unplanned retrospective analysis revealed that PFS benefits was similar in 39% (n=131) of bevacizumab patients who received either 6 X 10⁶ IU or 3 X 10⁶ IU instead of 9 X 10⁶ IU due to treatment related toxicity. The ORR for the reduced-dose group and full-dose group were 34% vs. 31% respectively and median duration of tumour response in turn was 13.6 months vs. 13.5 months respectively. This suggested that the dose of IFN-α could be reduced without compromising efficacy in patients who could not treatment related toxicities of IFN-α. (Melichar *et al*, 2008)

At the time of final OS analysis, only a trend towards OS was seen (23 months vs. 21.3 months, p = 0.1291). The effects of crossover to the bevacizumab arm, as well as the availability of second-line therapies where at least 35% received the TKIs (sunitinib and sorafenib) in both treatment arms, could well have compounded the results. An exploratory analysis showed that median OS was longer in patients receiving subsequent TKI therapy after bevacizumab plus IFN-α (n=113) compared with patients receiving TKIs after IFN plus placebo (n = 120) 38.6 months vs. 33.6 months respectively. (Escudier *et al*, 2007a)

In the Intergroup CALBG 90206, the ORR for active arm versus the control arm was 25.5% vs. 13.1% (p<0.0001) and the median PFS was in turn 8.4 months vs. 4.9 months (p<0.0001) respectively. (Rini *et al*, 2008) Only a trend in improved median OS was noted (18.3 months vs. 17.4 months, *p* = 0.097) and the trial did not achieve its primary end point, OS. The HR for progression was 0.71, which overlap with the AVOREN trial.

Stratification by MSKCC risk factors revealed the median PFS to be 11.1 months vs. 5.7 months in patients with absent risk factors (26%), 8.4 months vs. 5.3 months in patients with one or two risk factors (64%), and 3.3 months vs. 2.6 months in patients with three or more risk factors (10%), for the bevacizumab combination and INF-α monotherapy treatment groups, respectively. When stratified by the MKSCC risk factors, the median OS for bevacizumab / INF-α respectively was 32.5 months vs. 33.5 months for the favourable-risk group (26% of patients, p=0.524); 17.7 months vs. 16.1 months for the intermediate-risk group (64% of patients, p = 0.174) and lastly 6.6 months vs. 5.7 months for the poor risk group (p =0.25). (McDermott & George 2011, Rini *et al*, 2010)

Whilst no cross-over was allowed for the IFN-α monotherapy arm, 56% of study patients proceeded to at least one subsequent further systemic therapy in the form of a TKI. The patients who received second-line therapy were subsequently analysed and showed a median OS of 31.4 months vs. 26.8 months (p=0.079) in the bevacizumab/IFN-α and IFN-α monotherapy arms respectively. Amongst the patients who did not, the survival duration were 13.1 months vs. 9.1 months (p=0.059) respectively. (Rini *et al*, 2010)

Both trials were statistically robust and showed clear benefits in the median PFS arms with an overlapping HR and doubling of PFS when comparing the placebo/IFN-α arm with bevacizumab/IFN-α arm. (McDermott & George, 2010) The effects of crossover to the active bevacizumab arm in the AVOREN trial, as well as the permission of second-line therapies in both trials would account for the dilution of the actual overall survival benefits in both trials. (McDermott & George, 2010) Despite the lack of overall survival benefit and the notable toxicity of IFN-α with a large percentage of patients in the phase III trials undertaking dose reduction (40 – 60%), the combination of bevacizumab and IFN- α received Food and Drug Administration (FDA) approval for use as frontline of metastatic RCC.

4.2 mTOR Inhibitors

The mammalian target of rapamycin (mTOR) is a serine-threonine kinase that plays a crucial role in angiogenesis and regulation of cell cycle through a series of complex tightly regulated pathways. (Amato, 2011) mTOR activity is affected by a host of factors that influence cell functioning including nutrients (glucose, amino acid), energy depletion, as well as external signals such as cytokines, hormones, and growth factors. It also reacts to cellular stresses such as hypoxia, heat shock, oxidative stress, DNA damage and lastly a change in the microenvironment (pH or osmostic cell pressure). (Amato, 2011) The key pathway is via the phsophotidylinositol 3 kinase-protein kinase (P13K – AKT) pathway which is dysregulated in many cancers. (Amato, 2011; Beuvink *et al*, 2005) Activation of mTOR leads to phosphorylation of down-stream substrates (4E-binding protein-1 and protein S6 kinase) which in turn promotes mRNA translation, stimulation of protein synthesis and entry into the G_1 phase of cell cycle as illuastrated in figure 2. (Beuvink *et al*, 2005) Another important role of mTOR is the encoding and subsequent production of HIF-1α which drives angiogenesis, growth and survival of the cancer cells. The selective inhibition of this complex pathway by the mTOR inhibitors is achieved by binding to the intracellular protein FK506 binding protein 12 (FKBP-12) and causing inhibition of the kinase activity of the mTOR. (Amato, 2011) The two mTOR inhibitors, registered for the treatment of metastatic RCC are temsirolimus and everolimus.

4.2.1 Temsirolimus

The mTor inhibitor temsirolimus is similar to sirolimus (rapamycin) which has been used as an immunosuppressant in renal transplantation for many years. (Hudes *et al*, 2007) It affects cell division by inhibition of mTOR dependent protein translation, via binding to an intracellular protein (FK506 Binding Protein 12; FKBP12) resulting in a protein-drug complex. Temsirolimus is administered as a weekly intravenous infusion at 25mg. It is metabolised by CYP3A4 to active metabolite sirolimus and has a half-life of about 9 to 27 hours. (Hudes *et al*, 2007)

It was approved in 2007 by FDA as a first-line therapy in treatment-naïve metastatic RCC with poor prognostic features. Phase I and II trials of temsirolimus alone, or combined with IFN-α, found anti-tumour effects and stable disease in patients refractory to cytokine therapies. (Hidalgo *et al*, 2006; Raymond *et al*, 2004) In addition to that, another phase II trial on heavily pre-treated patients observed a median survival of 15 months. (Atkins *et al*, 2004) These encouraging results subsequently led to the development of an international multicentre phase III trial where 626 treatment-naïve patients with poor prognostic factors were randomized to temsirolimus (25 mg i.v. weekly), IFN-α (3×10^6 units, with an increase to 18×10^6 units s.c. thrice weekly) or the combination of temsirolimus (15 mg weekly) and IFN-α (6×10^6 thrice weekly). (Atkins *et al*, 2004) This was a pivotal trial that enrolled patients with poor prognostic factors only unlike previous studies with VEGF inhibitors which only recruited patients with good and intermediate risk features. The poor prognostic patients consisted of at least three or more of the 6 poor MSKCC prognostic factors. Another notable characteristic of recruitment is the enrolment of up to 20% of non-clear cell renal cell histological subtype. This is the only randomised study available so far for patients with the non-clear cell histology. (Atkins *et al*, 2004)

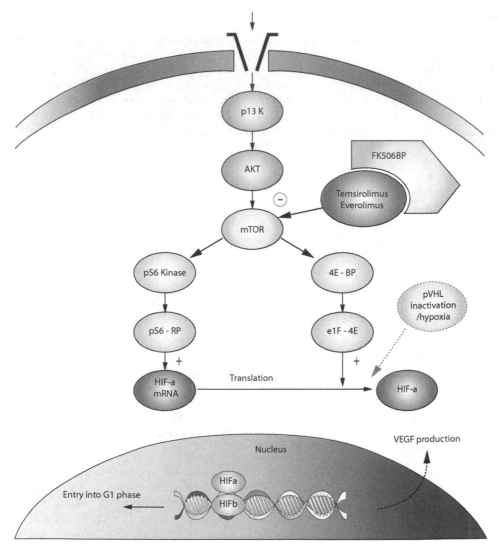

Fig. 2. External stimuli (growth factors)

Patients who received temsirolimus alone experienced a longer median OS (10.9 vs. 7.3 months; $p = 0.008$) and PFS (3.8 vs. 1.9 months; $p < 0.001$) compared with those who received INF-α alone. (Hudes *et al*, 2007) Patients in the combination therapy group had the most grade 3 or 4 adverse events leading to more dose reductions or delays. Their mean temsirolimus dose intensity was 10.9 mg per week vs. 23.1 mg per week for patients on temsirolimus alone. The median PFS in the temsirolimus, temsirolimus and IFN-α and IFN-α alone were 3.8, 3.7 and 1.9 months, respectively, and the median OS in turn was 10.9 months, 8.4 months and 7.3 months. (Hudes *et al*, 2007) Notably, older patients and patients with a higher serum LDH (> 1.5 fold the upper limit of normal) had better OS. (Hudes *et al*, 2007)

Clinicians are now faced with the challenge of treating patients who are refractory to VEGF targeted therapy as there is paucity of data in this area. The only published prospective randomised trial looking at this cohort of patients was RECORD-1 looking at everolimus vs. placebo. (Motzer et al, 2008) The few abstracts published on second line treatment with temsirolimus are all single institution case series confirming a modest activity in the second line setting with a median PFS of up to almost 4 months.

4.2.2 Everolimus

Everolimus is a derivative of rapamycin used in transplant medicine. Everolimus is an orally administered mTOR inhibitor with activity in patients with advanced clear-cell RCC who have failed VEGF-targeted therapies (sorafenib, sunitinib or both). (Motzer et al, 2008) Everolimus is converted to a main metabolite hydroxy everolimus is converted to a main metabolite hydroxy everolimus by the cytochrome 3A4 enzyme. The 30-hour half-life maintains a relative steady state achievable with the daily dosage regimen of 10mg/day. (Amato, 2011)

In RECORD-1, a double-blind placebo-controlled phase III trial, 410 patients with advanced clear-cell RCC which had progressed after sunitinib, sorafenib or both, were randomized in a 2:1 ratio to everolimus 10 mg once daily or placebo plus best supportive care. Regardless of age, gender, prognostic group, previous treatment with sorafenib, sunitinib or both, prolongation of PFS (4.9 vs. 1.9 months; $p< 0.0001$) was found with everolimus over placebo. (Motzer et al, 2008) However there was lack of difference for median OS (14.8 months vs. 14.4 months) as majority (80%) of patients in the placebo plus best supportive arm were allowed to cross over after the unbinding at the second interim analysis. This important landmark phase III trials proved the efficacy of mTOR inhibitors following VEGF therapy and as such received FDA registration for patients who have progressed following therapy with sunitinib and sorafenib. (Motzer et al, 2008)

5. New agents in clinical development

A number of second generation small molecule multi-targeted agents have been investigated in Phase II and III studies treating patients with metastatic RCC. (Fisher et al, 2011) These include axitinib and tivozanib which are in advanced clinical development, as well as dovitinib and others. (Fisher et al, 2011)

5.1 Axitinib

Axitinib is a potent oral agent that inhibits VEGFR-1, -2 and -3. It is rapidly absorbed with peak plasma concentration occurring 1 - 2 hours after administration on an empty stomach, terminal half-life of 3 - 5 hours, and bioavailability of 58%. (Pithavala et al, 2010) Dose-limiting toxicities seen in phase I studies were hypertension and mucositis, and in a phase II study, common adverse events also included diarrhoea and fatigue. ((Rixe et al, 2007b)

Axitinib has been investigated in a number of different cancers including cytokine-refractory metastatic RCC. A second line study in 52 patients using starting doses of axitinib 5 mg twice daily, resulted in two complete and 21 partial responses (ORR of 44.2%). The median response duration was 23 months and median overall survival was 29.9 months.

(Rixe *et al*, 2007b) Updated 5 year OS data from this study were presented in abstract form in 2011. (Motzer *et al*, 2011a) The 5 year survival rate was 20.6%. The ten patients surviving for more than five years had ORR 100% compared with 30% in <5 year survivors, took axitinib for longer (median 5.8 years vs. 0.67 years) and were fitter, with baseline ECOG PS of 0 in 80% of the longer term survivors compared with 53% in <5 year survivors. However they were all similar age, gender and risk factors. No unexpected new toxicities were seen with prolonged use of axitinib.

In a phase III second line study (AXIS), patients received axitinib at doses titrated up to 10mg BD or sorafenib 400mg BD. (Rini *et al*, 2011b) The 723 patients had progressive disease after one prior first line treatment (sunitinib, bevacizumab, temsirolimus or cytokines). The ORR was 19.4% for axitinib vs. 9.4% for sorafenib (p=0.0001) and significantly longer PFS (12.1 versus 6.5 months, p<0.0001) was seen in patients on the axitinib arm. Patients who had previously received cytokines were found to have significantly (p<0.0001) better PFS with axitinib (12.1 months) than sorafenib (6.5 months). This also occurred in those having prior sunitinib (4.8 vs. 3.4 months, p=0.0107). As part of the same trial, patient-reported kidney specific symptom and function assessments were secondary endpoints. (Cella *et al*, 2011) Outcomes according to validated tools were similar for both drugs during treatment, however as patients had a PFS with axitinib, this delayed worsening of the composite endpoint of cancer symptoms, progression or death compared with sorafenib.

5.2 Tivozanib

Tivozanib is an oral quinoline urea derivative small molecule TKI. It is a potent and selective inhibitor of VEGFR-1, -2 and -3 as well as inhibiting c-kit and PDGFR at higher concentrations. In 272 patients with advanced or metastatic RCC who had not received prior VEGF targeted therapy, tivozanib has shown promising efficacy and acceptable safety and tolerability in a phase II study reported in abstract form in 2011. (Nosov *et al*, 2011) All patients initially took tivozanib 1.5 mg daily for 16 weeks, and were then stratified according to response into stopping or continuing tivozanib, or if disease had stabilized, being randomised between tivozanib and placebo. Patients receiving placebo that developed progressive disease, or completed the double blind phase were allowed to restart tivozanib. Overall, 84% of patients demonstrated PR or SD by Week 16, ORR was 30%, disease control rate (DCR) was 85% and median PFS 11.7 months. Highest efficacy for tivozanib was in patients with clear-cell histology who had undergone a nephrectomy, who achieved an ORR of 36%, DCR of 88% and median PFS of 14.8 months. Commonest adverse effects included hypertension (45%) which was grade 3/4 in 12%, and dysphonia (22%). A low incidence of drug-related diarrhoea (12%), asthenia (10%), fatigue (8%), dyspnoea (6%), cough (5%), anorexia (5%), stomatitis (4%), hand-foot syndrome (4%) and proteinuria (3%) was reported. Overall median PFS, DCR and ORR were 11.7 months, 85% and 30%, respectively. Patients with clear-cell RCC who had undergone nephrectomy had PFS of 14.8 months and ORR of 36% with tivozanib. Phase III evaluation of tivozanib in nephrectomised patients with advanced clear cell RCC is on-going.

A phase Ib open-label study found tivozanib could be combined with temsirolimus at full dose/schedule in patients with advanced RCC (with clear cell component) who had failed up to one prior VEGF-targeted therapy. (Kabbinavar *et al*, 2011) Tivozanib was given orally daily for 3 weeks on, 1 week off (1 cycle) and IV temsirolimus was given once weekly. A standard 3+3 dose escalation design was used at four levels from 0.5 mg to 1.5 mg per day and 15 to 25 mg per week of tivozanib and temsirolimus, respectively. There were 28 patients (26 male) of median age 62 years and Karnofsky Performance Status from 100 to 80. Median duration of treatment was 21.1 weeks. Treatment-related adverse events seen in ≥10% of patients were: fatigue (20 all grades/4 grade 3), decreased appetite (14/0), stomatitis (13/2), thrombocytopenia (10/4), diarrhoea (16/2), nausea (13/1), constipation (10/1), and dypsnoea (10/1). There were no grade 4 events, and no dose limiting toxicities. The MTD for the combination of tivozanib and temsirolimus was 1.5 mg/day and 25 mg/week, respectively. PR was seen in 28%, SD in 64% and DCR (PR and SD>24weeks) of 48%. The combination of tivozanib with temsirolimus was well tolerated and showed encouraging clinical activity in patients with advanced RCC.

5.3 Dovitinib

Dovitinib is a potent oral inhibitor of angiogenic factors, including the fibroblast growth factor (FGFR) and VEGF receptors. The maximum tolerated dose of dovitinib is 500 mg daily on a 5 day on/ 2 day off dosing schedule in 28 day cycles. A phase II study of dovitinib in clear-cell metastatic RCC patients previously treated with a VEGFR inhibitor and/or mTOR inhibitor was reported in 2011. (Angevin et al, 2011) (NCT1217931, 2011) In 51 patients best overall responses were PR in 8%, and SD ≥ 4 months in 37%. Median PFS and OS were 6.1 and 16 months respectively. Fifty nine patients median age 60 years and ECOG PS 0 or 1 were evaluable for safety. The most common adverse events were nausea (73%; grade 3 : 9%), diarrhoea (64%; grade 3: 9%), vomiting (56%; grade 3: 5%), decreased appetite (48%; grade 3: 7%), asthenia (36%; grade 3: 12%), and fatigue (36%; grade 3: 10%). An on-going phase 3 trial is comparing dovitinib with sorafenib in patients who have had one previous VEFR- and mTOR-targeted therapy.

6. Combination therapy in metastatic RCC

Despite being in the era where increasing numbers of VEGF and mTOR inhibitors are at the clinician's disposal, their optimal use in patients with metastatic RCC has not been fully ascertained. Undeniably these agents have conferred significant survival benefits compared to historical series, however most patients eventually develop resistance and relapse after 6 months to 3 years of therapy. (Jonasch et al, 2011) This underscores the strong need to develop novel treatment strategies to achieve better clinical outcomes. This could be achieved by the use of combinations of anti-angiogenic agents or with mTOR inhibitors, chemotherapy or immunotherapy. Sequencing treatment with different anti-VEGF agents as well as with mTOR inhibitors and immunotherapeutic agents could be another solution which will be discussed subsequently. (Jonasch et al, 2011)

The concept of combining two (or more) targeted agents is biologically plausible as each agent may affect different targets simultaneously potentially resulting in additive or synergistic effects and achieving better clinical outcomes. (Hutson, 2011) Using a combination of drugs which target the same pathway (e.g. VEGF) at two or more different levels, has been termed "vertical blockade". In contrast, "horizontal blockade" occurs when the different pathways are blocked simultaneously by one or multiple agents in combination. (Hutson, 2011) It should be noted that combination therapy is often undertaken at the cost of increased toxicities as evidenced by some of the phase I trials where sunitinib was combined with temsirolimus, bevacizumab or everolimus. (Feldman *et al*, 2009; Rini *et al*, 2009)

6.1 VEGF-ligands or receptor inhibitors / mTOR plus immunotherapy combination

This is best illustrated by the two single arm phase II studies combining sorafenib with standard dose of IFN-α which conferred higher ORR (approximately 30%) and longer PFS (7 – 12 months) when compared with phase III data of sorafenib monotherapy. (Gollob *et al*, 2007; Ryan *et al*, 2007) However, in a randomised phase II study comparing sorafenib monotherapy with sorafenib /low-dose IFN-α combination, a very similar response rates and longer PFS were demonstrated equally in both arms. Interpretation of these phase II data required caution given the small number of patients recruited in comparison with the more robust phase III sorafenib vs. placebo trial. (Jonasch *et al*, 2010)

The AVOREN and CALBG 90206 trial demonstrated that the bevacizumab / IFN-α combination had achieved better clinical outcome when compared with IFN-α alone. (Escudier *et al*, 2007c; Rini *et al*, 2008) Unfortunately, the lack of bevacizumab as a control arm did not help address the question as to whether the addition of IFN-α to bevacizumab was able to achieve a more superior outcome compared to bevacizumab alone. A small randomised phase II study comparing erlotinib and bevacizumab with bevacizumab alone reported a non-statistical small PFS difference of 0.5 months (9.0 months vs. 8.5 months; p=0.58). Although this is small benefit may be clinically irrelevant, this trial provided insight into the clinical efficacy of bevacizumab as monotherapy. (Bukowski *et al*, 2007b)

A randomised three-arm trial was undertaken comparing temsirolimus (25mg) / bevacizumab (10mg/kg) combination with sunitinib alone and with IFN-α (9X 10^6 IU thrice weekly) / bevacizumab (10mg/kg) combination in patients with advanced RCC (TORAVA). A total of 171 treatment naïve patients were recruited in a 2:1:1 ratio and was equally distributed into the three arms. The reported median FPS was similar (8.2 months) for both temsirolimus (25mg) / bevacizumab (10mg/kg) (experimental) arm and sunitinib (comparator) arm. The duration for bevacizumab / IFN-α was however up to 16.8 months. The patients in the experimental arm experienced a high number of discontinuation from treatment for reasons other than progression (51%) when compared to the sunitinib arm (12%) and bevacizumab / IFN-α arm (38%). (Negrier *et al*, 2011) Furthermore up to 77% in the experimental arm experienced a grade 3 or higher toxicity. The trial again highlighted the lack of survival benefit due to a toxic combination that is poorly tolerated and the investigators appropriately commented that this combination would not be recommended for first-line treatment in patients with metastatic RCC. (Negrier *et al*, 2011) Similarly, when temsirolimus was prescribed in conjunction with IFN-α in a phase III trial for patients with poor prognostic advanced RCC, the overall survival benefit was worst in the tmesirolimus / IFN-α arm compared to temsirolimus monotherapy arm. Once again, toxicity prevailed in the combination arm and therefore the temsirolimus / IFN-α combination is not recommended as standard practice yet outside a clinical trial for treatment of advanced RCC. (Hudes *et al*, 2007)

6.2 VEGF-ligands or receptor inhibitors / mTOR combination

Sorafenib like sunitinib was also investigated in combination with bevacizumab in two phase I studies. In one the study of patients with metastatic RCC, the median time to progression was 11.2 months and the partial response rate was 46%. (Sosman *et al*, 2008) In the second trial which included 39 patients with solid tumours (with 3 patients with RCC), PR or disease stabilisation of ≥4 months was observed in 59% of the assessable patients, and a PR was achieved in one of the 3 patients with RCC. (Azad *et al*, 2008) The combination arm required dose reduction of both agents and resulted in a considerably lower maximum tolerated dose compared to maximal tolerated dose of the single agent. It is postulated that bevacizumab most likely enhanced the side-effects of sorafenib such as hypertension and hand-foot syndrome. (Azad *et al*, 2008; Sosman *et al*, 2008) When sunitinib was combined with bevacizumab, a high incidence of haematological and vascular toxicities (including microangiopathic haemolytic anaemia) and hypertension were observed. (Feldman *et al*, 2009) Again bevacizumab was likely responsible for the exaggeration of the side-effects of sunitinib which would have been otherwise manageable.

Finally, a phase II trial examining the feasibility, tolerability, and efficacy of multiple combinations of currently available therapies are being tested in the Eastern Cooperative Oncology BeST trial. The four arms are bevacizumab (10mg/kg), bevacizumab (5mg/kg) /temsirolimus (25 mg), bevacizumab (5mg/kg) and sorafenib (200mg twice daily)/ temsirolimus (25mg). (NCT00378703, 2006) This trial will provide insight into the efficacy of bevacizumab monotherapy and the clinical tolerability and efficacy of lowered dose of bevacizumab and sorafenib dose in conjunction with temsirolimus where previously significant toxicities was noted on the earlier phase II studies.

7. Sequencing therapy in metastatic RCC

Sequencing the systemic treatment of metastatic RCC has several potential benefits. Sequential treatment is less toxic than combination therapy and thus allowing patients to be exposed to a more optimal dose (and subsequent higher total accumulative dose) resulting in improved clinical efficacy. It also creates a treatment continuum with the goal of maintain responding patients on treatment for as long as clinically feasible. Lastly, targeting the different pathway at different point in time theoretically offers the benefit of overcoming the resistance to the individual agents. (Bellmunt, 2009)

7.1 Antiangiogenic therapy after immunotherapy

A phase II study published in 2003 examined the role of bevacizumab (10mg/kg) post progression on immunotherapy demonstrated a time-to-progression (TTP) of 4.8 months. (Yang *et al*, 2003) Two phase II trials mentioned earlier on similarly examined the efficacy of sunitinib post immunotherapy revealed promising survival benefits which subsequent led to the landmark phase III trial comparing sunitinib with IFN-α. (Motzer *et al*, 2006; Motzer *et al*, 2007b) The phase III sorafenib trial vs. placebo (TARGET) also recruited patient who had cytokine therapy and observed a doubling of PFS benefit of 2.8 to 5.6 months. (Escudier *et al*, 2007b) More recently, in a phase II trial examined the use of axitinib post cytokine therapy demonstrated a TTP of 15.7 months. (Rixe *et al*, 2007b) Whilst it is possible to compare the results of each individual phase II trials and rank them to their clinical benefit, a proper conducted phase III is essential to determine the best anti-angiogenic agent to use post-cytokine therapy.

7.2 mTOR blockade after anti-angiogenic therapy

The best illustrating example is the RECORD-1 trial which investigated the benefits of everolimus vs. placebo with best supportive care post progression on sunitinib, sorafenib or both. Of note 71% of patients had received prior sunitinib whilst 55% sorafenib. Patient that received everolimus achieved an additional of 3-month of PFS benefit regardless whether they received sunitinib or sorafenib. No overall survival benefits were noted due to large numbers of patients from placebo crossing over to everolimus arm (80%). (Motzer *et al*, 2008)

An on-going trial (RECORD-3) will randomly assign patients between either everolimus or sunitinib where at first sign of progression, patients would cross over to sunitinib if they were on everolimus and vice versa. The primary end point of this trial is to assess whether PFS after first-line treatment for patients who received everolimus will be non-inferior to patients who receive sunitinib after first-line therapy. (NCT00720941, 2011)

7.3 Serial anti-angiogenic agents

Axitinib has been investigated in both phase II and III second-line trials in advanced RCC. The results of the survival benefits have so far been encouraging especially in the phase III trial comparing with sorafenib. (Dutcher *et al*, 2008) Further trials will be undertaken clarify the outcomes. Specifically, in the Sequential Two-agent Assessment in Renal Cell Carcinoma Therapy (START)   two hundred and forty treatment-naïve patients with clear-cell component mRCC will be randomly assigned to receive bevacizumab, pazopanib, or everolimus. On first progression or intolerance to therapy, patients will be randomly assigned to one of two of the remaining agents. The primary end point is the detection of the longest combination of the TTP. (NCT1217931, 2011)

A retrospective study described the efficacy of sorafenib or sunitinib in the first-line setting in 49 patients with metastatic RCC as well as the subsequent derived benefit after switching to the alternative agent on progression. (Dudek *et al*, 2009) The TTP for patients treated with sunitinib or sorafenib (after initial treatment) was 5.8 and 5.1 months respectively (p=0.299). However, sequential treatment with sorafenib followed by suntinib resulted in a trend toward improved TTP (p = 0.115). Similarly, the median OS was better for patients who received sorafenib followed by sunitinib (23.5 months) than if they received sunitinib after sorafenib (10.4 months; p=0.061). This analysis of median survival did not include patients who did not need to cross over. This retrospective study suggested the benefit of utilizing sorafenib as first line may improve duration of disease control if a subsequent agent is used and certainly warrants further investigation. (Dudek *et al*, 2009) The SWITCH trial is a prospective phase III trial which will randomize patients to upfront sunitinib and switching to sorafenib on progression versus switching from sorafenib to sunitinib on progression. The primary end point is the PFS and hopefully this trial will show further insight into which anti-VEGF treatment sequence will confer better clinical outcome in patients with metastatic RCC. (NCT00732914, 2010)

8. Systemic treatment for non-clear-cell RCC

The treatment for advanced non-clear-cell RCC is less well established than the clear-cell variants and the evidence to guide treatment is limited. Majority of the data is derived from expanded access trials, retrospective series, and subset analyses of major trials. (Tazi el *et al*, 2011) The phase III sunitinib trial virtually excluded all patients with non-clear-cell RCC. In spite of this, sunitinib was made available to all patients with clear-cell and non-clear-cell histology in a subsequent multi-centre, international, non-randomized expanded access compassionate trial. (Motzer *et al*, 2007a) A total of 588 patients with non-clear cell histology (not characterized further) received sunitinib and of that, 437 evaluable patients demonstrated an ORR of 11% (n=48) with 46 partial responders and 2 complete responders) and 57% had stable disease (n=250) for at least 3 months. (Gore *et al*, 2009) The median OS was 13.4 months. The ORR of 11% was lower than the original phase III study and was thought to due to the non-mandatory reporting of the disease response and the reliance of local practice to detect any change in the disease burden. The authors of the study therefore concluded that sunitinib is active in subjects with non-clear- cell histology amongst other subsets of patients (poor performance status, brain metastasis and patients of ≥ 65 years old) which were not enrolled in the original trial. (Motzer *et al*, 2002)

One of the largest retrospective series for papillary RCC was a multi-centre review consisting of 41 patients treated with either sunitinib or sorafenib. The response rate was disappointing with an ORR of 5% for all comers but was higher at 17% for sunitinib. The PFS was statistically longer for patients treated with sunitinib (11.9 months) when compared with sorafenib (5.1 months; p <0.001). The PFS for sunitinib was comparable to the phase III clear-cell trial suggesting clinical efficacy in sunitinib for papillary carcinoma. (Choueiri *et al*, 2008) In contrast, two small phase II studies showed little-to-no clinical response and disease stability being the best clinical response for only a short duration of 1.4 to 3 months. (Plimack *et al*, 2010; Ravaud *et al*, 2009)

The efficacy of sorafenib in the treatment of advanced papillary variant is best demonstrated in the Advance Renal cell Carcinoma Sorafenib Expanded Access Program in North America. One hundred and fifty eight patients with papillary RCC were enrolled. Of the 107 patients with papillary RCC that could be evaluated, 84% (n=90) demonstrated 3 PR and 87 SD for a duration of 8 weeks or more. Sixteen percent (n=17) of patients showed early progression of disease. (Beck *et al*, 2008)

The phase III international, multicentre trial, comparing temsirolimus, IFN-α, or combination of both, is the first trial that prospectively recruited all histological subtypes of RCC. Twenty percent (n=120) were classified as non-clear cell RCC without further subclassification at the outset due to the absence central pathology review. (Hudes *et al*, 2007) An improvement in the median OS and median PFS were seen in the temsirolmus monotherapy arm compared to the combination temsirolimus/IFN-α or IFN-α monotherapy arm. Subsequent exploratory subset analyses based on tumour histology determined that 55 patients that had papillary RCC also demonstrated an OS and PFS benefit when treated with temsirolimus. (Schmidt *et al*, 2001) The OS and PFS for temsirolimus vs. IFN-α were 11.6 months vs. 4.3 months and 7.0 months vs. 1.8 months respectively. These results led to the subsequent FDA approval of temsirollimus as treatment for non-clear-cell histology in advanced RCC. Everolimus has demonstrated efficacy in the pivotal trial for patients with clear-cell RCC, post progression on sunitinib, sorafenib or both in the RECORD-1 trial. (Motzer *et al*, 2008) This has prompted the development of an open-label, single arm, multi-centre phase II examining the efficacy of everolimus as first-line systemic therapy for patients with advanced papillary RCC. (Amato,

2011) Central confirmation of histology and subclassification into type I and II will be undertaken. This trial which is still recruiting will hopefully show further insight into the treatment of papillary RCC which thus far has been disappointing.

Erlotinib was examined in a phase II study in treatment naïve patients with locally advanced or metastatic papillary RCC. (Gordon *et al*, 2009) Of the 52 registered patients, 45 were evaluable. The ORR was 11% (n=5) and the DCR was 64% with five partial responders and 24 patients with stable disease. The median OS time was 27 months with a 29% probability of freedom from treatment failure at 6 months. The presence of EGFR receptors scores and staining intensity determined by immunohistochemistry showed no correlation with TTP or OS. The estimated median survival was estimated to be 27 months. (Gordon *et al*, 2009) Combination of erlotinib with bevacizumab is currently underway designed to further evaluate the efficacy of erlotinib. (2010)

As with papillary variant of RCC, the chromophobe variant has also been excluded from many of the initial targeted therapy trials. Not surprisingly the data is even more limited. Furthermore, with the low incidence of 4% and the low likelihood of chromophobe to metastasize, any attempts to recruit patients of this type into a clinical trial is a difficult process. In the sorafenib access program described earlier, an overall DCR of 90% was noted with 5% (n=1) demonstrating partial response and 85% (n=17) of the patients experiencing disease stability for at least 2 months. (Stadler *et al*, 2010) The chromophobe variant were also included in the phase III temsirolimus versus IFN-α trial but the subgroup analysis only focused on papillary variant and the data for chromophobe was therefore not published. Nevertheless the PFS and OS were prolonged in the non-clear cell subgroup, therefore hinting some weak evidence of efficacy in this group of tumour. (Tazi el *et al*)

The strongest treatment evidence for treatment of the rare collecting duct renal cell carcinoma stemmed from a phase II multi-centre trial of 23 treatment-naïve patients who received cisplatin or carboplatin if inadequate renal function with gemcitabine. This variant is very aggressive and patient often presents with more advanced stage and succumbed earlier. This combination was selected based on some similarities in the histological features comparing with transitional cell carcinoma of the urinary bladder. In the trial, there was an observed ORR of 26%. The median PFS and OS were 7.1 months and 10.5 months. (Oudard *et al*, 2007a) To date, there is very little data to support the use of anti-VEGF therapies in this very bad prognostic cancer.

9. Side effects of targeted therapies used in renal cell carcinoma

The clinical benefit of newer targeted agents in metastatic RCC over previous conventional treatment has been shown in Sections 1 to 5 in this chapter. However as with any new treatment, sideeffects must be carefully measured and evaluated against older treatments and supportive or pharmacologic interventions developed for their prevention or control. (di Lorenzo *et al*, 2011) This is essential when considering patients' quality of life (see Section 11) and should allow patients to stay on beneficial treatment for as long as possible. (Bellmunt, 2007) Safety data from clinical trials and post-marketing surveillance have identified that many of the targeted therapies have toxicities that are different from those usually seen with conventional anticancer drugs. (di Lorenzo *et al*, 2011; Ravaud, 2011)

These angiogenesis inhibitors directly or indirectly target the VEGF pathway, and their individual mechanisms are pointers to their toxicities. (Schmidinger & Bellmunt, 2011) They share several adverse effects in common, including hypertension, fatigue, gastrointestinal, skin, and bone marrow effects. The mTOR inhibitors can cause metabolic alterations, immunosuppression and interstitial pneumonitis, whereas hypothyroidism is seen in patients taking sunitinib, potentially sorafenib and pazopanib. (di Lorenzo et al, 2011) Suggestions for management are shown below. The importance of patient education with respect to self-management strategies has been emphasized. (Ravaud, 2011)

9.1 Hypertension

Hypertension is a well recognised class side effect commonly observed in cancer patients treated with angiogenesis inhibitors that target the VEGF pathway, but not with mTOR inhibitors. (Izzedine et al 2009, diLorenzo 2011) Hypertension is reported with axitinib, bevacizumab, sorafenib, sunitinib and pazopanib. (Escudier et al, 2007b; Motzer et al, 2007a; Rini et al, 2011a; Rixe et al, 2007a; Sternberg et al, 2010) Hypertension has occurred whether or not the patient has a history of high blood pressure, however incidence may be higher in patients with pre-existing cardiovascular disease. Reversible posterior leukoencephalopathy syndrome is a rare association with hypertension seen with sunitinib and sorafenib where patients in addition experienced seizures and impaired vision thought to be attributed to capillary leakage and vasogenic oedema of the brain. This is reversible with cessation of the implicated agent. (Kapiteijn et al, 2007) Hypertension is an independent risk factor for the onset of cardio- and renovascular disease. In patients with metastatic disease, the goal of optimizing blood pressure is to allow continuous and safe administration of the anti-VEGF agents. (Izzedine et al, 2009; Keefe et al, 2011) Blood pressure monitoring (either daily or multiple times per week) is recommended and the use of antihypertensive medication may be required to avoid potential cardiovascular complications. Algorithms for hypertension management have been developed, (di Lorenzo et al, 2011) and treatment should be individualised to the patient. (Izzedine et al, 2009) The best anti-hypertensive agents is yet to be determined, however an angiotensin-converting enzyme (ACE) inhibitors is a logical choice if bevacizumab is the underlying cause as they may improve the associated proteinuria. (Keefe et al, 2011) Angiotensin II inhibitors, diuretics, hydropyridine calcium channel blockers (CCBs), and β-blockers are also possible anti-hypertensive agents. In patients on anti-hypertensive medications at baseline, an increase in the dose of pre-existing antihypertensive medications may be required. Temporary suspension of therapy may be required to allow for better control of the hypertension. In some cases, severe hypertension with life-threatening consequences (e.g. malignant hypertension, transient or permanent neurologic deficit, hypertensive crisis) has led to permanent discontinuation. (Keefe et al, 2011) The relationship between hypertension and anti-tumour effect is postulated with several of the drugs used for renal cell cancer and this will be addressed in Section 10.

9.2 Fatigue

Fatigue is the commonest of the constitutional side effects seen with the targeted agents used in metastatic RCC, but is less common than with cytokine treatment. (Adams & Leggas, 2007; di Lorenzo et al, 2011; Hutson, 2011; Motzer et al, 2007a) The incidence of fatigue in Phase III studies ranged from 14% to 51% for all grades, up to 11% for grade 3–4.

(di Lorenzo *et al*, 2011) Patients with cancer-related fatigue experience a chronic feeling of tiredness or lack of energy that is not relieved by rest. Fatigue can be caused by the targeted therapy and/or aggravated by other factors, such as anaemia, anxiety, hypothyrodism or depression, nutritional status, side effects of other medications or even organ dysfunction. (di Lorenzo *et al*, 2011; Ravaud, 2009) Patients may find it useful to record a daily fatigue diary to see when their energy levels are highest during the day in order to allow themselves time and energy for activities they enjoy. Evidence-based pharmacological interventions remain scarce, but monitoring and treating patients for any aggravating factors may help. If grade 3–4 fatigue persist, it may be necessary to dose reduce or stop treatment. (di Lorenzo *et al*, 2011; Ravaud, 2009)

9.3 Gastrointestinal side effects

Gastrointestinal toxicities are common to most of the targeted therapies for RCC but rarely lead to dose interruptions. (di Lorenzo *et al*, 2011) These include diarrhoea, nausea and to a lesser degree vomiting. Standard protocols used in prevention and treatment of these toxicities in patients having cytotoxic chemotherapy are suitable for use in this setting. Supportive medications will include loperamide (up to 16mg per day) for diarrhoea; dopamine antagonists such as metoclopramide or where necessary 5HT3 receptor antagonists for nausea and vomiting. (di Lorenzo *et al*, 2011)(di Lorenzo 2011)   Oral mucositis is also reported with the mTOR inhibitors everolimus and temsirolimus, and the tyrosine kinase receptor inhibitors. Evidence-based guidelines advise good oral hygiene, local anaesthetic mouthwashes or systemic analgesics if required for mouth pain, and avoidance of alcohol based mouthwashes. (see www.mascc.org)

9.4 Dermatological side effects

Various dermatological side effects can be seen with all of the agents used in metastatic RCC. Prevention and management is important to maintain patients' health-related quality of life as well as treatment dose intensity. (Lacouture *et al*, 2011) Toxicities seen include papulopustular (acneiform) rash, hair changes (including alopecia, colour changes), dermatitis enhancement, pruritus, xerosis, skin fissures, paronychia and hand-foot skin reactions (HFSR). (di Lorenzo *et al*, 2011; Lacouture *et al*, 2011) HFSR appears as plaques or blisters with painful tingling or burning sensations in the soles of the feet or palms of the hands, and these effects are particularly common with sorafenib and sunitinib. (di Lorenzo) Avoiding tight shoes, and using moisturiser, emollient creams and topical treatment containing urea or salicyclic acid is suggested. (di Lorenzo *et al*, 2011; Ravaud, 2009) Evidence-based treatment guidelines for managing skin toxicities have recently been published by the MASCC Skin Toxicity Study Group (Lacouture *et al*, 2011) Topical hydrocortisone cream (1 %) and oral antibiotics (doxycycline or minocycline) are the mainstay of prevention of papulopustolar rash or if they are painful. (Lacouture *et al*; Ravaud, 2009)

9.5 Other reported adverse effects

Clinical hypothyroidism defined as a decrease in free thyroxine index with elevated thyroid stimulating hormone levels has been reported in patients taking sunitinib, pazopanib and sorafenib (the latter specifically in Japanese subjects). (di Lorenzo *et al*, 2011) Screening pretreatment and on days 1 and 28 each cycle, and use of thyroxine is advised. (di Lorenzo *et al*, 2011)

Heart failure is seen with a number of targeted agents including sunitinib, bevacizumab and sorafenib. (Jarkowski *et al*, 2011) Patients, especially those with pre-existing cardiovascular disease, should be closely monitored especially if they have cardiac risk factors. (Ravaud, 2011) If heart failure occurs it should be managed according to standard protocols, and the offending agent ceased. (Jarkowski *et al*, 2011) Myocardial ischaemia or infarction was significantly more frequent in patients taking sorafenib group (3%) than placebo.

Severe and fatal hepatotoxicity (boxed warning) and grade 3 or 4 proteinuria have occurred with pazopanib treatment which necessitates routine monitoring of liver function tests, and urinalyses. (Ravaud, 2011)

Venous and arterial thromboses have been reported in patients on bevacizumab. (Escudier *et al*, 2007c; Rini *et al*, 2008) Both sunitinib and sorafenib are also associated with thromboembolic events although the rates are lower to bevacizumab. (Keefe *et al*, 2011) The role of therapeutic anticoagulation for venous thrombosis and aspirin for arterial thrombosis are currently being undertaken given the increased use of the anti-VEGF agents not only in metastatic RCC but in other advance cancers such as non-small cell lung cancer and colorectal carcinoma. (Keefe *et al*, 2011) Pazopanib has also been associated with arterial thrombotic events including myocardial infarction or ischaemia, cerebrovascular accidents and transient ischaemic attacks. Incidence was 3% of patients on pazopanib compared with none in patients taking placebo. (Sternberg *et al*, 2010) The incidence of haemorrhagic events (all grades) in the pazopanib arm was 13% compared with 5% with placebo. (Sternberg *et al*, 2010)

Other agent-specific side effects include adrenal insufficiency, especially in the setting of increased physical stressors with sunitinib; (Desai *et al*, 2007) hyperglycaemia, hyperlipidaemia and acute infusion reactions with temsirolimus (Hudes *et al*, 2007); and non-infectious pneumonitis in patients receiving everolimus, or temsirolimus. (Ravaud, 2011) Patients with pneumonitis may exhibit few if any symptoms and the diagnosis is radiological. Monitoring is advisable although pneumonitis resolves spontaneously when the mTOR inhibitor is ceased and rarely requires use of corticosteroids. (Hudes *et al*, 2007)

Lastly, thrombotic microangiopathy has been reported in association with suntinib, sorafenib, and bevacizumab, either as combined or as single agents. The manifestations included thrombocytopenia, haemolytic anaemia with schistocytosis, and renal dysfunction. (Kapiteijn *et al*, 2007; Patel *et al*, 2008) The treatment of this condition would involve the cessation of the implicated agent and plasma exchange. (Frangie *et al*, 2007)

10. Hypertension as biomarker of efficacy of sunitinib

Data from the two second-line phase II trials, one first-line phase III trial, and an expanded access study of sunitinib were retrospectively analysed to determine whether there was a relationship between hypertension and anti-tumour effect. (Rini *et al*, 2011a) Hypertension in this context was defined by either maximum or mean systolic blood pressure (SBP) of ≥140 mmHg or diastolic blood pressure (DBP) of ≥ 90 mmHg, measured on days 1 and 28 of each 6-week treatment cycle at any time during the study after the first dose of sunitinib. (Rini *et al*, 2011a) The ORR was 54.8% in hypertensive patients vs. 8.7% in patients without a maximum SBP of at least 140 mmHg. Median PFS was 12.5 months vs. 2.5 months, and median OS was 30.9 months vs. 7.2 months in the same two cohorts respectively. (Rini *et al*, 2011a) Overall, a better clinical outcome was demonstrated in patients who experienced hypertension and indeed a direct correlation between SBP and DBP and clinical outcome was observed. To determine whether or not antihypertensive medications reduced the anti-tumour efficacy of sunitinib, clinical outcomes were compared in patients using medications with those that were not at baseline, after cycle 1 and cycle 2. No statistical differences were noted in the ORR or the PFS between the two cohorts regardless of the presence of anti-hypertensive treatments at baseline. The median PFS in the treated and not on antihypertensive were 11.3 months and 10.6 months respectively (p=0.20). There was however a significant difference in median OS of more than 10 months with patients on anti-hypertensive medications demonstrating a 31.8 month survival vs. 21.4 months for patients not taking anti-hypertensive agents (p <0.001). The results of median PFS and median OS measured in patients with or without hypertension at the end of cycle 1 and 2 mirrored those obtained at baseline. (Rini *et al*, 2011a) To illustrate, median PFS measured at the end of cycle 1 for patients with and without anti-hypertensive agents were 13.4 months vs. 10.8 months respectively (p=0.31) and at the end of cycle 2, the median PFS were 13.6 months vs. 10.8 months respectively (p=0.15). (Rini *et al*, 2011a)The overall survival benefit at the end of cycle 1 for patients on anti-hypertensive and not on anti-hypertensive were 30.1 months vs. 23.3 months (p=0.155) and for cycle 2 was 31.1 months vs. 23.0 months (p=0.013) respectively. When analysed according to the prognostic factors (ECOG performance status, time from diagnosis to treatment, LDH, platelet count, corrected calcium), treatment induced hypertension remained a statistically significant predictor of survival benefit (p<0.001). (Rini *et al*, 2011a) In spite of these results supporting the hypothesis that hypertension may be a viable biomarker of anti-tumour efficacy, the development of hypertension during sunitinib treatment was neither necessary nor sufficient for clinical benefit in all patients.(Rini *et al*, 2011a)

11. Drug interactions

The targeted agents are predominantly metabolized by the hepatic cytochrome P450 enzyme CYP3A4 which raises the possibility of drug- drug interactions with concomitant medications that are strong inducers or inhibitors of CYP3A4 (Table 1). (Adams & Leggas, 2007; di Lorenzo *et al*, 2011; Kollmannsberger *et al*, 2007b) For example, the CYP3A4 inhibitors that would potentially increase toxicity of targeted agents include antiretroviral agents such as ritonavir, indinavir and nelfinavir, and antibiotics/antifungals such as clarithromycin, ketoconazole, fluconazole, itraconazole and voriconazole. Potent CYP3A4 inducers that decrease therapeutic efficacy of the targeted agents would include antiepileptic medications such as phenytoin and carbamazepine; antibiotics such as rifampicin and rifabutin. (Kollmannsberger *et al*, 2007a) If the interacting concomittant agent cannot be stopped, doses of the targeted agents may need upward or downward adjustment. It is not only drug-to-drug interactions that are of concern, as many patients take supplements or complementary and alternative medicines (CAM) which they may not mention to their treating physicians. (Lees & Chan, 2011) *Hypericum perforatum*, commonly

Targeted agent	Possible clinical effect	Recommended management
sunitinib		
carbamazepine phenytoin primidone	Decreased blood levels of sunitinib, potential for reduced effect	Avoid concurrent use, choose a non-interacting anti-epileptic agent or consider increasing sunitinib dose; monitor closely for effect and tolerability
St John's Wort	Decreased blood levels of sunitinib, potential for reduced effect	Avoid concurrent use
sorafenib		
carbamazepine phenytoin primidone	Decreased blood levels of sunitinib, potential for reduced effect	Avoid concurrent use, choose a non-interacting anti-epileptic agent or consider increasing sorafenib dose; monitor closely for effect and tolerability
warfarin	Increased INR, bleeding	Monitor patient's INR closely
everolimus		
ketoconazole itraconazole fluconazole voriconazole	Increased blood levels of everolimus; potential for toxicity	Avoid concurrent use or consider reducing everolimus dose; monitor closely for effect and tolerability
phenytoin	Decreased blood levels of everolimus, potential for reduced effect	
St John's Wort	Decreased blood levels of everolimus, potential for reduced effect	Avoid concurrent use

Table 1. Selected examples of drug interactions with some targeted agents

known as St John's Wort is a herbal preparation cancer patients may well be taking for its supposed antidepressant benefits. As it is a CYP3A4 enzyme inducer if taken with sunitinib, sorafenib or everolimus, for example, their effects may be decreased. Grapefruit juice is known to be a CYP3A4 enzyme inhibitor and as such may lead to unexpected toxicity if taken with sunitinib. (Kollmannsberger *et al*, 2007a) A comprehensive full medication history incuding prescribed, self-prescribed over the counter and CAM should be taken when any patient is about to start treatment. (di Lorenzo *et al*, 2011; Lees & Chan, 2011) Drug interaction databases should be utilised, since more reports of interactions may appear as experience with these newer therapies increases.

12. Quality of life in patients with renal cell carcinoma receiving targeted therapies

Health-related quality of life (QoL) has been assessed in a number of studies of patients taking newer targeted therapies for RCC (or kidney cancer). Questionnaires used have included the Functional Assessment of Cancer Therapy-General (FACT-G), the FACT-Kidney Symptom Index-15 item (FKSI-15), the FACT-Kidney Symptom Index-Disease related Symptoms (FKSI-DRS), the European Organisation for Research and Treatment of Cancer Quality of Life Questionnaire (EORTC QLQ-C30 and the Euro QOL 5D (Index and Visual Analogue Scale) utility score (EQ-5D) Index.

Sunitinib has shown improvement over IFN-α with clinically meaningful differences both in kidney cancer related symptoms and overall QoL. (Motzer *et al*, 2007a) Sorafenib when compared with placebo, showed no difference in QoL based on the FACT-G or FKSI-15 mean scores in a sub-analysis of the TARGET trial. However certain symptoms such as fevers, ability to enjoy life, dyspnoea and cough as well as concerns for well being were reported less in the patients on sorafenib. (Bukowski *et al*, 2007a) Quality of life was assessed as a secondary end point in the pazopanib vs. placebo phase III trial (EORTC-QLQ-C30 Version 3) and EQ-5D Index. Patients on pazopanib did not have a clinically different QoL compared with placebo, despite the toxicities that may be expected with pazopanib. (Sternberg *et al*, 2010)

More recently, patient-reported kidney-specific symptom and function assessments as secondary endpoints of the AXIS trial (axitinib vs. sorafenib) were reported at ASCO 2011 (Cella *et al*, 2011). Over 700 patients randomised to axitinib or sorafenib completed FKSI-15 and its disease-related symptoms subscale FKSI-DRS with a completion rate of about 90%. (Cella *et al*, 2011) Overall estimated means in the FKSI-15 and FKSI-DRS mixed-effects models were similar between treatments. The composite time to deterioration (TTD) endpoint, using FKSI-15 or FKSI-DRS, showed a 25% risk reduction for axitinib vs. sorafenib (p=0.0001 for both comparisons). Axitinib treatment resulted in patient reported outcomes comparable to sorafenib in patients being treated for second-line metastatic RCC. The PFS benefit demonstrated by axitinib is accompanied by a delay in worsening of the composite endpoint of advanced RCC symptoms, progression, or death compared with sorafenib.

These data reporting on improved or unchanged QoL during treatment with anti-VEGF tyrosine kinase inhibitors (TKIs) are reassuring and may well allay any fears that patient may have and in fact encourage them to proceed on with the treatment. Indeed, the improvement of QoL with some of the TKIs may be attributed to the resolution of their cancer-related-symptoms from the treatment.

In a double-blind, placebo-controlled trial, everolimus 10 mg daily was evaluated using FKSI-DRS and EORTC QLQ-C30. (Beaumont *et al*, 2011) Longitudinal trends for FKSI-DRS scores did not differ between everolimus and placebo. For physical functioning and global QoL, a small but statistically significant decrease was seen with everolimus. All three measures were significantly related to PFS. The authors reported that even when progression of disease was delayed by the new treatment, it did not affect patients' symptoms, functioning, or their QoL, which they proposed is something patients, their family and healthcare providers might expect. (Beaumont *et al*, 2011) Furthermore,

Beaumont and colleagues suggest that for patients receiving first line treatment with a targeted agent, the prospect for clinical benefit may outweigh concerns about health-related QoL. However, in contrast, when these agents are being used in the second- and third-line settings, health-related quality of life may be of more importance to all concerned groups. Continued research is needed into the positive and negative outcomes associated with new treatments for metastatic RCC. (Beaumont et al, 2011)

13. Pharmacoeconomics

It is important to determine the optimal setting and sequence of new targeted agents in metastatic RCC to improve patient survival outcomes whilst considering cost-effectiveness. Comparative cost-effectiveness in the first- and second-line setting should be assessed with respect to life years gained. (Molina & Motzer, 2011) For example, Benedict and colleagues utilized a Markov model simulating disease progression, adverse events and survival to assess economic value of first-line treatments in the US and Sweden. Their analyses suggested sunitinib is cost-effective compared with sorafenib, or bevacizumab plus IFN-α for first line metastatic RCC treatment. (Benedict et al, 2011) In 2011 NICE, the UK National Institute for Health and Clinical Effectiveness, was unable to approve everolimus for second-line metastatic RCC as it was too expensive for the benefit provided. (http://guidance.nice.org.uk/TA219/Guidance/pdf/English accessed August 1st 2011)

14. Conclusion

The treatment landscape for metastatic RCC has dramatically changed with the development of targeted therapy. Metastatic RCC, once considered a dismal disease to treat has been transformed into a treatable cancer in the era of targeted therapy. These agents are now being investigated either in a sequential or combination fashion in an attempt to search for improved clinical efficacy. The side-effects profile is unique to each agent although there are some common class adverse effects. Careful monitoring and management of side-effects are warranted for patients on these agents to ensure good adherence and effective therapy. Further understanding and insight into the intracellular molecular signaling pathways to both clear-cell and non-clear cell RCC will hopefully lead to the discovery of agents that would confer more durable response and improved prognosis.

15. References

(1999) Interferon-alpha and survival in metastatic renal carcinoma: early results of a randomised controlled trial. Medical Research Council Renal Cancer Collaborators. Lancet 353: 14-7

(2010) National Institutes of Health: A phase II study of bevacizumab and erlotinib in subsets with advanced hereditary leiomyomatosis and renal cell cancer (HLRCC) or sporadic papillary renal cell cancer. Accessed Oct 2010. Available from: http://clinicaltrials.gov/ct2/show/NCT01130519?term=bevacizumab+and+erlotinib&rank=2

Abrams TJ, Murray LJ, Pesenti E, Holway VW, Colombo T, Lee LB, Cherrington JM, Pryer NK (2003) Preclinical evaluation of the tyrosine kinase inhibitor SU11248 as a single agent and in combination with "standard of care" therapeutic agents for the treatment of breast cancer. *Mol Cancer Ther* 2: 1011-21

Adams VR, Leggas M (2007) Sunitinib malate for the treatment of metastatic renal cell carcinoma and gastrointestinal stromal tumors. *Clin Ther* 29: 1338-53

Amato R (2011) Everolimus for the treatment of advanced renal cell carcinoma. *Expert Opin Pharmacother* 12: 1143-55

Angevin E, Grünwald V, Castellano DE, Lin CC, Gschwend JE, Harzstark AL, cHang J, Want Y, Shi MM, Escudier BJ (2011) A phase II study of dovitinib (TKI258), an FGFR- and VEGFR-inhibitor, in patients with advanced or metastatic renal cell cancer (mRCC). *J Clin Oncol* 29: (abstr 4551)

Atkins MB, Hidalgo M, Stadler WM, Logan TF, Dutcher JP, Hudes GR, Park Y, Liou SH, Marshall B, Boni JP, Dukart G, Sherman ML (2004) Randomized phase II study of multiple dose levels of CCI-779, a novel mammalian target of rapamycin kinase inhibitor, in patients with advanced refractory renal cell carcinoma. *J Clin Oncol* 22: 909-18

Azad NS, Posadas EM, Kwitkowski VE, Steinberg SM, Jain L, Annunziata CM, Minasian L, Sarosy G, Kotz HL, Premkumar A, Cao L, McNally D, Chow C, Chen HX, Wright JJ, Figg WD, Kohn EC (2008) Combination targeted therapy with sorafenib and bevacizumab results in enhanced toxicity and antitumor activity. *J Clin Oncol* 26: 3709-14

Barkholt L, Bregni M, Remberger M, Blaise D, Peccatori J, Massenkeil G, Pedrazzoli P, Zambelli A, Bay JO, Francois S, Martino R, Bengala C, Brune M, Lenhoff S, Porcellini A, Falda M, Siena S, Demirer T, Niederwieser D, Ringden O (2006) Allogeneic haematopoietic stem cell transplantation for metastatic renal carcinoma in Europe. *Ann Oncol* 17: 1134-40

Beaumont JL, Butt Z, Baladi J, Motzer RJ, Haas T, Hollaender N, Kay A, Cella D (2011) Patient-reported outcomes in a phase iii study of everolimus versus placebo in patients with metastatic carcinoma of the kidney that has progressed on vascular endothelial growth factor receptor tyrosine kinase inhibitor therapy. *Oncologist* 16: 632-40

Beck J, Procopio E, Verzoni S, Bajetta E, Escudier B (2008) Large open label non-comparative clinical experience trial of the multi-targeted kinase inhibitor sorafenib in European patients with advanced RCC *J Clin Oncol* 26: (Abstract 1621)

Beck J, Procopio G, Bajetta E, Keilholz U, Negrier S, Szczylik C, Bokemeyer C, Bracarda S, Richel DJ, Staehler M, Strauss UP, Mersmann S, Burock K, Escudier B (2011) Final results of the European Advanced Renal Cell Carcinoma Sorafenib (EU-ARCCS) expanded-access study: a large open-label study in diverse community settings. *Ann Oncol* 22: 1812-1813

Beck SD, Patel MI, Snyder ME, Kattan MW, Motzer RJ, Reuter VE, Russo P (2004) Effect of papillary and chromophobe cell type on disease-free survival after nephrectomy for renal cell carcinoma. *Ann Surg Oncol* 11: 71-7

Bellmunt J (2007) The Oncologist's View: Targeted Therapies in Advanced Renal Cell Carcinoma. *Eur Urol Suppl* 7: 55-62

Bellmunt J (2009) Future developments in renal cell carcinoma. *Ann Oncol* 20 Suppl 1: i13-17

Benedict A, Figlin RA, Sandstrom P, Harmenberg U, Ullen A, Charbonneau C, Sandin R, Remak E, Hariharan S, Negrier S (2011) Economic evaluation of new targeted therapies for the first-line treatment of patients with metastatic renal cell carcinoma. *BJU Int*

Beuvink I, Boulay A, Fumagalli S, Zilbermann F, Ruetz S, O'Reilly T, Natt F, Hall J, Lane HA, Thomas G (2005) The mTOR inhibitor RAD001 sensitizes tumor cells to DNA-damaged induced apoptosis through inhibition of p21 translation. *Cell* 120: 747-59

Bukowski R, Cella D, Gondek K, Escudier B (2007a) Effects of sorafenib on symptoms and quality of life: results from a large randomized placebo-controlled study in renal cancer. *Am J Clin Oncol* 30: 220-7

Bukowski RM, Kabbinavar FF, Figlin RA, Flaherty K, Srinivas S, Vaishampayan U, Drabkin HA, Dutcher J, Ryba S, Xia Q, Scappaticci FA, McDermott D (2007b) Randomized phase II study of erlotinib combined with bevacizumab compared with bevacizumab alone in metastatic renal cell cancer. *J Clin Oncol* 25: 4536-41

Cebe-Suarez S, Zehnder-Fjallman A, Ballmer-Hofer K (2006) The role of VEGF receptors in angiogenesis; complex partnerships. *Cell Mol Life Sci* 63: 601-15

Cella D, Escudier B, Rini BI, Chen HX, Bhattacharyya JC, Tarazi JC, Rosbrook B, Kim S, Motzer RJ (2011) Patient-reported outcomes (PROs) in a phase III AXIS trial of axitinib versus sorafenib as second-line therapy for metastatic renal cell carcinoma (mRCC) *J Clin Oncol* 29 (suppl) abstr 4504

Cheville JC, Lohse CM, Zincke H, Weaver AL, Blute ML (2003) Comparisons of outcome and prognostic features among histologic subtypes of renal cell carcinoma. *Am J Surg Pathol* 27: 612-24

Choi JS, Kim MK, Seo JW, Choi YL, Kim DH, Chun YK, Ko YH (2006) MET expression in sporadic renal cell carcinomas. *J Korean Med Sci* 21: 672-7

Choueiri TK, Plantade A, Elson P, Negrier S, Ravaud A, Oudard S, Zhou M, Rini BI, Bukowski RM, Escudier B (2008) Efficacy of sunitinib and sorafenib in metastatic papillary and chromophobe renal cell carcinoma. *J Clin Oncol* 26: 127-31

Cindolo L, de la Taille A, Schips L, Zigeuner RE, Ficarra V, Tostain J, Artibani W, Gallo A, Salzano L, Patard JJ (2005) Chromophobe renal cell carcinoma: comprehensive analysis of 104 cases from multicenter European database. *Urology* 65: 681-6

Cohen HT, McGovern FJ (2005) Renal cell carcinoma. *N Engl J Med* 353: 2477-90

Coppin C, Porzsolt F, Awa A, Kumpf J, Coldman A, Wilt T (2005) Immunotherapy for advanced renal cell cancer. *Cochrane database of systematic reviews (Online)*: CD001425

Costa LJ, Drabkin HA (2007) Renal cell carcinoma: new developments in molecular biology and potential for targeted therapies. *The oncologist* 12: 1404-15

Desai J, Gurney H, Pavlakis N, McArthur GA, Davis ID (2007) Sunitinib malate in the treatment of renal cell carcinoma and gastrointestinal stromal tumor: Recommendations for patient management. *Asia-Pac J Clin Oncol* 3: 167-176

Dharmawardana PG, Giubellino A, Bottaro DP (2004) Hereditary papillary renal carcinoma type I. *Curr Mol Med* 4: 855-68

di Lorenzo G, Porta C, Bellmunt J, Sternberg C, Kirkali Z, Staehler M, Joniau S, Montorsi F, Buonerba C (2011) Toxicities of targeted therapy and their management in kidney cancer. *Eur Urol* 59: 526-40

Dudek AZ, Zolnierek J, Dham A, Lindgren BR, Szczylik C (2009) Sequential therapy with sorafenib and sunitinib in renal cell carcinoma. *Cancer* 115: 61-7

Dutcher JP, Wilding G, Hudes GR, Stadler WM, Kim S, Tarazi JC, Rosbrook B, Rini BI (2008) Sequential axitinib (AG-013736) therapy of patients (pts) with metastatic clear cell renal cell cancer (RCC) refractory to sunitinib and sorafenib, cytokines and sorafenib, or sorafenib alone. *J Clin Oncol* 26: abstr 5127

Eisenhauer EA, Therasse P, Bogaerts J, Schwartz LH, Sargent D, Ford R, Dancey J, Arbuck S, Gwyther S, Mooney M, Rubinstein L, Shankar L, Dodd L, Kaplan R, Lacombe D, Verweij J (2009) New response evaluation criteria in solid tumours: revised RECIST guideline (version 1.1). *Eur J Cancer* 45: 228-47

Elaraj DM, White DE, Steinberg SM, Haworth L, Rosenberg SA, Yang JC (2004) A pilot study of antiangiogenic therapy with bevacizumab and thalidomide in patients with metastatic renal cell carcinoma. *J Immunother* 27: 259-64

Escudier B, Bellmunt J, Negrier S, Bajetta E, Melichar B, Bracarda S, Ravaud A, Golding S, Jethwa S, Sneller V (2007a) Phase III trial of bevacizumab plus interferon alfa-2a in patients with metastatic renal cell carcinoma (AVOREN): final analysis of overall survival. *J Clin Oncol* 28: 2144-50

Escudier B, Eisen T, Stadler WM, Szczylik C, Oudard S, Siebels M, Negrier S, Chevreau C, Solska E, Desai AA, Rolland F, Demkow T, Hutson TE, Gore M, Freeman S, Schwartz B, Shan M, Simantov R, Bukowski RM (2007b) Sorafenib in advanced clear-cell renal-cell carcinoma. *N Engl J Med* 356: 125-34

Escudier B, Eisen T, Stadler WM, Szczylik C, Oudard S, Staehler M, Negrier S, Chevreau C, Desai AA, Rolland F, Demkow T, Hutson TE, Gore M, Anderson S, Hofilena G, Shan M, Pena C, Lathia C, Bukowski RM (2009a) Sorafenib for treatment of renal cell carcinoma: Final efficacy and safety results of the phase III treatment approaches in renal cancer global evaluation trial. *J Clin Oncol* 27: 3312-8

Escudier B, Pluzanska A, Koralewski P, Ravaud A, Bracarda S, Szczylik C, Chevreau C, Filipek M, Melichar B, Bajetta E, Gorbunova V, Bay JO, Bodrogi I, Jagiello-Gruszfeld A, Moore N (2007c) Bevacizumab plus interferon alfa-2a for treatment of metastatic renal cell carcinoma: a randomised, double-blind phase III trial. *Lancet* 370: 2103-11

Escudier B, Roigas J, Gillessen S, Harmenberg U, Srinivas S, Mulder SF, Fountzilas G, Peschel C, Flodgren P, Maneval EC, Chen I, Vogelzang NJ (2009b) Phase II study of sunitinib administered in a continuous once-daily dosing regimen in patients with cytokine-refractory metastatic renal cell carcinoma. *J Clin Oncol* 27: 4068-75

Escudier B, Szczylik C, Hutson TE, Demkow T, Staehler M, Rolland F, Negrier S, Laferriere N, Scheuring UJ, Cella D, Shah S, Bukowski RM (2009c) Randomized phase II trial of first-line treatment with sorafenib versus interferon Alfa-2a in patients with metastatic renal cell carcinoma. *J Clin Oncol* 27: 1280-9

Faivre S, Delbaldo C, Vera K, Robert C, Lozahic S, Lassau N, Bello C, Deprimo S, Brega N, Massimini G, Armand JP, Scigalla P, Raymond E (2006) Safety, pharmacokinetic, and antitumor activity of SU11248, a novel oral multitarget tyrosine kinase inhibitor, in patients with cancer. *J Clin Oncol* 24: 25-35

Feldman DR, Baum MS, Ginsberg MS, Hassoun H, Flombaum CD, Velasco S, Fischer P, Ronnen E, Ishill N, Patil S, Motzer RJ (2009) Phase I trial of bevacizumab plus escalated doses of sunitinib in patients with metastatic renal cell carcinoma. *J Clin Oncol* 27: 1432-9

Fisher R, Pickering L, Larkin J (2011) New targeted therapies for renal cell carcinoma. *Expert Opin Investig Drugs* 20: 933-45

Frangie C, Lefaucheur C, Medioni J, Jacquot C, Hill GS, Nochy D (2007) Renal thrombotic microangiopathy caused by anti-VEGF-antibody treatment for metastatic renal-cell carcinoma. *Lancet Oncol* 8: 177-8

Furge KA, MacKeigan JP, Teh BT (2010) Kinase targets in renal-cell carcinomas: reassessing the old and discovering the new. *Lancet Oncol* 11: 571-8

Fyfe G, Fisher RI, Rosenberg SA, Sznol M, Parkinson DR, Louie AC (1995) Results of treatment of 255 patients with metastatic renal cell carcinoma who received high-dose recombinant interleukin-2 therapy. *J Clin Oncol* 13: 688-96

Gollob JA, Rathmell WK, Richmond TM, Marino CB, Miller EK, Grigson G, Watkins C, Gu L, Peterson BL, Wright JJ (2007) Phase II trial of sorafenib plus interferon alfa-2b as first- or second-line therapy in patients with metastatic renal cell cancer. *J Clin Oncol* 25: 3288-95

Gommersall L, Hayne D, Lynch C, Joseph JV, Arya M, Patel HR (2004) Allogeneic stem-cell transplantation for renal-cell cancer. *Lancet Oncol* 5: 561-7

Gordon MS, Hussey M, Nagle RB, Lara PN, Jr., Mack PC, Dutcher J, Samlowski W, Clark JI, Quinn DI, Pan CX, Crawford D (2009) Phase II study of erlotinib in patients with locally advanced or metastatic papillary histology renal cell cancer: SWOG S0317. *J Clin Oncol* 27: 5788-93

Gore ME, Szczylik C, Porta C, Bracarda S, Bjarnason GA, Oudard S, Hariharan S, Lee SH, Haanen J, Castellano D, Vrdoljak E, Schoffski P, Mainwaring P, Nieto A, Yuan J, Bukowski R (2009) Safety and efficacy of sunitinib for metastatic renal-cell carcinoma: an expanded-access trial. *Lancet Oncol* 10: 757-63

Harris DT (1983) Hormonal therapy and chemotherapy of renal-cell carcinoma. *Semin Oncol* 10: 422-30

Hidalgo M, Buckner JC, Erlichman C, Pollack MS, Boni JP, Dukart G, Marshall B, Speicher L, Moore L, Rowinsky EK (2006) A phase I and pharmacokinetic study of temsirolimus (CCI-779) administered intravenously daily for 5 days every 2 weeks to patients with advanced cancer. *Clin Cancer Res* 12: 5755-63

Hudes G, Carducci M, Tomczak P, Dutcher J, Figlin R, Kapoor A, Staroslawska E, Sosman J, McDermott D, Bodrogi I, Kovacevic Z, Lesovoy V, Schmidt-Wolf IG, Barbarash O, Gokmen E, O'Toole T, Lustgarten S, Moore L, Motzer RJ (2007) Temsirolimus, interferon alfa, or both for advanced renal-cell carcinoma. *N Engl J Med* 356: 2271-81

Hurwitz HI, Dowlati A, Saini S, Savage S, Suttle AB, Gibson DM, Hodge JP, Merkle EM, Pandite L (2009) Phase I trial of pazopanib in patients with advanced cancer. *Clin Cancer Res* 15: 4220-7

Hutson TE (2011) Targeted therapies for the treatment of metastatic renal cell carcinoma: clinical evidence. *Oncologist* 16 Suppl 2: 14-22

Hutson TE, Davis ID, Machiels JP, De Souza PL, Rottey S, Hong BF, Epstein RJ, Baker KL, McCann L, Crofts T, Pandite L, Figlin RA (2010) Efficacy and safety of pazopanib in patients with metastatic renal cell carcinoma. *J Clin Oncol* 28: 475-80

Isaacs JS, Jung YJ, Mole DR, Lee S, Torres-Cabala C, Chung YL, Merino M, Trepel J, Zbar B, Toro J, Ratcliffe PJ, Linehan WM, Neckers L (2005) HIF overexpression correlates with biallelic loss of fumarate hydratase in renal cancer: novel role of fumarate in regulation of HIF stability. *Cancer Cell* 8: 143-53

Izzedine H, Ederhy S, Goldwasser F, Soria JC, Milano G, Cohen A, Khayat D, Spano JP (2009) Management of hypertension in angiogenesis inhibitor-treated patients. *Ann Oncol* 20: 807-15

Jarkowski A, 3rd, Glode AE, Spangenthal EJ, Wong MK (2011) Heart failure caused by molecularly targeted therapies for cancer. *Pharmacotherapy* 31: 62-75

Jonasch E, Corn P, Pagliaro LC, Warneke CL, Johnson MM, Tamboli P, Ng C, Aparicio A, Ashe RG, Wright JJ, Tannir NM (2010) Upfront, randomized, phase 2 trial of sorafenib versus sorafenib and low-dose interferon alfa in patients with advanced renal cell carcinoma: clinical and biomarker analysis. *Cancer* 116: 57-65

Jonasch E, Hutson TE, Harshman LC, Srinivas S (2011) Advanced Renal Cell Carcinoma: Overview of Drug Therapy fro the Practicing Physician. *J Clin Oncol* ASCO Education Book: 145-151

Kabbinavar FF, Srinivas S, Hauke RJ, Amato RJ, Esteves WB, Cotreau MM, Strahs AL, Bhargava P, Fishman MN (2011) Results from a phase I trial of tivozanib (AV-951) combined with temsirolimus therapy in patients (pts) with renal cell carcinoma (RCC). *J Clin Oncol* 29: abstr 4549

Kamura T, Sato S, Iwai K, Czyzyk-Krzeska M, Conaway RC, Conaway JW (2000) Activation of HIF1alpha ubiquitination by a reconstituted von Hippel-Lindau (VHL) tumor suppressor complex. *Proc Natl Acad Sci U S A* 97: 10430-5

Kapiteijn E, Brand A, Kroep J, Gelderblom H (2007) Sunitinib induced hypertension, thrombotic microangiopathy and reversible posterior leukencephalopathy syndrome. *Ann Oncol* 18: 1745-7

Keefe D, Bowen J, Gibson R, Tan T, Okera M, Stringer A (2011) Noncardiac vascular toxicities of vascular endothelial growth factor inhibitors in advanced cancer: a review. *Oncologist* 16: 432-44

Kim DW, Jo YS, Jung HS, Chung HK, Song JH, Park KC, Park SH, Hwang JH, Rha SY, Kweon GR, Lee SJ, Jo KW, Shong M (2006) An orally administered multitarget tyrosine kinase inhibitor, SU11248, is a novel potent inhibitor of thyroid oncogenic RET/papillary thyroid cancer kinases. *J Clin Endocrinol Metab* 91: 4070-6

Kim WY, Kaelin WG (2004) Role of VHL gene mutation in human cancer. *J Clin Oncol* 22: 4991-5004

Klatte T, Han KR, Said JW, Bohm M, Allhoff EP, Kabbinavar FF, Belldegrun AS, Pantuck AJ (2008) Pathobiology and prognosis of chromophobe renal cell carcinoma. *Urol Oncol* 26: 604-9

Kollmannsberger C, Soulieres D, Wong R, Scalera A, Gaspo R, Bjarnason G (2007a) Sunitinib therapy for metastatic renal cell carcinoma: recommendations for management of side-effects. *Can Urol Assoc J* 1 (Suppl 2): S41-S54

Kollmannsberger C, Soulieres D, Wong R, Scalera A, Gaspo R, Bjarnason G (2007b) Sunitinib therapy for metastatic renal cell carcinoma: recommendations for management of side effects. *Can Urol Assoc J* 1: S41-54

Lacouture ME, Anadkat MJ, Bensadoun RJ, Bryce J, Chan A, Epstein JB, Eaby-Sandy B, Murphy BA (2011) Clinical practice guidelines for the prevention and treatment of EGFR inhibitor-associated dermatologic toxicities. *Support Care Cancer* 19: 1079-95

Lees J, Chan A (2011) Polypharmacy in elderly patients with cancer: clinical implications and management. *Lancet Oncol* Epub 7 July

Linehan WM, Pinto PA, Srinivasan R, Merino M, Choyke P, Choyke L, Coleman J, Toro J, Glenn G, Vocke C, Zbar B, Schmidt LS, Bottaro D, Neckers L (2007) Identification of the genes for kidney cancer: opportunity for disease-specific targeted therapeutics. *Clin Cancer Res* 13: 671s-679s

Margulis V, Tamboli P, Matin SF, Swanson DA, Wood CG (2008) Analysis of clinicopathologic predictors of oncologic outcome provides insight into the natural history of surgically managed papillary renal cell carcinoma. *Cancer* 112: 1480-8

Maxwell PH, Wiesener MS, Chang GW, Clifford SC, Vaux EC, Cockman ME, Wykoff CC, Pugh CW, Maher ER, Ratcliffe PJ (1999) The tumour suppressor protein VHL targets hypoxia-inducible factors for oxygen-dependent proteolysis. *Nature* 399: 271-5

McDermott DF, George DJ (2010) Bevacizumab as a treatment option in advanced renal cell carcinoma: an analysis and interpretation of clinical trial data. *Cancer Treat Rev* 36: 216-23

McDermott DF, Regan MM, Clark JI, Flaherty LE, Weiss GR, Logan TF, Kirkwood JM, Gordon MS, Sosman JA, Ernstoff MS, Tretter CP, Urba WJ, Smith JW, Margolin KA, Mier JW, Gollob JA, Dutcher JP, Atkins MB (2005) Randomized phase III trial of high-dose interleukin-2 versus subcutaneous interleukin-2 and interferon in patients with metastatic renal cell carcinoma. *J Clin Oncol* 23: 133-41

Mekhail TM, Abou-Jawde RM, Boumerhi G, Malhi S, Wood L, Elson P, Bukowski R (2005) Validation and extension of the Memorial Sloan-Kettering prognostic factors model for survival in patients with previously untreated metastatic renal cell carcinoma. *J Clin Oncol* 23: 832-41

Melichar B, Koralewski P, Ravaud A, Pluzanska A, Bracarda S, Szczylik C, Chevreau C, Filipek M, Delva R, Sevin E, Negrier S, McKendrick J, Santoro A, Pisa P, Escudier B (2008) First-line bevacizumab combined with reduced dose interferon-alpha2a is active in patients with metastatic renal cell carcinoma. *Ann Oncol* 19: 1470-6

Mendel DB, Laird AD, Xin X, Louie SG, Christensen JG, Li G, Schreck RE, Abrams TJ, Ngai TJ, Lee LB, Murray LJ, Carver J, Chan E, Moss KG, Haznedar JO, Sukbuntherng J, Blake RA, Sun L, Tang C, Miller T, Shirazian S, McMahon G, Cherrington JM (2003) In vivo antitumor activity of SU11248, a novel tyrosine kinase inhibitor targeting vascular endothelial growth factor and platelet-derived growth factor receptors: determination of a pharmacokinetic/pharmacodynamic relationship. *Clin Cancer Res* 9: 327-37

Molina AM, Motzer R (2008) Current Algorithm and Prognostic Factors in the Treatment of Metastatic Renal Cell Carcinoma. *Clin Genitourinary Can* 6: S7-S13

Molina AM, Motzer RJ (2011) Clinical practice guidelines for the treatment of metastatic renal cell carcinoma: today and tomorrow. *Oncologist* 16 Suppl 2: 45-50

Motzer RJ, Bacik J, Mariani T, Russo P, Mazumdar M, Reuter V (2002) Treatment outcome and survival associated with metastatic renal cell carcinoma of non-clear-cell histology. *J Clin Oncol* 20: 2376-81

Motzer RJ, Bacik J, Mazumdar M (2004) Prognostic Factors for Survival of Patients with Stage IV Renal Cell Carcinoma. *Clin Cancer Research* 10: 6302S-6303S

Motzer RJ, Bander NH, Nanus DM (1996) Renal-cell carcinoma. *N Engl J Med* 335: 865-75

Motzer RJ, de La Motte Rouge T, Harzstark AL, michaelson MD, Liu G, Gruenwald V, Ingrosso A, Tortorici MA, Bycott PW, Kim S, Rini BI (2011a) Axitinib second-line therapy for metastatic renal cell carcinoma (mRCC): Five-year (yr) overall survival (OS) data from a phase II trial. *J Clin Oncol* 29: (suppl; abstr 4527)

Motzer RJ, Escudier B, Oudard S, Hutson TE, Porta C, Bracarda S, Grunwald V, Thompson JA, Figlin RA, Hollaender N, Urbanowitz G, Berg WJ, Kay A, Lebwohl D, Ravaud A (2008) Efficacy of everolimus in advanced renal cell carcinoma: a double-blind, randomised, placebo-controlled phase III trial. *Lancet* 372: 449-56

Motzer RJ, Hutson TE, Olsen MR, Hudes GR, Burke JM, Edenfield WJ, Wilding G, Martell B, Hariharan S, Figlin RA (2011b) Randomized phase II multicenter study of the efficacy and safety of sunitinib on the 4/2 versus continuous dosing schedule as first-line therapy of metastatic renal cell carcinoma: Renal EFFECT Trial. *J Clin Oncol* 29: (suppl 7; abstrc LBA308)

Motzer RJ, Hutson TE, Tomczak P, Michaelson MD, Bukowski RM, Oudard S, Negrier S, Szczylik C, Pili R, Bjarnason GA, Garcia-del-Muro X, Sosman JA, Solska E, Wilding G, Thompson JA, Kim ST, Chen I, Huang X, Figlin RA (2009) Overall survival and updated results for sunitinib compared with interferon alfa in patients with metastatic renal cell carcinoma. *J Clin Oncol* 27: 3584-90

Motzer RJ, Hutson TE, Tomczak P, Michaelson MD, Bukowski RM, Rixe O, Oudard S, Negrier S, Szczylik C, Kim ST, Chen I, Bycott PW, Baum CM, Figlin RA (2007a) Sunitinib versus interferon alfa in metastatic renal-cell carcinoma. *N Engl J Med* 356: 115-24

Motzer RJ, Mazumdar M, Bacik J, Berg W, Amsterdam A, Ferrara J (1999) Survival and prognostic stratification of 670 patients with advanced renal cell carcinoma. *J Clin Oncol* 17: 2530-40

Motzer RJ, Michaelson MD, Redman BG, Hudes GR, Wilding G, Figlin RA, Ginsberg MS, Kim ST, Baum CM, DePrimo SE, Li JZ, Bello CL, Theuer CP, George DJ, Rini BI (2006) Activity of SU11248, a multitargeted inhibitor of vascular endothelial growth factor receptor and platelet-derived growth factor receptor, in patients with metastatic renal cell carcinoma. *J Clin Oncol* 24: 16-24

Motzer RJ, Michaelson MD, Rosenberg J, Bukowski RM, Curti BD, George DJ, Hudes GR, Redman BG, Margolin KA, Wilding G (2007b) Sunitinib efficacy against advanced renal cell carcinoma. *J Urol* 178: 1883-7

Murray LJ, Abrams TJ, Long KR, Ngai TJ, Olson LM, Hong W, Keast PK, Brassard JA, O'Farrell AM, Cherrington JM, Pryer NK (2003) SU11248 inhibits tumor growth and CSF-1R-dependent osteolysis in an experimental breast cancer bone metastasis model. *Clin Exp Metastasis* 20: 757-66

NCT00378703 Cgi (2006) Bevacizumab, Sorafenib, and Temsirolimus in Treating Patients With Metastatic Kidney Cancer (BeST) *[cited 16 Dec 2010]*. Available from http://clinicaltrials.gov/ct2/show/NCT00378703

NCT00720941 Cgi (2011) Pazopanib Versus Sunitinib in the Treatment of Locally Advanced and/or Metastatic Renal Cell Carcinoma (COMPARZ) *[cited 21 July 2011]*. Available from: http://clinicaltrials.gov/ct2/show/NCT00720941

NCT00732914 Cgi (2010) Sequential Study to Treat Renal Cell Carcinoma *[cited 18 Oct 2010]*. Available from:
   http://clinicaltrials.gov/ct2/show/NCT00732914?term=NCT00732914&rank=1

NCT1217931 Cgi (2011) Sequential Two-agent Assessment in Renal Cell Carcinoma Therapy *[cited 17 May 2011]*. Available from:

http://clinicaltrials.gov/ct2/show/NCT01217931?term=NCT01217931&rank=1

Negrier S, Gravis G, Perol D, Chevreau C, Delva R, Bay JO, Blanc E, Ferlay C, Geoffrois L, Rolland F, Legouffe E, Sevin E, Laguerre B, Escudier B (2011) Temsirolimus and bevacizumab, or sunitinib, or interferon alfa and bevacizumab for patients with advanced renal cell carcinoma (TORAVA): a randomised phase 2 trial. *Lancet Oncol* 12: 673-80

Nosov D, Bhargava P, Esteves WB, Strahs AL, Lipatov ON, Lyulkp OO, Anischenko AO, Chacki RT, Doval D, Slichenmyer WJ (2011) Final analysis of the phase II randomized discontinuation trial (RDT) of tivozanib (AV-951) versus placebo in patients with renal cell carcinoma (RCC). *J Clin Oncol* 29: (suppl; abstr 4503)

O'Farrell AM, Abrams TJ, Yuen HA, Ngai TJ, Louie SG, Yee KW, Wong LM, Hong W, Lee LB, Town A, Smolich BD, Manning WC, Murray LJ, Heinrich MC, Cherrington JM (2003) SU11248 is a novel FLT3 tyrosine kinase inhibitor with potent activity in vitro and in vivo. *Blood* 101: 3597-605

Ohh M, Park CW, Ivan M, Hoffman MA, Kim TY, Huang LE, Pavletich N, Chau V, Kaelin WG (2000) Ubiquitination of hypoxia-inducible factor requires direct binding to the beta-domain of the von Hippel-Lindau protein. *Nat Cell Biol* 2: 423-7

Oudard S, Banu E, Vieillefond A, Fournier L, Priou F, Medioni J, Banu A, Duclos B, Rolland F, Escudier B, Arakelyan N, Culine S (2007a) Prospective multicenter phase II study of gemcitabine plus platinum salt for metastatic collecting duct carcinoma: results of a GETUG (Groupe d'Etudes des Tumeurs Uro-Genitales) study. *J Urol* 177: 1698-702

Oudard S, George D, Medioni J, Motzer R (2007b) Treatment options in renal cell carcinoma: past, present and future. *Ann Oncol* 18 Suppl 10: x25-31

Parton M, Gore M, Eisen T (2006) Role of cytokine therapy in 2006 and beyond for metastatic renal cell cancer. *J Clin Oncol* 24: 5584-92

Patard JJ, Leray E, Rioux-Leclercq N, Cindolo L, Ficarra V, Zisman A, De La Taille A, Tostain J, Artibani W, Abbou CC, Lobel B, Guille F, Chopin DK, Mulders PF, Wood CG, Swanson DA, Figlin RA, Belldegrun AS, Pantuck AJ (2005) Prognostic value of histologic subtypes in renal cell carcinoma: a multicenter experience. *J Clin Oncol* 23: 2763-71

Patel TV, Morgan JA, Demetri GD, George S, Maki RG, Quigley M, Humphreys BD (2008) A preeclampsia-like syndrome characterized by reversible hypertension and proteinuria induced by the multitargeted kinase inhibitors sunitinib and sorafenib. *J Natl Cancer Inst* 100: 282-4

Pavlovich CP, Walther MM, Eyler RA, Hewitt SM, Zbar B, Linehan WM, Merino MJ (2002) Renal tumors in the Birt-Hogg-Dube syndrome. *Am J Surg Pathol* 26: 1542-52

Pithavala YK, Tortorici M, Toh M, Garrett M, Hee B, Kuruganti U, Ni G, Klamerus KJ (2010) Effect of rifampin on the pharmacokinetics of Axitinib (AG-013736) in Japanese and Caucasian healthy volunteers. *Cancer Chemother Pharmacol* 65: 563-70

Plimack ER, Jonasch E, Bekele bN, Qiao W, Ng CS, Tannir NM (2010) Sunitinib in papillary renal cell carcinoma (pRCC): Results from a single-arm phase II study. *J Clin Oncol* 28: (suppl; abstr 4604)

Ratain MJ, Eisen T, Stadler WM, Flaherty KT, Kaye SB, Rosner GL, Gore M, Desai AA, Patnaik A, Xiong HQ, Rowinsky E, Abbruzzese JL, Xia C, Simantov R, Schwartz B,

O'Dwyer PJ (2006) Phase II placebo-controlled randomized discontinuation trial of sorafenib in patients with metastatic renal cell carcinoma. *J Clin Oncol* 24: 2505-12

Ravaud A (2009) How to optimise treatment compliance in metastatic renal cell carcinoma with targeted agents. *Ann Oncol* 20 (Suppl 1): i7-12

Ravaud A (2011) Treatment-Associated Adverse Event Management in the Advanced Renal Cell Carcinoma Patient Treated with Targeted Therapies. *Oncologist* 16(suppl 2): 32-44

Ravaud A, Oudard S, Gravis-Mescam G, Sevin E, Zanetta S, Théodore C, de Fromont M, Mahier-Aït Oukhatar C, Chêne G, Escudier B (2009) First-line sunitinib in type I and II papillary renal cell carcinoma (PRCC): SUPAP, a phase II study of the French Genito-Urinary Group (GETUG) and the Group of Early Phase trials (GEP). *J Clin Oncol* 27: (suppl; abstr 5146)

Raymond E, Alexandre J, Faivre S, Vera K, Materman E, Boni J, Leister C, Korth-Bradley J, Hanauske A, Armand JP (2004) Safety and pharmacokinetics of escalated doses of weekly intravenous infusion of CCI-779, a novel mTOR inhibitor, in patients with cancer. *J Clin Oncol* 22: 2336-47

Rini B, Al-Marrawi MY (2011) Pazopanib for the treatment of renal cancer. *Expert Opin Pharmacother* 12: 1171-89

Rini BI, Cohen DP, Lu DR, Chen I, Hariharan S, Gore ME, Figlin RA, Baum MS, Motzer RJ (2011a) Hypertension as a biomarker of efficacy in patients with metastatic renal cell carcinoma treated with sunitinib. *J Natl Cancer Inst* 103: 763-73

Rini BI, Escudier B, Tomczak P, Kaprin A, Hutson TE, Szczylik C, Tarazi JC, Rosbrook B, Kim S, Motzer RJ (2011b) Axitinib versus sorafenib as second-line therapy for metastatic renal cell carcinoma (mRCC): Results of phase III AXIS trial. *J Clin Oncol* 29: (suppl; abstr 4503)

Rini BI, Garcia JA, Cooney MM, Elson P, Tyler A, Beatty K, Bokar J, Mekhail T, Bukowski RM, Budd GT, Triozzi P, Borden E, Ivy P, Chen HX, Dolwati A, Dreicer R (2009) A phase I study of sunitinib plus bevacizumab in advanced solid tumors. *Clin Cancer Res* 15: 6277-83

Rini BI, Halabi S, Rosenberg JE, Stadler WM, Vaena DA, Archer L, Atkins JN, Picus J, Czaykowski P, Dutcher J, Small EJ (2010) Phase III trial of bevacizumab plus interferon alfa versus interferon alfa monotherapy in patients with metastatic renal cell carcinoma: final results of CALGB 90206. *J Clin Oncol* 28: 2137-43

Rini BI, Halabi S, Rosenberg JE, Stadler WM, Vaena DA, Ou SS, Archer L, Atkins JN, Picus J, Czaykowski P, Dutcher J, Small EJ (2008) Bevacizumab plus interferon alfa compared with interferon alfa monotherapy in patients with metastatic renal cell carcinoma: CALGB 90206. *J Clin Oncol* 26: 5422-8

Rini BI, Zimmerman T, Stadler WM, Gajewski TF, Vogelzang NJ (2002) Allogeneic stem-cell transplantation of renal cell cancer after nonmyeloablative chemotherapy: feasibility, engraftment, and clinical results. *J Clin Oncol* 20: 2017-24

Rixe O, Billemont B, Izzedine H (2007a) Hypertension as a predictive factor of Sunitinib activity. *Ann Oncol* 18: 1117

Rixe O, Bukowski RM, Michaelson MD, Wilding G, Hudes GR, Bolte O, Motzer RJ, Bycott P, Liau KF, Freddo J, Trask PC, Kim S, Rini BI (2007b) Axitinib treatment in patients with cytokine-refractory metastatic renal-cell cancer: a phase II study. *Lancet Oncol* 8: 975-84

Ryan CW, Goldman BH, Lara PN, Jr., Mack PC, Beer TM, Tangen CM, Lemmon D, Pan CX, Drabkin HA, Crawford ED (2007) Sorafenib with interferon alfa-2b as first-line treatment of advanced renal carcinoma: a phase II study of the Southwest Oncology Group. *J Clin Oncol* 25: 3296-301

Schmidinger M, Bellmunt J (2011) Plethora of agents, plethora of targets, plethora of side effects in metastatic renal cell carcinoma. *Cancer Treat Rev* 36: 416-24

Schmidt LS, Warren MB, Nickerson ML, Weirich G, Matrosova V, Toro JR, Turner ML, Duray P, Merino M, Hewitt S, Pavlovich CP, Glenn G, Greenberg CR, Linehan WM, Zbar B (2001) Birt-Hogg-Dube syndrome, a genodermatosis associated with spontaneous pneumothorax and kidney neoplasia, maps to chromosome 17p11.2. *Am J Hum Genet* 69: 876-82

Sosman JA, Flaherty KT, Atkins MB, McDermott DF, Rothenberg WL, Vermeulen WL, Harlacker K, Hsu A, Wright JJ, Puzanov I (2008) Updated results of phase I trial of sorafenib (S) and bevacizumab (B) in patients with metastatic renal cell cancer (mRCC). *J Clin Oncol* 26 (May 20 Suppl): Abstr 5011

Stadler WM, Figlin RA, McDermott DF, Dutcher JP, Knox JJ, Miller WH, Jr., Hainsworth JD, Henderson CA, George JR, Hajdenberg J, Kindwall-Keller TL, Ernstoff MS, Drabkin HA, Curti BD, Chu L, Ryan CW, Hotte SJ, Xia C, Cupit L, Bukowski RM (2010) Safety and efficacy results of the advanced renal cell carcinoma sorafenib expanded access program in North America. *Cancer* 116: 1272-80

Sternberg CN (2010) Randomised, double-blind phase III study of pazopanib in patients with advaced/metastatic renal cell carcinoma (MRCC), ESMO: Pazopanib in advanced MRCC - late breaker published 11/10/2011 by cancer reported Jo Armstrong.

Sternberg CN, Davis ID, Mardiak J, Szczylik C, Lee E, Wagstaff J, Barrios CH, Salman P, Gladkov OA, Kavina A, Zarba JJ, Chen M, McCann L, Pandite L, Roychowdhury DF, Hawkins RE (2010) Pazopanib in locally advanced or metastatic renal cell carcinoma: results of a randomized phase III trial. *J Clin Oncol* 28: 1061-8

Sudarshan S, Linehan WM (2006) Genetic basis of cancer of the kidney. *Semin Oncol* 33: 544-51

Tan TH, Pranavan G, Haxhimolla HZ, Yip D (2010) New systemic treatment options for metastatic renal-cell carcinoma in the era of targeted therapies. *Asia Pac J Clin Oncol* 6: 5-18

Tazi el M, Essadi I, Tazi MF, Ahellal Y, M'Rabti H, Errihani H (2011) Advanced treatments in non-clear renal cell carcinoma. *Urol J* 8: 1-11

Vaupel P (2004) The role of hypoxia-induced factors in tumor progression. *Oncologist* 9 Suppl 5: 10-7

Yagoda A, Bander NH (1989) Failure of cytotoxic chemotherapy, 1983-1988, and the emerging role of monoclonal antibodies for renal cancer. *Urol Int* 44: 338-45

Yamazaki K, Sakamoto M, Ohta T, Kanai Y, Ohki M, Hirohashi S (2003) Overexpression of KIT in chromophobe renal cell carcinoma. *Oncogene* 22: 847-52

Yang JC, Haworth L, Sherry RM, Hwu P, Schwartzentruber DJ, Topalian SL, Steinberg SM, Chen HX, Rosenberg SA (2003) A randomized trial of bevacizumab, an anti-vascular endothelial growth factor antibody, for metastatic renal cancer. *N Engl J Med* 349: 427-34

Zbar B, Alvord WG, Glenn G, Turner M, Pavlovich CP, Schmidt L, Walther M, Choyke P, Weirich G, Hewitt SM, Duray P, Gabril F, Greenberg C, Merino MJ, Toro J, Linehan WM (2002) Risk of renal and colonic neoplasms and spontaneous pneumothorax in the Birt-Hogg-Dube syndrome. *Cancer Epidemiol Biomarkers Prev* 11: 393-400

8

Contemporary Management in Metastatic Renal Cell Carcinoma

Murat Lekili

Celal Bayar University, Medical Faculty, Urology Department, Manisa
Turkey

1. Introduction

In addition to advancing our understanding of RCC, improved abdominal imaging technology has caused a migration of tumor stage and alteration of surgical strategies, with tumors commonly being diagnosed at an earlier stage. Despite these advances, the prognosis for patients with metastatic RCC is poor. Of the total number of patients with renal cancer, approximately a third either presents with or later develops metastatic disease. Unfortunately, for these patients, contemporary systemic therapies are generally ineffective—median survival is less than 1 year. Despite adjuvant systemic chemotherapy, hormonal or cytokine therapies, used alone or in combination, overall response rates rarely exceed 20% and durable, complete responses are rare. Targeted therapy in the management of metastatic renal cell cancer is newly introduced to urology practise. These drugs were used in very limited number of patients and only for clear cell histology. No recommendation to use these drugs for other than clear cell histology was seen in the literature. Nevertheless, there is a encouraging responses in trials with limited number of patients in the literature. Future advances are expected.

Spontaneous remissions in 0.8–7.0% of patients are reported in surgical series of clinical trials with previous surgical intervention. The role of surgical intervention in patients with metastatic renal cancer can be twofold. First, to render a patient clinically free of all sites of metastases ('metastasectomy'). Second, to resect the primary tumor prior to initiation of systemic therapy ('cytoreductive nephrectomy').

Studies that examine combinations of surgery and systemic therapy aim to improve survival in this high-risk group. In an attempt to address this important clinical issue, two randomized, prospective clinical trials were organized in the US (Southwest Oncology Group [SWOG]) and Europe (European Organization for Research and Treatment of Cancer [EORTC]) under similar entry criteria. The trials compared treatment of metastatic renal cancer with cytoreductive nephrectomy plus IFNα-2b versus IFNα-2b alone. Median survival of patients that underwent cytoreductive nephrectomy plus IFNα-2b was significantly greater than that of those treated with IFNα-2b only.

More recent metastasectomy studies also identified favorable clinical and surgical characteristics that were associated with a positive enhancement of outcome, but metastasectomy has never been assessed in a randomized clinical trial. It is not certain that metastasectomy can be curative, but operative intervention can provide effective palliation for symptomatic metastases in sites such as bone, the brain, and the adrenal gland. Ultimately a prospective clinical trial comparing metastasectomy to best standard systemic therapy will define the exact role of this approach.The occasionally unpredictable natural history of renal cancer and varying patient selection criteria can make the interpretation of outcomes from different centers difficult. As a conclusion although there is a tendency in favor of surgery, operative intervention for metastatic renal cancer is still controversial.

The aim of this review is more recent management modalities in the management of metastatic renal cell carcinoma. In addition, the role of surgery in metastatic RCC have been emphasised.

2. The role of nephrectomy

Although it is a part of multidisciplinary approach in the management of metastatic renal cell carcinoma (RCC), the role of Cytoreducive nephrectomy is still controversial in urologic literature. Recently according to some multicentric prospective randomized trials, because of providence little survival advantage, cytoreductive nephrectomy has gained some popularity. The objectives of nephrectomy in metastatic disease are avoidance of local symptoms and negative effects of primary tumor on immunological system (asynergy) and obtaining suitable nominee for immunotherapy, increasing patient quality of life and probably increased response to systemic therapy and finally increased overall survival. On the other hand, to prevent new metastases from primary tumor, capture of circulating immune cells, especially lymphocytes, which absorbed from primary tumor and so properties of immune pressure of primary tumor on immune system. Decreasing tumor burden may help the effectiveness of systemic therapy on tumor.

Surgical mortality rates are reported as 2-11%. In NCI trial, 62% patients can take immunotherapy and response rate is 18% in 195 patients. In this trial 38% patients cannot take immunotherapy because of complications of nephrectomy or rapid deterioration in general performance after progression of the disease (6). Some oncological centers recommend primary immunotherapy in order to avoid surgical morbidity especially in patients with clinical regression in metastatic sites (7,8).

Actually, two points provide that nephrectomy is a safe procedure; one is observation of spontaneous regression phenomena in metastatic sites after nephrectomy which is very rare. Freed has reported that 51 patients presented spontaneous regression after nephrectomy in literature (9). Similarly, NCI reported 4 patients (4.4%) have demonstrated spontaneous regression in 99 patients (10). In these 4 patients have only lung metastases and they were in remission for mean 24.3 months. Although spontaneous remission rates are very low, it is still very objective data in favor of nephrectomy. The other point for nephrectomy is unresponsiveness of primary tumor to systemic therapy. Radical nephrectomy may help to increase objective responses to systemic therapy. It has been obtained 32% objective response with immunotherapy after nephrectomy in 55 patients, but 4.7% response rate has been observed with same immunotherapeutic regimen in insitu tumor (11). Recently, surgical technique for cytoreductive nephrectomy is getting importance. Minimal invasive techniques gain popularity. While laparoscopic experience increased, laparoscopic radical nephrectomy performance is increasing in literature. The surgery time is longer, but postoperative analgesic requirements and hospital stay are decreasing. Therefore patients can take systemic therapy earlier than open surgery (Mean 35 vs 67 day). Patients without immunotherapy in case of disease progression are 13-77 % in literature (16). The shared conclusion of all the reports in literature is that the patients for cytoreductive nephrectomy have to be selected and they have to be in good ECOG performance status.

The last clues for nephrectomy are quality of life. Hematuri, pain and paraneoplastic syndromes including anemia, anorexia, hypertension, hypocalcaemia etc. can be controlled with nephrectomy.

In conclusion, multidisciplinary approach including surgery stands in the forefront. But some questions are on the agenda. Timing and coordination. Which one should be the first, nephrectomy or systemic therapy?

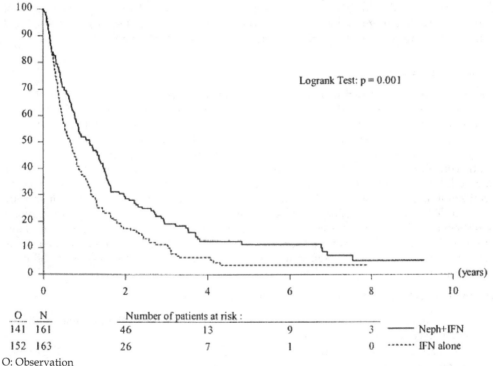

Fig. 1. SWOG and EORTC trials

O: Observation
N: Nephrectomy

3. Metastasectomy

For a long time, if possible excision of metastases is recommended. Complete metastasectomy was performed in Kierney" report. 59% and 31% 3 and 5 years survival was obtained in 77 patients with metastatic RCC. These survivals were significantly different from patients within conservative follow (20,21). In another retrospective study with 278 patients, complete and incomplete metastasis resection can provide 44% vs 14% 5-years survival advantage (22).

In conclusion, the presence of solitary metastases and localization are important factors for clinical improvement. Resection of solitary metastases is recommended for survival and also quality of life.

4. Systemic treatments

4.1 Cytotoxic drugs

Standard cytotoxic drugs are generally ineffective. Response rates were reported below 10%. Response rate was reported 17% with Gemcitabine and 5-Florourasil combination in phase II study. Gemcitabine and capecitabine combination is effective as 20%. But grade 3-4 toxicity was reported. Same regimen reported by CALGB, Survival was 12% and stable disease rate was 59% in this study. Nevertheless toxicity was always a problem. 36% of patients could not continue the treatment protocol. The main problem is neutropenie and hand-food syndrome. Therefore, phase III studies can not be conducted.

4.2 Immunotherapy

Standard theurepathic regimen is still lack in the management of metastatic RCC. But interferon and interleukin therapy is in management list in many centers. Histological type is the most important factor for the response. The only histological type which is sensitive to immunotherapy is clear cell RCC. Granular, papillary or sarcomatoid type variants are resistant to immunotherapy. The main mechanism of cytokines is still contraversial. Cytokines are binding to specific receptors on tumor cells and initiate intracellular and intercellular signal mechanism. IL-2 is a potent stimulator of T cell proliferation. Anti-tumor T cells rapidly begin to proliferation, then tumor-specific cytotoxic T lymphocytes=CTL, natural killer lymphocytes=NK and probably intratumoral lymphocytes=TIL become active and try to kill tumor cell. However, interferons have some antiangiogenetic effects. Absence of anemia and hypocalcaemia, normal lactic dehydrogenase, prior nephrectomy and good performance status increase possibility of positive response.

The main expectations for immunotherapy in metastatic RCC

- Overhelming of T-lymphocite dysfunction, dendrtic cell dysfunction, soluble inhibitory factors secreted from tumor cells (IL-10),
- The changes of T-lymphocite antigen receptors and transmission of signals (TCRdelta, decreasing p56 levels, NFkappaB compliment changes)
- Identification of unique tumor surface antigens
- Vaccination manuplations for immun tolerence

Current immunotheraupeutic cytokines are;

- Interferons
- İnterleukins
- Colony-stimulating factors (CSF)
- Tumor necrosis factor (TNF)

4.3 Interferon

IFN-alpha is approved for the management of metastatic RCC in Europe and it is used routinely in Urological practise. Response rates are 10-25%. Recently, with recombinant forms response rates are increased to 29%. Survival advantage is 3-5 months. Toxicities are flu-like syndromes, dryness in skin and mucosal membranes, mental changes and depression. Combination with IL-2 is frequently applied in many centers. Dosage scheme is controversial.

IFN-beta and gamma are ineffective.

4.4 Interleukin-2 (IL-2)

A group of cytocine which are activated and regulated lymphocite growing and/ or differantiation

First described one is IL-2.

It is produced by activated CD4+ lymphocites.Cytotoxic T cells are stimulated by IL-2. CD8+ T cells, monocytes, lymphocyte activated killer lymphocytes (LAK) are activated and tumor necrosis factor is secreted. It is reported that IL-2 is as effective as 15% in many series. Rekombinant IL-2 (rIL-2)

- Bolus high-dose *i.v.* infusion= highly toxic
- İnhalation
- Response rate 7-27%
- Only clear cell type is respondable

Recently, there are more than 10 interleukin described other than IL-2 (IL-4; IL-7; IL-12 have been still investigating)

4.5 Cytokine combination therapy

Class I MHC Ag expression + T-lymphocite activation

- Synergy
- Mean 22% response
- Similar response rate as seen in high-dose IL-2

Phase 1 and 2 studies showed that response rates were 6-30%. Retrospective series showed that 15% and 20% response rates, but these results are not statistically significant. Nevertheless, mean survival is a little bit meaningful (9.1 vs 13 mos).

4.6 Targeted therapies

Since more new agents have been produced and limited number of prospective, randomized, placebo-controlled studies have been reported, Therefore, we have evaluated only;

1. Sorafenib (Nexavar®)
2. Sunitinib (Sutent®)
3. Bevasizumab (Avastin®) + IFN-alfa

4.   Temsirolimus (Torisel®) in this review

Sorafenib and/or sunitinib, a multikinase inhibitor of tumor-cell prolferation and angiogenesis, have been shown some activity, in two double blind, placebo-controlled trial in patients with metastatic renal cell ca. All the patients' histology were clear cell ca (24,25). Renal cell carcinoma is most aggressive and mortal genitourinary cancer with more than 40% of patients dying of cancer (26). Unfortunately, no reliable treatment alternative has been still conducted for especially metastatic RCC. Recently, investigations in targeted therapy including multikinase inhibition and antiangioenesis encouraged the clinicans that they have some activity in the management of metastatic RCC. Survival benefit with the targeted therapy was demonstrated in two double blind, placebo-controlled study in the treatment of metastatic disease (24,25). Nevertheless, there are still many unresponded questions. Response rate in different histological type is not clear. We have administered sorafenib in a patient with metastatic RCC with sarcomatoid differentiation and obtained excellent result.

This case report might be an evidence that antiangiogenic agents can be used in any histologic type of renal cell carcinoma.

Additional data on the durability of the response may further clarify the complete response and survival benefit

Inactive VHL gene

↓
HIF-1-alfa↑
↓
HIF-alpha/HIF-beta complex ↑
↓
Hypoxia induced gene transcription
↓   ↓   ↓   ↓
VGEF↑ PDGF-beta↑ TGF-alpha↑ Erythropoietin ↑

Fig. 2. Loss of VHL gene and pathways

Small molecule inhibitors have mainly targeted growth factor signals, cell cycle regulatory factors and angiogenesis. Growth factors like VGEF and PDGF have been effective by transmembrane tyrzin kinase receptors which expressed in endothelial cells. They have triggered autophosphorilazition of intracellular tyrozin kinase receptors and protein activation link with the attachment of extracellular parts of receptors. Recently many small molecule inhibitors have been discovered (27,28,29). Raf kinase inhibitors like sorafenib and sunitinib, multiple kinase like VEGFR-2, VEGFR-3 and PDGFR inhibitors or mTOR inhibitors like temsirolimus, everolimus and epidermal growth factor receptor tyrosine kinase inhibitors like erlotinib and lapatinib are the most popular molecules nowadays

(30,31). Nevertheless, still prospective, placebo-controlled studies are significantly lacking in describing the most effective treatment modality in the management of metastatic RCC (32).

5. Conclusion

Cytotoxic chemotherapy and immunotherapy are less effective treatment modalities in the management of metastatic RCC. However, better understanding of promotion of RCC caused newly produced many targeted therapies. Now, it is early to say that newly introduced drugs can solve the problem, but they are encouraging. .Due to SWOG and EORTC studies which are the most reliable studies in the literature, still primary nephrectomy and combination immunotherapy modalities are the only acceptable choice in patients with good performance status for the treatment of metastatic RCC.

6. References

[1] Russo P. Renal cell carcinoma: Presentation, staging and surgical treatment. Semin Oncol 2000; 27: 160-176.

[2] Russo P. Partial nephrectomy: The contemporary gold standard operation for T1 renal masses. Am J Urol Rev 2004; 2: 214-222.

[3] Chan DY, Marshall FF. Surgery in advanced and metastatic renal cell carcinoma. Curr Opin Urol 1998; 8(5): 369-373.

[4] Motzer RJ, Russo P. Systemic therapy for renal cell carcinoma. J Urol 2000; 163: 408-417.

[5] Russo P. Surgical intervention in patients with metastatic renal cancer: current status of metastasectomy and cytoreductive nephrectomy. Nat Clin Prac Urol 2004; 1(1): 26-30.

[6] Walther MM, Yang JC, Pass HI et al. Cytoreductive surgery before high dose IL-2 based therapy in patients with metastatic renal cell carcinoma. J Urol, 1997; 158:1675-78

[7] Rackley R, Novick AC, Klein EA. The impact of adjuvant nephrectomy on multimodality treatment of metastatic renal cell carcinoma J Urol. 1994; 152:1399-403

[8] Sella A et al Surgery following response to interferon-alpha-based therapy for residual renal cell carcinoma. J Urol 1993; 149 (1): 19-21.

[9] Freed SZ, Halperin JP, Gordon M. Idioppathic regression of metastases from renal cell carcinoma. J Urol 1977; 118 (4): 538-542.

[10] Marcus SG et al. Regression of metastatic renal cell carcinoma after cytoreductive nephrectomy. J Urol 1993; 150 (2): 463-466.

[11] Mickisch GHJ. Rational selection of a control arm for randomized trials in metastatic renal cell carcinoma. Eur Urol 2003; 43: 670-9.

[12] Wagner JR et al. Interleukin-2 based immunotherapy for metastatic renal cell carcinoma with the kidney in place. J Urol 1999; 162 (1): 43-45.

[13] Bennett RT, Lerner SE, Taub HC. Cytoreductive surgery for stage IV renal cell carcinoma J Urol, 1995; 154: 32-4.

[14] Krishnamurthi V, Novick AC, Bukowski RM. Efficacy of multimodality therapy in advanced RCC. Urology 1998; 51:933-7.

[15] Finelli A, Kaouk JH, Fergany AF et al. BJU International 2004; 94(3): 291-4.

[16] Wood CG. The role of cytoreductive nephrectomy in the management of metastatic renal cell carcinoma. Urol Clin N Am 2003; 30:581-588.

[17] Mickisch G, Garin A, van Poppel H et al. Radical nephrectomy plus interferon-alfa-based immunotherapy compared with interferon-alfa alone in metastatic renal cell carcinoma: a randomized trial. Lancet 2001; 358: 966-970.

[18] Flanigan RC, Salmon SE, Blumenstein BA et al. Nephrectomy followed by interferon-alfa-2b compared with interferon alfa-2b alone for metastatic renal cell cancer. N Eng J Med, 2001; 345: 1655-9.

[19] Flanigan RC, Mickisch G, Sylvester R et al. Cytoreductive nephrectomy in patients with metastatic renal cancer: A combined analysis. J Urol, 2004; 171:1071-1076.

[20] Kierney PC, van heerden JA, Segura JW et al. Surgeon`s role in the management of solitary renal cell carcinoma metastases occuring subsequent to initial curative nephrectomy: an institutional review. Ann Surg Oncol 1994; 1:345-352.

[21] Han KR, Pantuck AJ, Bui MH et al. Number of metastatic sites rather than location dictates overall survival of patients with node-negative metastatic renal cell carcinoma. Urology 2003; 61: 314-9.

[22] Kavolius JP, Mastrorakos DP, Pavlovich C et al. Resection of metastatic renal cell carcinoma J Clin Oncol 1998; 16: 2261-6.

[23] Swanson DA. Surgery for metastases of renal cell carcinoma. Scand J Surg 2004; 93: 150-5.

[24] Pirrotta MT, Bernardeschi P, Fiorentini G. Targeted-therapy in advanced renal cell carcinoma..Curr Med Chem. 2011;18(11):1651-7.

[25] Hutson TE. Targeted therapies for the treatment of metastatic renal cell carcinoma: clinical evidence.. Oncologist. 2011;16 Suppl 2:14-22.

[26] Facchini G, Perri F, Caraglia M, Pisano C, Striano S, Marra L, Fiore F, Aprea P, Pignata S, Iaffaioli RV New treatment approaches in renal cell carcinoma.. Anticancer Drugs. 2009 Nov;20(10):893-900.

[27] Escudier B Signaling inhibitors in metastatic renal cell carcinoma.. Cancer J. 2008 Sep-Oct;14(5):325-9.

[28] Mizutani Y Recent advances in molecular targeted therapy for metastatic renal cell carcinoma.. Int J Urol. 2009 May;16(5):444-8.

[29] Motzer RJ, Bukowski RM Targeted therapy for metastatic renal cell carcinoma.. J Clin Oncol. 2006 Dec 10;24(35):5601-8.

[30] Di Lorenzo G, Scagliarini S, Di Napoli M, Scognamiglio F, Rizzo M, Carteni' G Targeted therapy in the treatment of metastatic renal cell cancer.. Oncology. 2009;77 Suppl 1:122-31.

[31] Motzer RJ, Escudier B, Oudard S, Hutson TE, Porta C, Bracarda S, Grünwald V, Thompson JA, Figlin RA, Hollaender N, Urbanowitz G, Berg WJ, Kay A, Lebwohl D, Ravaud A; RECORD-1 Study Group Efficacy of everolimus in advanced renal cell carcinoma: a double-blind, randomised, placebo-controlled phase III trial. Lancet. 2008 Aug 9;372(9637):449-56.

[32] Patard JJ, Pouessel D, Bensalah K, Culine S Targeted therapy in renal cell carcinoma. World J Urol. 2008 Apr;26(2):135-40.

9

Prognostic Factors in Renal Cell Carcinoma: An Evaluation of T-Stage, Histopathological Grade, p53, Ki-67, COX-2, and Her-2 Expressions

Minna Kankuri-Tammilehto
Department of Oncology and Radiotherapy,
Turku University Hospital,
Finland

1. Introduction

Kidney cancer[1] represents 2-3% of all diagnosed malignancies worldwide although in some Northern and Central European countries the incidence is higher, even 4-5% (Ferlay, 2010). Kidney cancer is responsible for approximately 116,000 deaths per year worldwide (Ferlay, 2010). In the European Union (EU), the annual number of new kidney cancers was 73 171 in 2008 (Ferlay, 2010). The majority of renal cell carcinomas (RCCs) arise from the cells of renal proximal tubules of nephrons, but 5% of cases from the cells of the collecting ducts (Chao *et al.* 2002, Kovacs *et al.* 1997, Störkel *et al.* 1997) (Figure 1.). Renal tumors are members of a complex family with unique histology, cytogenetic defects and variable metastatic potential (Linehan *et al.* 2003, Thoenes *et al.* 1986). Of all RCCs, 70-80% is of conventional type, also known as clear cell RCCs. Of these, approximately 75% have a mutation in the von Hippel-Lindau tumor suppressor gene (*VHL*), in the short arm of chromosome 3 (Maxwell *et al.* 1999, Gnarra *et al.* 1994).

The annual increase in RCC incidence has been 2-4% since the 1970s (Finnish Cancer Registry 2007, American Cancer Society 2004, Mathew *et al.* 2002). This has been attributed to the use of radiological imaging which is able to find presymptomatic RCC lesions (Jayson and Sanders 1998), as well as the increased prevalence of etiologic risk factors, such as obesity (Chow *et al.* 2000) and cigarette smoking (Hunt *et al.* 2005). The increase has been highest in localized disease, especially in tumors with less than 4 cm in diameter (Hollingsworth *et al.* 2006). 30-60% of RCC tumors are found incidentally in abdominal imaging performed for some other reason than suspected renal tumor, such as the evaluation of non-specific musculoskeletal or abdominal complaints (Jayson and Sanders 1998). Macroscopic hematuria, palpable tumor and pain, together called the classic triad in RCC, indicate metastatic disease (Cunningham 1938). Metastatic disease is seen in 20-30% of RCC patients at diagnosis (Janzen *et al.* 2003, Mc

---

[1] In epidemiological statistics, RCC and renal pelvis cancer are usually not reported separately, but combined under the heading of kidney cancer (Parkin *et al.* 2003).

Nichols *et al.* 1981). Half of the patients diagnosed with local RCC will later have a recurrence of their cancer: two thirds within the first year (Janzen *et al.* 2003), and the majority within five years (Lam *et al.* 2005, McNichols *et al.* 1981). The risk for late recurrence, at over 10 years from nephrectomy, is at least 10% (McNichols *et al.* 1981).

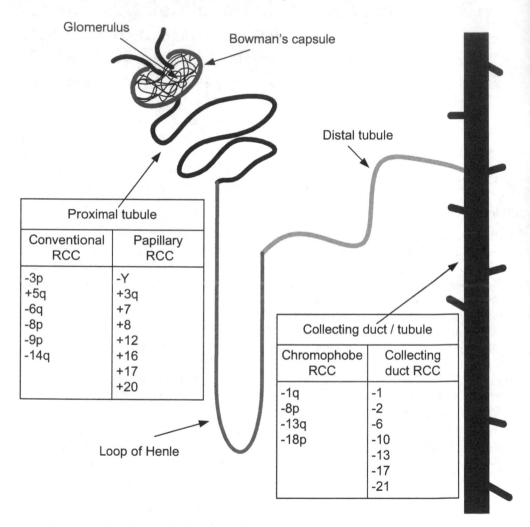

Proximal tubule	
Conventional RCC	Papillary RCC
-3p	-Y
+5q	+3q
-6q	+7
-8p	+8
-9p	+12
-14q	+16
	+17
	+20

Collecting duct / tubule	
Chromophobe RCC	Collecting duct RCC
-1q	-1
-8p	-2
-13q	-6
-18p	-10
	-13
	-17
	-21

The number reflects the chromosome in which its genetic aberration is located.

- means loss of function.
+ means gain of function.
p is the short arm of the chromosome.
q is the long arm of the chromosome.

Fig. 1. The genetic changes that characterize the different RCC subtypes according to the Heidelberg classification (Modified from Bodmer *et al.* 2002).

Prognostic Factors in Renal Cell Carcinoma: An Evaluation of T-Stage, Histopathological Grade, p53, Ki-67, COX-2, and Her-2 Expressions

159

For those RCC patients with performance status enabling current treatments the expected five-year survival rate is slightly higher than 60% (Parkin et al. 2003). According to a few previous studies on long-term outcome for metastatic RCC (mRCC), the five-year survival is from 3% to 16% (Atzpodien et al. 2002, Motzer et al. 2000, Minasian et al. 1993) if metastasectomy has not been a possible treatment. For localized RCC, nephrectomy is the only curative treatment (Robson et al. 2002), and currently there is no adjuvant therapy in RCC. Possible treatments for mRCC, in addition to cytoreductive nephrectomy (Flanigan et al. 2001, Mickisch et al. 2001), are immunomodulators, such as interferon-α (IFN-α) (Kankuri et al. 2001, Pyrhönen et al. 1999), interleukin-2 (IL-2) (Négrier et al. 2007), and more recently tyrosine kinase inhibitors, such as sunitinib (Motzer et al. 2007), sorafenib (Escudier et al. 2007), and mTOR inhibitor temsirolimus (Hudes et al. 2007). Everolimus, another mTOR inhibitor, has an encouraging antitumor activity against mRCC (Motzer et al. 2008). The efficacy of bevacizumab, an antiangiogenesis monoclonal antibody, has also been shown when used with IFN-α (Bracarda et al. 2011, Rini et al. 2010, Yang et al. 2003). The Food and Drug Administration (FDA) and EU have also approved pazopanib, an angiogenesis inhibitor, with advanced RCC due to the efficacy of it in RCC (Sternberg et al. 2010). Ongoing clinical trials are addressing the role of targeted agents in adjuvant therapy in RCC (Choueiri et al. 2011). The efficacy of many potent novel targeted agents in RCC is under investigation in phase II and III trials, among these axitinib, a multitargeted tyrosine kinase receptor inhibitor (Goldstein et al. 2010), tivozanib, a pan-VEGFR tyrosine kinase inhibitor (De Luca and Normanno 2010), and ipilimumab, an anti-CTLA4 antibody (Yang et al. 2007). Additionally, vaccine therapy in RCC is being studied (Rini et al. 2011). The stabilization of the disease has been shown to be beneficial for the survival of mRCC patients (Thiam et al. 2010, Kankuri et al. 2001).

2. Staging and prognostic factors in RCC

2.1 Pathological tumor staging

In the 1960's, Robson et al, created the staging system based on physical characteristics and tumor spread with the addition of tumor venous invasion (Robson et al. 2002). The poor correlation between the different Robson stages and survival led to the recommendation to use the TNM (tumor, node, metastases) staging system. Since 1978, the TNM classification system for the extent of the tumor spread has integrated characteristics such as tumor size, vascular involvement, nodal spread and distant metastases (Bassil et al. 1985, Harmen 1978). pTNM classification system was updated by the Union Internationale Contre le Cancer (UICC) and the American Joint Committee on Cancer (AJCC) in 1997 when the cut-off between T1 and T2 tumors was increased from 2.5 cm to 7 cm, in order to increase the difference in survival from these two tumor types. Analysis of outcome in nephrectomized patients showed that the 1997 TNM-system cut-off point between T1 and T2 tumors is too high, and a cut-off point of 4.5 – 5.0 cm has been suggested (Elmore et al. 2003, Zisman et al. 2001). In 2002, the pTNM classification system was revised: T1 was divided into T1a and T1b by a cut-off point of 4 cm, according to the suitability for partial nephrectomy, and prognostication (Sobin and Wittekind 2002, Guinan et al. 1997). A uniform staging classification, the TNM staging system, has improved the division of patients into radical or partial nephrectomy candidates. Additionally, it has increased the co-operation between oncologists and pathologists concerning the outcome of RCC patients (Janzen et al. 2003, Javidan et al. 1999). Howerer, modifications in the TNM system may cause difficulty in comparing outcome data in different studies (Belldegrun et al. 1999, Störkel et al. 1989).

Pathological tumor stage (T-stage) has been observed to be the most important factor for locally confined RCC in predicting the survival of patients who have undergone nephrectomy (Kankuri et al. 2006, Delahunt et al. 2002). The observed five-year survival is approximately 75-80% for stage T1, 55% for T2, 40% for T3, and 20-30% for T4 (Sunela et al. 2009, Tsui et al. 2000). For patients with stage I disease (tumor confined to the kidney) the five-year survival is approximately 90%, and for those with stage I and histologic of chromophobe type it is almost 100% (Zisman et al. 2001). The five-year survival rate for stage III disease is approximately 50% (Zisman et al. 2001). There is an 80% difference in survival rates between patients with local disease compared to those with advanced disease and distant metastases (American Cancer Society 2004). In a retrospective review of 2 473 RCC patients from 1975 - 1985, regardless of T-stage, tumor size was observed to have an inverse association with survival (Guinan et al. 1995). In the study of Kankuri et al. (2006), in the analysis of those RCC patients who later developed metastatic disease, high T-stage caused twice the risk of metastatic disease and three times the risk of death compared with low T-stage which indicates that as the tumor size increases, the more aggressive its growth becomes and the more probable is tumor cell dissemination. T-stage is a prognostic factor for both metastases-free and overall survival in RCC patients.

T-stage can be used in estimating the correct duration and frequency of surveillance of RCC patients after nephrectomy. RCC with a diameter of less than 3.0 cm grows slowly; only 2.5% have metastases during the first three years (Bosniak et al. 1995). Therefore, in the treatment of those in whom surgery is contraindicated, careful monitoring (watchful waiting) by computed tomography (CT scan) may be used (Roberts et al. 2005, Bosniak et al. 1995). Previously, it has been suggested that T-stage is not an important prognostic factor in the survival of patients who have neither lymph node nor distant metastases (Giuliani et al. 1990). The therapeutic value of lymph node dissection remains unproven (Mickish 1999). T-stage alone has been pointed to be a valuable prognostic factor for survival, even when the status of lymph nodes is unknown (Kankuri et al. 2006). Additionally, a high T-stage has been used as an inclusion criterion for adjuvant treatments in trials (Atzpodien et al. 2005, Repmann et al. 2003).

Moreover, T-stage is an independent prognostic factor in mRCC patients (Kankuri-Tammilehto et al. 2010). In the study of Kankuri-Tammilehto et al. (2010) high T-stage caused twice the risk of death compared with low T-stage in mRCC. The association between T-stage and overall survival was also found in those with primary metastases at the time of nephrectomy (Kankuri et al. 2006). T-stage is not typically used in prognostic models in mRCC, a UCLA model (Zisman et al. 2002) being an exception. T-stage seems to be a good tool in prognostic evaluation in mRCC patients and could be included in prognostic models.

2.2 Histopathological tumor grading

In grading systems, the major criteria are nuclear and nucleolar appearances, while in some systems, tumor architecture and cell type is also included (Mostofi et al. 1998, Goldstein 1997, Fuhrman et al. 1982, Syrjänen and Hjelt 1978, Skinner et al. 1971). The WHO grading system is based on the size and prominence of nucleoli (Eble et al. 2004, Mostofi et al. 1998), while the Fuhrman grading system is based on nuclear size, shape, and presence or absence of nucleoli (Fuhrman et al. 1982). The WHO grading system contains three grades, whereas the Fuhrman contains four.

Prognostic Factors in Renal Cell Carcinoma: An Evaluation of T-Stage, Histopathological Grade, p53, Ki-67,
COX-2, and Her-2 Expressions

161

Several studies have failed to demonstrate any statistically significant differences in the survival of patients with different grades, when all three or four grades are analyzed separately (Kankuri et al. 2006, Rioux-Leclercq et al. 2000, Usubutyn et al. 1998, Selli et al. 1983) although when analyzing only the highest and the lowest grades the statistically significant difference in survival have been found (Kankuri et al. 2006). This is partly because, as yet, no consensus has been reached on a universal tumor grading system (Kanamaru et al. 2001, Medeiros et al. 1997). The observed five-year disease-specific survival (DSS) rate is approximately 90% for G1, 70-85% for G2, 45-60% for G3, and 15-30% for G4 (Gudbjartsson et al. 2005, Ficarra et al. 2001). Currently, different grading systems are utilized at different institutions. Tumor-grading systems have been criticized because of their subjectivity in tumor evaluations (Lanigan et al. 1994), and comparison of different patient cases with respect to histopathological grade is difficult. More quantitative measures which describe the size or the shape of the nuclei have been requested by pathologists. In 1997, an international consensus conference on RCC by UICC and AJCC outlined recommendations for the grading of RCC (Goldstein 1997): the grading system should be based on standardized and reproducible criteria that reflect the heterogeneity of nuclear and nucleolar features within a tumor, and each grade should result in significant differences in patient outcome. Recently again, a joint group of urologists and pathologists has published a proposal that the criteria for nuclear grading should be different for the different histopathologic subtypes of RCC according to the Heidelberg classification (Paner et al. 2006). Additionally, reducing the grades in the Fuhrman system has been proposed, for better outcome stratification (Rioux-Leclercq et al. 2007, Lohse et al. 2002, Bretheau et al. 1995). Overall, histopathological grade seem to be imprecise for prognostic evaluation in RCC patients (Uchida et al. 2002, Rioux-Leclercq et al. 2000, Lanigan et al. 1994).

2.3 Heidelberg and WHO classifications for typing of renal tumors

In Heidelberg, in October 1996, the morphology was combined with genetic findings for a new classification, called the Heidelberg classification of renal tumors, in a workshop organized by the UICC and the AJCC (Kovacs et al. 1997, Störkel et al. 1997). In addition to this, in 2004, WHO published the reassessed classification which is now based on both genetic and pathological abnormalities (Eble et al. 2004). Progress in our knowledge of genetic alterations leads to new suggestions for RCC entities (Eble 2003). With the progress of research, the Heidelberg classification may lead to more specific treatments in different subgroups of RCC patients. The 5-year DSS for locally confined RCC is for chromophobe RCC approximately 87-100%, for papillary RCC 87%, and for conventional RCC 70-75% (Cheville et al. 2003, Amin et al. 2002). In the case of sarcomatoid change, the survival decreases with the 5-year DSS of 35% (Amin et al. 2002). A very rare entity of collecting duct RCC is highly aggressive with highly decreased prognosis (Antonelli et al. 2003). The prognostic power of the Heidelberg classification has been investigated. The current Heidelberg classification does not have independent prognostic ability, and thus it should not be considered as a major prognostic variable comparable to T-stage and histopathological tumor grade (Patard et al. 2005). However, Heidelberg classification associates with metastases development, indicating that unclassified tumor type metastasizes with high probability (Kankuri et al. 2006). In future, with the progress of research, the Heidelberg classification may lead to more specific treatments in different subgroups of RCC patients (Störkel et al. 1997).

2.4 Prognostic models in RCC

The heterogeneity of RCC within the same T-stage and grade (Tsui et al. 2000) has resulted in a need for prognostic models for prognostication and treatment modality selection. Prognostic models, anagrams and nomograms, have been developed to find those nephrectomized RCC patients who potentially have a long-term recurrence-free interval and survival, as well as those mRCC patients who have long-term survival (Table 1.). The most often represented as an independent prognostic factors in metastatic RCC (mRCC) are performance status, time to metastases, number of metastatic sites, and prior nephrectomy. Therapies for mRCC cause a wide variety of adverse effects, which reduce the quality of life. Determining the prognostic factors for survival in mRCC patients is valuable in directing therapy for those patients who would benefit from it. Several models have been developed for predicting the likelihood of response to therapy and to predict survival. However, novel biomarkers are hoped to specify the diagnosis, staging, and prognosis and to guide targeted cancer therapies. Molecular tumor markers are expected to revolutionize the staging of RCC in the future (Srigley et al. 1997), as nowadays stratifying the patients into risk groups is largely done on the basis of clinopathological factors, e.g. clinical stage of the disease. Still, all the molecular mechanisms that affect the development, progression and clinical behavior of RCC are not known. Advances in the understanding of the pathogenesis, behavior, and molecular biology of RCC may help to better predict tumor prognosis, and thus improve survival of RCC carcinoma patients when a more tailored therapy can be given to each individual patient. Molecular biomarkers, such as p53, Ki-67 and COX-2, are candidates for defining prognostic subgroups (Delahunt et al. 2002), and for guiding targeted therapies (Masters 2007), as shown in the studies, where p53, Ki-67 and COX-2 had prognostic value in predicting survival. The following chapters describe in more detail about the value of them in the prognosis in RCC.

3. Biomarkers related to molecular mechanism in RCC

3.1 pVHL, von Hippel-Lindau protein, mudulator of hypoxic response

pVHL, a tumor suppressor gene product, is expressed especially in the kidney's proximal renal tubule (Corless et al. 1997, Iliopoulos et al. 1995). Approximately 61-75% of sporadic conventional RCCs contain mutations in VHL, in the short arm of chromosome 3 (3p25-26) (van Houwelingen et al. 2005, Maxwell et al. 1999, Gnarra et al. 1994,), of which 50% show loss of heterozygosity (LOH) (Kovacs et al. 1997, Gnarra et al. 1994) and 10-20% silencing of the wild-type allele by promoter hypermethylation (Herman et al. 1994). VHL is associated with carcinogenesis. The function of pVHL is ubiquitylation of hypoxia-inducible factor (HIF); therefore, it modulates the hypoxic response; VHL protein can bind to hypoxia inducible factor-1 alpha (HIF-1α) and target this factor for destruction in the presence of oxygen. HIF in turn controls the expression of several proteins, including carbonic anhydrase 9 (CA9) and proteins involved in angiogenesis, i.e. vascular endothelial growth factor (VEGF) and EPO, via oxygen-dependent ubiquitination (van Houwelingen et al. 2005, George and Kaelin 2003). Normally, VHL down regulates vascular endothelial growth factor (VEGF) by different pathways. In VHL-defective cancer cells, increased concentrations of VEGF and EPO are observed.

Reference	Year	No. of Patients	Therapy Administered	Tumor Subtype	Prognostic Factors	Prognostic Information
Motzer *et al.* (MSKCC)	2002	463	IFN-α	All	Performance status, time from diagnosis to start of therapy, LDH, hemoglobin, corrected calcium	Survival
Zisman *et al.* (UCLA)	2002	262	IL-2 or IFN-α (197 pts), other (65 pts)	All	T-stage, nodal involvement, nuclear grade, no. of symptoms, immunotherapy	Survival
Négrier *et al.* (Group Francais d'Immunother apie)	2002	782	IFN-α ± IL-2	All	Performance status, no. of metastatic sites, disease-free interval, signs of inflammation, hemoglobin	Survival, rapid progression
Atzpodien (Medizinische Hochschule Hannover)	2003	425	IFN-α + IL-2 ± 5-FU ± 13CRA	All	Neutrophil count , LDH, CRP, time from diagnosis to start of therapy, no. of metastatic sites, bone metastases	Survival
Motzer *et al.* (MSKCC)	2004	251	New agents	All, if cytokine refractory disease	Performance status, hemoglobin, corrected calcium	Survival for those who enter clinical trials of new agents
Choueiri *et al.* (Cleveland Clinic Foundation)	2007	358	IFN-α ± IL-2 ± chemotherapy	All	Performance status, hemoglobin, no. of metastatic sites, involved kidney of primary tumor	Long-term survival
Cho et al (Yonsei University)	2008	197	Immunotherapy	All	Performance status, N stage, no. of metastatic sites, sarcomatoid differentiation, liver metastasis	Survival
Motzer *et al.* (MSKCC)	2008	375	Sunitinib	Conventional RCC	Performance status, time from diagnosis to start of therapy, nephrectomy status, no. of metastatic sites, presence of liver or lung metastases, LDH, corrected calcium, hemoglobin, alkaline phosphatase, thrombosytosis	Probability of 12-month progression-free survival

LDH=lactate dehydrogenase
MSKCC = Memorial Sloan Kettering Cancer Center
UCLA = University of California

Table 1. Prognostic algorithms and nomograms for survival in mRCC between 2000 and 2008.

3.2 CA9, hypoxia associated enzyme

CA9, a member of the carbonic anhydrase family, is suggested to play a role in the regulation of cell proliferation in response to hypoxic conditions. Low CA9 expression associates with the absence of VHL mutation and aggressive tumor characteristics in conventional RCC (Pantuck *et al.* 2007). CA9 may indicate those patients who benefit from IL-2, as low CA9 expression associates with lower survival compared to high CA9 expression in mRCC patients who receive IL-2 (Atkins *et al.* 2005, Bui *et al.* 2003). It has also been suggested that CA9 may indicate those patients who benefit from CA9-targeted therapies. It is also being investigated whether CA9 may indicate those patients who are potential candidates for adjuvant therapy.

3.3 p53, biomarker of cell cycle point

p53, a tumor suppressor gene product, is a promoter of cell growth arrest and apoptosis (Choisy-Rossi and Yonish-Rouach 1998). Activated p53 elicits several cellular responses, including apoptosis and cell cycle arrest (Reich and Levine 1984), and responds to DNA damage at the restriction checkpoint of the G1 phase of the cell cycle (May and May 1999). In normal cells, p53 is usually undetectable (Finlay *et al.* 1988). Mutant p53 accumulates in cell nuclei and can be immunostained (Reich and Levine 1984), whereas wild-type p53, because of its short half-life, is usually undetectable by routine immunohistochemistry (Reich and Levine 1984). p53 accumulation and increased cell proliferative activity are parallel phenomena in RCC (Kankuri *et al.* 2006, Pinto *et al.* 2005). p53 may be upregulated in part by VHL, accounting for some of the tumor suppressive functions of VHL in RCC (Galban *et al.* 2003). p53 seems to associate weakly with tumor grade, as the association was seen only in univariate analysis. Nor was an association between p53 and grade observed in a previous microarray study (Zigeuner *et al.* 2004). In both studies, the nuclear grade was determined according to the WHO guidelines.

Published results on the association of p53 with survival have been controversial, some studies suggesting positive p53 associating with poor survival (Shvarts *et al.* 2005 , Zigeuner *et al.* 2004, Uchida *et al.* 2002, Haitel *et al.* 2000), while others have observed no association (Itoi *et al.* 2004, Olumi *et al.* 2001, Rioux-Leclercq *et al.* 2000, Hofmockel *et al.* 1996). In the study of Phuoc *et al.* (2007), p53 was significantly associated with survival in univariate analysis, but the association was not independent. In a tissue array study on metastasized patients, overexpression of p53 was associated with impaired DSS in renal carcinoma (Kim *et al.* 2004). In some studies, the association of p53 and survival has been investigated in a group of RCC patients with both locally confined and primary metastatic RCC; thus, patient selection varies in different studies (Olumi *et al.* 2001). The study of Kankuri *et al.* (2006) indicates that p53 is not able to predict which patients will develop metastatic disease after nephrectomy, but interestingly, they predict poor survival in mRCC patients (Figure 2.). Therefore, p53 can help in determining metastatic patients with a poor prognosis and, e.g. those who might benefit from aggressive treatment, such as high-dose interleukin-2 (Spanknebel *et al.* 2005) or temsirolimus (Hudes *et al.* 2007).

3.4 Ki-67, proliferation marker

Ki-67, a proliferation biomarker, is expressed throughout the active phases of the cell cycle, and serves as a good marker for proliferative activity in cell nuclei (Gerdes *et al.* 1984). Ki-67 accumulates during the cell cycle from G1 to mitosis, and is at its lowest level after mitosis (du Manoir *et al.* 1991). The percentage of nuclei staining by immunohistochemistry reflects Ki-67 expression (Olumi *et al.* 2001). An association between Ki-67 and high T-stage and metastases development have been observed

Prognostic Factors in Renal Cell Carcinoma: An Evaluation of T-Stage, Histopathological Grade, p53, Ki-67, COX-2, and Her-2 Expressions

165

(Kankuri *et al.* 2006, Dudderidge *et al.* 2005, Rioux-Leclercq *et al.* 2000), indicating that Ki-67 is a marker for aggressive disease in RCC with an increased risk of early metastases development. Ki-67 has been reported to independently predict survival following nephrectomy in many studies (Dudderidge *et al.* 2005, Bui *et al.* 2004, Itoi *et al.* 2004, Rioux-Leclercq *et al.* 2000, Aaltomaa *et al.* 1997). Ki-67 has been observed to increase in sarcomatoid change (Kanamaru *et al.* 1999), indicating different protein expression profiles in different entities according to the Heidelberg classification.

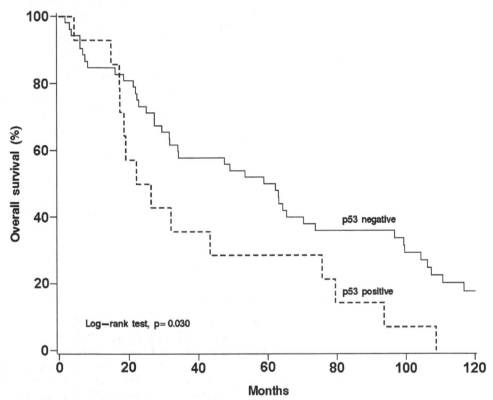

Fig. 2. Kaplan-Meier survival curve for p53 in mRCC (n=66) (Kankuri *et al.* 2006).

Dudderidge *et al.* (2005) found Ki-67 to be an independent prognostic factor for disease-free survival in nephrectomized RCC, but opposite results have also been published (Donskov *et al.* 2004, Kim *et al.* 2004, Yildiz *et al.* 2004). No association between Ki-67 alone and survival in locally confined RCC patients was found in the study of Kankuri *et al.* (2006). The differences in the classification of metastases are seen: Kim and coworkers (2004) classified both distant and local lymph node metastases as metastatic disease, whereas in the study of Kankuri *et al.* (2006), only tumors with distant metastases were classified as metastatic. However, Ki-67 predicts poor survival in mRCC patients (Figure 3.). Therefore, in addition to p53, Ki-67 can help in determining metastatic patients with a poor prognosis and, e.g. those who might benefit from aggressive treatment.

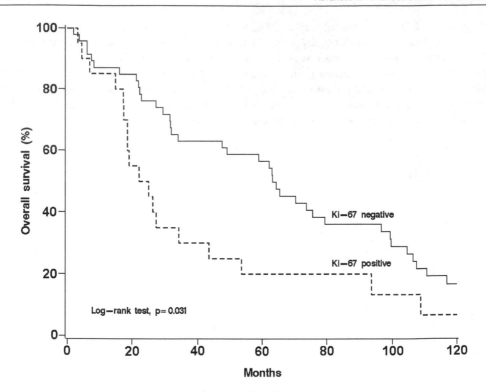

Fig. 3. Kaplan-Meier survival curve for Ki-67 in mRCC (n=66) (Kankuri *et al.* 2006).

3.5 COX-2, biomarker for inflammation and neoplasia

Cyclo-oxygenase-2 (COX-2), an isoform of the COX[3] enzyme, is an inducible form of an enzyme involved in the first steps of prostaglandins and thromboxane synthesis. COX-2 converts arachidonic acid first into prostaglandin G2, and afterwards by peroxidase activity into prostaglandin H_2, a precursor of the prostaglandins (Taketo 1998). COX-2 is suggested to play a physiological role in fetal nephrogenesis (Khan *et al.* 2001). COX-2 increases in inflammation and neoplasia (Miyata *et al.* 2003, Hara *et al.* 2002, Nose *et al.* 2002, *et al.* Taketo 1998), and is undetectable in most normal tissues (Mungan *et al.* 2006, Yoshimura *et al.* 2004). The conversion of procarcinogens to proximate carcinogens is catalyzed by the peroxidase activity of COX-2 (Elinq *et al.* 1990). COX-2 is highly induced by stimulus of oncogenes, cytokines, growth factors, and tumor promoters (Smith *et al.* 2000, Herschman 1996, Subbaramaiah *et al.* 1996). Associations between COX-2 over-expression and antiapoptotic ability, tumor invasiveness, tumor growth, angiogenesis, and immunosuppression, as well as multidrug resistance in cancer have been reported (Cao and Prescott 2002, Masferrer *et al.* 2000, Subbramaiah *et al.* 1996, Tsujii and DuBois 1995).

Cytoplasmic/membranous COX-2 staining by immunohistochemistry reflects COX-2 protein expression (Cho *et al.* 2005). The study results on associations of COX-2 with tumor stage, grade, and survival have been contradictory. Yoshimura *et al.* (2004) demonstrated that COX-2 was expressed at its highest in G1, as well as in pT1 RCC tumors, compared to other RCC tumors in grade and T-stage, while in Hashimoto *et al*'s study (2004), more COX-2 was found at the higher tumor grade, as well as stage. Kankuri-Tammilehto *et al*. (2010) found no association between COX-2 and tumor grade or T-stage. A significant association has been observed between COX-2 and Ki-67 expression in the study of Miyata *et al*. (2003), whereas Kankuri-Tammilehto *et al*. (2010) found no association between them. No association between COX-2 and p53 has been found in studies (Kankuri-Tammilehto *et al*. 2010, Cho *et al*. 2005).

Kankuri-Tammilehto *et al*. (2010) found that the proportion of COX-2 positive tumors is highest in RCC with the ability to develop later metastases, when compared to both RCC without metastatic potential and RCC with primary metastases. This finding was new. Previously, Miyata *et al*. (2003) observed that positive COX-2 expression associated with primary metastases in univariate analysis (when M0-patients were compared to M1-patients). Cho *et al*. (2005) found no association between positive COX-2 expression and metastases (when M0-patients were compared to M1-patients, or appearance of metastatic disease was compared to non-metastatic disease). In those studies, the method of analysis differs from that of the study of Kankuri-Tammilehto *et al*. (2010), where patients were divided into three categories according to the appearance of metastases. According to the study of Kankuri-Tammilehto *et al*. (2010), metastases-free survival is longer in patients with COX-2 positive tumors. The median metastases-free survival was 46 months in RCC with COX-2 positivity compared to 15 months in RCC with COX-2 negativity (Figure 4.). These

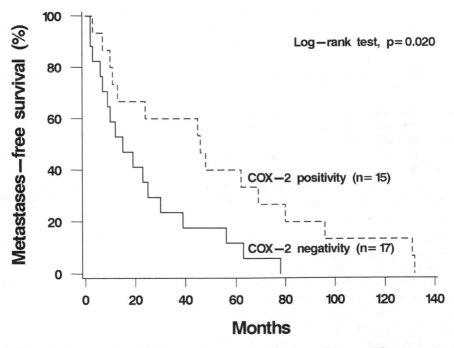

Fig. 4. The prognostic value of COX-2 for metastases-free survival from nephrectomy in RCC patients who later developed metastatic disease (n=32, Kaplan-Meier method): the median metastases-free survival time was 46 months with COX-2 positivity, and 15 months with COX-2 negativity (Kankuri-Tammilehto *et al*. 2010).

results indicate that COX-2 positivity associates with the delay of metastatic formation in RCC patients who do not have disseminated disease at presentation, and that COX-2 negativity associates with an aggressive phenotype in mRCC disease.

Few studies have reported the results of an association between COX-2 expression and survival in RCC patients. Previously, Miyata *et al.* (2003) found that the five-year survival of patients with COX-2 positive tumors from nephrectomy was 66%, and of COX-2 negative patients 91% (Miyata *et al.* 2003). In Miyata's study, the patients were 86% M0 and 14% M1 at nephrectomy. Previously, no results of COX-2 and overall survival in mRCC patients have been published. The study of Kankuri-Tammilehto *et al.* (2010) indicates that COX-2 positivity predicts improved overall survival in patients with mRCC treated with IFN-α. This is in line with the previous study of Rini *et al.* (2006), in which COX-2 positivity associated with longer time to progression in the patients treated with celecoxib plus interferon-α. Kankuri-Tammilehto *et al.* (2010) observed no association between COX-2 staining and response to IFN-α alone, while Rini *et al.* (2006) reported that all the RCC patients with objective responses to celecoxib plus interferon-α expressed COX-2 staining. Additionally, COX-2 does not associate with the Heidelberg classification (Kankuri-Tammilehto *et al.* 2010, Yoshimura *et al.* 2004).

3.6 Her-2, biomarker of proto-oncogene product

Her-2, a proto-oncogene product, is a member of the ErbB family of receptor tyrosine kinases. Her-2 functions in secretory epithelial tissues, and regulates intracellular signaling cascades (Arteaga *et al.* 2001, Olayioye *et al.* 2000). Her-2 is over-expressed in approximately 20-30% of human adenocarcinomas (Latif *et al.* 2002, Lipponen *et al.* 1994, Slamon *et al.* 1989), and the over-expression is associated with metastatic phenotype and poorer prognosis, e.g. in breast and ovarian cancer (Slamon *et al.* 1989).

Gene amplification of *Her-2* can be investigated by cytogenetic analyses, such as fluorescent *in situ* hybridization (FISH), chromogenic *in situ* hybridization (CISH), and polymerase chain reaction (PCR). In breast cancer, FISH and CISH positivity are accurate predictors of response to trastuzumab (anti-Her2 therapy) (Isola *et al.* 2004, Lebeau *et al.* 2001). Receptor-mediated targeted tumor therapy with Herceptin® (RhuMAb HER-2), a recombinant humanized monoclonal anti-Her-2 antibody, has improved the survival of breast carcinoma patients both in adjuvant therapy and in therapy for metastatic disease (Smith *et al.* 2007, Montemurro *et al.* 2003).

Membranous staining of HER-2 in immunohistochemistry reflects HER-2 protein expression (Zhang *et al.* 1997). Her-2 receptor-specific tumor toxin, in an animal model, effectively reduced pulmonary tumors of advanced RCC (Maurer-Gebhard *et al.* 1998). Parallel associations of Her-2 expression between tumor stage and grade in RCC patients have been observed in many studies (Zhang *et al.* 1997, Stumm *et al.* 1996), although in the study of Seliger *et al.* (2000) no such association was found. In the study of Hofmockel *et al.* (1997), higher tumor grades were seen when Her-2 expression was low, and higher T-stage associated with high Her-2. In the study of Phuoc *et al.* (2007), Her-2 protein expression did not correlate with Ki-67 protein expression.

In most *HER-2* gene amplification studies, *Her-2* gene amplification was observed neither by FISH analysis (Latif *et al.* 2002), messenger ribonucleic acid (mRNA) analysis (Stumm *et al.*

Prognostic Factors in Renal Cell Carcinoma: An Evaluation of T-Stage, Histopathological Grade, p53, Ki-67, COX-2, and Her-2 Expressions

169

1996), nor PCR analysis (Selli *et al.* 1997, Zhang *et al.* 1997). Selli *et al.* (1997) found *HER-2* gene amplification in collecting duct RCC cases (45%). Therefore, *HER-2* gene amplification may be more pronounced in collecting duct RCC, than in other more common RCC types (Matei *et al.* 2005, Zhang *et al.* 1997). The association of *HER-2* gene amplification and HER-2 protein expression with the prognosis of RCC patients has been estimated in few studies and the results have been contradictory (Phuoc *et al.* 2007, Lipponen *et al.* 1994). Further studies are needed to determine whether HER-2 protein expression or *HER-2* gene amplification may be used as prognostic factors in RCC patients.

3.7 Incidence of p53, Ki-67, and COX-2 expressions

The incidence of p53- and Ki-67-positive expression in RCC tumors was low in RCC studies (Kankuri-Tammilehto *et al.* 2010, Kirkali *et al.* 2001, Haitel *et al.* 2000, Rioux-Leclercq *et al.* 2000). It is known that in addition to melanoma, RCC belongs to tumors with a low incidence of *p53* mutations compared to, e.g. prostate and bladder cancer (Haitel *et al.* 2000, Kirkali *et al.* 2001, Rioux-Leclercq *et al.* 2000). The low *p53* mutation in different cancers (Olivier *et al.* 2002) and the low immunohistochemical staining of RCC tissue blocks for the p53 protein in studies (Haitel *et al.* 2000, Rioux-Leclercq *et al.* 2000) suggest that mutations in *p53* result in an accumulation of the p53 protein. In the study of Oda *et al.* (1995), p53 expression was found only in those components with *p53* mutations, mainly in the sarcomatoid components. The 10% cut-off value of p53 and Ki-67 was often selected to achieve statistically reliable results, and in accordance with previous studies on the subject (Kankuri *et al.* 2006, Olumi *et al.* 2001). Previously published reports indicate that the proportion of COX-2 positive cells varies in human RCCs (Cho *et al.* 2005, Miyata *et al.* 2003). In the study of Kankuri-Tammilehto *et al.* (2010), weak intensity of COX-2 staining was considered as COX-2 negative, which resulted in a lower number of positive COX-2 cells than in some other RCC studies (Tuna *et al.* 2004, Cho *et al.* 2005). For comparison, in the study of Miyata *et al.* (2003), the criterion for positive COX-2 expression was 5%, whereas in the study of Kankuri-Tammilehto *et al.* (2010), it was considered to be 10%. Also different antibodies have been used in other studies (Rini *et al.* 2006, Cho *et al.* 2005, Hashimoto *et al.* 2004). This fact and the criteria for immunohistochemical classification may contribute to the difference in the results. Validation of immunohistochemical methods is needed before the methods could be widely adopted for in clinical use.

3.8 Combining markers

In multivariate analysis, COX-2 and Ki-67 were independent variables, indicating that they are both stronger biomarkers than p53 for the development of metastases in RCC. However, combining markers may specify prognostic subgroups better than observing a single marker. As shown in a study by Haitel *et al.* (2000), p53 was not an independent predictor for survival, but p53 and mdm2, a negative regulator of p53, showed a strong association with poor survival. In the study of Kankuri *et al.* (2006), in RCC patients, double positivity for p53 and Ki-67 expression seems to indicate a higher probability of metastases than either marker alone. Additionally, combining COX-2 and Ki-67 increases their ability to predict survival in mRCC (Figure 5.). In this study, median overall survival time of RCC with COX-2 negativity/Ki-67 positivity was 19 months, which was almost five times shorter than of RCC with COX-2 positivity/Ki-67 negativity. Median overall survival time of RCC with

COX-2 negativity alone was 28 months, which was three times shorter than that of RCC with COX-2 positivity.

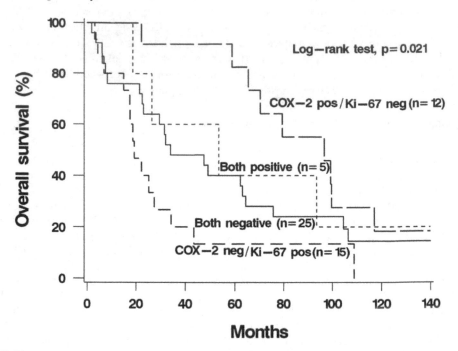

Fig. 5. The prognostic value of covariation of COX-2/Ki-67 for overall survival from nephrectomy in RCC patients with metastases (either primary presentation or later) (n=57, Kaplan-Meier method): the median overall survival time was 97 months with COX-2 positivity/Ki-67 negativity, and 19 months with COX-2 negativity/Ki-67 positivity (p=0.004) (Kankuri-Tammilehto *et al.* 2010).

Prognostic markers can be used in patient counseling, to select treatment modalities, and to determine eligibility for clinical trials. Different prognostic models have been created to specify the prognosis of RCC patients; they typically include conventional prognostic markers. However, combining biomarkers and conventional clinical markers seems to predict DSS more accurately than grade or TNM stage alone, both in locally confined and metastatic RCC (Kim *et al.* 2004).

3.9 Trends in the use of biomarkers

Prospective clinical trials on the clinical use of p53, Ki-67, and COX-2 protein expression in predicting overall survival could answer the question of whether the expression of these biomarkers can be reliably used in mRCC. These biomarkers cannot predict response to IFN-α (Kankuri-Tammilehto *et al.* 2010). Whether these biomarkers can predict response to novel targeted therapies should be investigated in trials. The new era of genetic cancer studies shows great promise in terms of patient evaluation for new targeted therapies or immunotherapy. By means of the tissue microarray technique, thousands of tumors can be

Prognostic Factors in Renal Cell Carcinoma: An Evaluation of T-Stage, Histopathological Grade, p53, Ki-67, COX-2, and Her-2 Expressions

171

investigated simultaneously to determine the protein expression profile. However, creating a consensus in the tissue microarray construction protocol is challenging, as RCC is a relatively large-size tumor of a highly heterogenous nature (Signoretti *et al.* 2008). At current, whole tissue sections are considered the gold standard, but the more cores per tumor are sampled the fewer errors are introduced by limited sampling. Using gene chips to profile kidney tumors defines the genes that determine patient survival and response to therapy, thus enabling precise prognosis determination and individual treatment planning (Tan *et al.* 2008). Additionally, tissue microarrays enable the analysis of protein expression profiles in specimens to determine their potential clinical significance and role in RCC biology.

4. Conclusion

RCC is an extremely heterogeneous disease, with patients having an overall survival from a few months to several years. For those RCC patients with performance status enabling current treatments, such as nephrectomy, immunomodulators, and more recently targeted therapies, the expected five-year survival rate has been slightly higher than 60%. Metastatic disease is seen in 20-30% of RCC patients at diagnosis. The five-year survival for metastatic RCC is from 3% to 16% if metastasectomy has not been a possible treatment. Currently, tumour (T)-stage is the best known prognostic factor for locally confined RCC. T-stage is a prognostic factor for both metastases-free and overall survival in locally confined RCC patients as well as in overall survival in metastatic RCC (mRCC). No consensus has been reached on a universal histopathologic tumor grading system. Several published reports have pointed out the differences in survival between the highest and the lowest tumor grades, even though when all three or four tumor grades were analyzed separatedly, the differences were no longer statistically significant. The heterogeneity of RCC within the same T-stage and grade has resulted in a need for more specific prognostic markers, related to molecular mechanisms of RCC, to specify diagnosis, staging and prognosis. Prognostic markers can also be used in to select treatment modalities, help in surveillance, and to determine eligibility for clinical trials. p53 associates weakly with tumor grade whereas Ki-67 associates with T-stage and metastatic development, indicating that Ki-67 is a marker for aggressive disease in RCC with an increased risk of early metastases development. The proportion of COX-2 positive tumors is highest in RCC with the ability to develop later metastases, when compared to both RCC without metastatic potential, and RCC with primary metastases. Metastases-free survival is longer in patients with COX-2 positive tumors compared to COX-2 negative tumors. These data show that COX-2 negativity associates with an aggressive phenotype in mRCC disease. COX-2 and Ki-67 alone are stronger biomarkers than p53 for the development of metastases in RCC. Her-2 seems to associate with p53 and Ki-67, but results of associations between Her-2 and survival have been contradictory. Few studies have been published on the significance of Her-2 protein expression or *Her-2* gene amplification in RCC, so more studies are warranted. p53 or Ki-67 alone are not valuable prognostic markers in locally confined RCC, but they can predict poor survival in mRCC. Therefore, p53 and Ki-67 can help in determining metastatic patients with a poor prognosis and, e.g. those who would benefit from high-dose IL-2 or temsirolimus. COX-2 positivity predicts improved overall survival in patients with mRCC treated with IFN-α. p53, Ki-67, and COX-2 cannot predict response to IFN-α. Investigating the ability of p53, Ki-67, and COX-2 protein expression to predict overall survival in a prospective clinical trial would answer the question of whether these biomarkers can be reliably used in mRCC. Combining the results of COX-2 and Ki-67 expression, may predict overall survival in mRCC. In predicting the development of metastases in nephrectomized RCC patients, COX-2 alone or a covariation of p53 and Ki-67 seem to have prognostic value. Combining p53 or COX-2 with Ki-67 may result in more specific prognosis staging in RCC than observing a single marker. In future, using the tissue microarray technique, the protein expression profile with several biomarkers can be determined quickly. Further investigations are needed on the reproducibility of staining of these novel biomarkers, and on validation of the ability of the expressions to discriminate clinical outcome in RCC. Findings on novel biomarkers have increased our understanding of the molecular biology of locally confined RCC patients and metastatic RCC patients. RCC is characterized by high resistance to radiation and chemotherapy, which may be due to the suppression of apoptotic mechanisms, such as the p53 tumour suppressor pathway. In RCC patients, Ki-67 expression is not very high, which may partly explain RCC's resistance to chemotherapy. Specification of the roles of novel tumor-related molecular prognostic factors might be translated into prognostic tools that could be used in clinical work.

5. References

Aaltomaa S et al. (1997). Prognostic value of Ki-67 expression in renal cell carcinomas. Eur Urol 31(3): 350-355

American Cancer Society (2004). Cancer facts and figures.

Amin MB et al. (2002). Prognostic impact of histologic subtyping of adult renal epithelial neoplasms: an experience of 405 cases. Am J Surg Pathol 26 (3):281-291.

Antonelli A et al. (2003). The collecting duct carcinoma of the kidney: a cytogenetical study. Eur Urol 43 (6): 680-685.

Arteaga CL et al. (2001) Inhibitors of HER2/neu (erbB-2) signal transduction. Semin Oncol 28 (6 Suppl 18): 30-35.

Atkins M et al. (2005). Carbonic anhydrase IX expression predicts outcome of interleukin 2 therapy for renal cancer. Clin Cancer Res 11: 3714-3721.

Atzpodien J et al. (2002). Thirteen-year, long-term efficacy of interferon 2alpha and interleukin 2-based home therapy in patients with advanced renal cell carcinoma. Cancer 95 (5): 1045-1050.

Atzpodien J et al.; DGCIN -- German Cooperative Renal Carcinoma Chemo-Immunotherapy Trials Group (2003).Metastatic renal carcinoma comprehensive prognostic system. Br J Cancer 88 (3): 348-353.

Atzpodien J et al.; German Cooperative Renal Carcinoma Chemo-Immunotherapy Trials Group (DGCIN) (2005). Adjuvant treatment with interleukin-2- and interferon-alpha2a-based chemoimmunotherapy in renal cell carcinoma post tumour nephrectomy: results of a prospectively randomised trial of the German Cooperative Renal Carcinoma Chemoimmunotherapy Group (DGCIN). Br J Cancer 92 (5): 843-846.

Bassil B et al. (1985).Validation of the tumor, nodes and metastasis classification of renal cell carcinoma. J Urol 134: 450-454.

Belldegrun A et al. (1999).Efficacy of nephron-sparing surgery for renal cell carcinoma: analysis based on the new 1997 tumor-node- metastasis staging system. J Clin Oncol 17: 2868-2875.

Prognostic Factors in Renal Cell Carcinoma: An Evaluation of T-Stage, Histopathological Grade, p53, Ki-67, COX-2, and Her-2 Expressions

173

Bodmer D et al. (2002). Understanding familial and non-familial renal cell cancer. Hum Mol Genet. 11 (20): 2489-2498.

Bosniak MA et al. (1995). Small renal parenchymal neoplasms: further observations on growth. Radiology 197: 589-597.

Bracarda S et al. (2011). Overall survival in patients with metastatic renal cell carcinoma initially treated with bevacizumab plus interferon-α2a and subsequent therapy with tyrosine kinase inhibitors: a retrospective analysis of the phase III AVOREN trial. BJU Int. 107(2): 214-219.

Bretheau D et al. (1995). Prognostic value of nuclear grade of renal cell carcinoma. Cancer 76 (12): 2543-2549.

Bui MH et al. (2003). Carbonic anhydrase IX is an independent predictor of survival in advanced renal clear cell carcinoma: implications for prognosis and therapy. Clin Cancer Res 9: 802-811.

Bui MH et al. (2004). Prognostic value of carbonic anhydrase IX and KI67 as predictors of survival for renal clear cell carcinoma. J Urol 171 (6 Pt 1): 2461-2466.

Cao Y and Prescott SM (2002) . Many actions of cyclooxygenase-2 in cellular dynamics and in cancer. J Cell Physiol 190(3): 279-286.

Chao D et al. (2002). Collecting duct renal cell carcinoma: clinical study of a rare tumor. J Urol 167: 71-74.

Cheville JC et al. (2003). Comparisons of outcome and prognostic features among histologic subtypes of renal cell carcinoma. Am J Surg Pathol 27 (5): 612-624.

Cho KS et al. (2008). A comprehensive prognostic stratification for patients with metastatic renal clear cell carcinoma. Yonsei Med J 49 (3): 451-458.

Cho DS et al. (2005). Cyclooxygenase-2 and p53 expression as prognostic indicators in conventional renal cell carcinoma. Yonsei Med J 46 (1): 133-140.

Choisy-Rossi C and Yonish-Rouach E (1998). Apoptosis and the cell cycle: the p53 connection. Cell Death Differ 5: 129-131.

Choueiri M et al (2011). Adjuvant and neoadjuvant therapy in renal cell carcinoma. Curr Clin Pharmacol. 6 (3): 144-50.

Choueiri TK et al. (2007). Prognostic factors associated with long-term survival in previously untreated metastatic renal cell carcinoma. Ann Oncol 18 (2): 249-255.

Chow WH et al. (2000). Obesity, hypertension, and the risk of kidney cancer in men. N Engl J Med 343: 1305-1311.

Corless CL et al. (1997). Immunostaining of the von Hippel-Lindau gene product in normal and neoplastic human tissues. Hum Pathol. 28 (4): 459-464.

De Luca A and Normanno N (2010). Tivozanib, a pan-VEGFR tyrosine kinase inhibitor for the potential treatment of solid tumors. Idrugs 13(9): 636-645.

Cunningham J (1938). The kidney: tumors. 1938 Year book of Urology 167-192.

Delahunt B et al. (2002). Prognostic importance of tumor size for localized conventional (clear cell) renal cell carcinoma: assessment of TNM T1 and T2 tumor categories and comparison with other prognostic parameters. Cancer 94: 658-664.

Donskov F et al. (2004). In vivo assessment of the antiproliferative properties of interferon-alpha during immunotherapy: Ki-67 (MIB-1) in patients with metastatic renal cell carcinoma. Br J Cancer 90 (3): 626-631.

du Manoir S et al. (1991). Ki-67 labeling in postmitotic cells defines different Ki-67 pathways within the 2c compartment. Cytometry 12:455-463.

Dudderidge TJ et al. (2005). Mcm2, Geminin, and KI67 define proliferative state and are prognostic markers in renal cell carcinoma. Clin Cancer Res 11: 2510-2517.

Eble JN (2003). Mucinous tubular and spindle cell carcinoma and post-neuroblastoma carcinoma: newly recognised entities in the renal cell carcinoma family. Pathology 35(6):499-504.

Eble JN et al., eds. (2004). World Health Organization Classification of Tumors. Pathology and Genetics of Tumors of the Urinary System and Male Genital Organs. IARC Press, Lyon, p360.

Elinq TE et al. (1990). Prostaglandin H synthase and xenobiotic oxidation. Ann Rev Pharmacol Toxicol 30: 1-45.

Elmore JM et al. (2003). Reassessment of the 1997 TNM classification system for renal cell carcinoma. Cancer 98 (11): 2329-2334.

Escudier B et al.; TARGET Study Group (2007). Sorafenib in advanced clear-cell renal-cell carcinoma. N Engl J Med 356(2):125-134. Erratum in: N Engl J Med. 2007 357 (2): 203.

Ferlay J et al (2010). GLOBOCAN 2008 v1.2, Cancer Incidence and Mortality Worldwide: IARC CancerBase No. 10 [Internet]. Lyon, France: International Agency for Research on Cancer; 2010.

Ficarra V et al. (2001). Prognostic value of renal cell carcinoma nuclear grading: multivariate analysis of 333 cases. Urol Int 67 (2): 130-134.

Finlay C et al. (1998). Activating mutations for transformation by p53 produce a gene product that forms an hsc70-p53 complex with an altered half-life. Mol Cell Biol 8: 531-539.

Finnish Cancer Registry (2007). Institute for Statistical and Epidemiological Cancer Research: Cancer in Finland 2004 and 2005. Cancer Statistics of the National Research and Development Centre for Welfare and Health (STAKES), publication No. 72. Cancer Society of Finland, Helsinki.

Flanigan RC et al. (2001). Nephrectomy followed by interferon alfa-2b compared with interferon alfa-2b alone for metastatic renal-cell cancer. N Engl J Med 345: 1655-1659.

Fuhrman SA et al. (1982). Prognostic significance of morphologic parameters in renal cell carcinoma. Am J Surg Pathol 6: 655-663.

Galban S et al. (2003). Influence of the RNA-binding protein HuR in pVHL-regulated p53 expression in renal carcinoma cells. Mol Cell Biol 23 (20): 7083-7095.

George DJ and Kaelin WG Jr (2003). The von Hippel-Lindau protein, vascular endothelial growth factor, and kidney cancer. N Engl J Med 349 (5): 419-421.

Gerdes J et al. (1984). Cell cycle analysis of a cell proliferation-associated human nuclear antigen defined by the monoclonal antibody Ki-67. J Immunol 133: 1710-1715.

Giuliani L et al. (1990). Radical extensive surgery for renal cell carcinoma: long-term results and prognostic factors. J Urol 143: 468-473.

Gnarra JR et al. (1994). Mutations of the VHL tumor suppressor gene in renal carcinoma. Nat Genet 7: 85-90.

Goldstein NS (1997). The current state of renal cell carcinoma grading. Union Internationale Contre le Cancer (UICC) and the American Joint Committee on Cancer (AJCC) Cancer 80 (5): 977-980.

Goldstein R et al. (2010). Does axitinib (AG-01376) have a future role in metastatic renal cell carcinoma and other malignancies? Expert Rev Anticancer Ther 10(10): 1545-1557.

Gudbjartsson T et al. (2005). Histological subtyping and nuclear grading of renal cell carcinoma and their implications for survival: a retrospective nation-wide study of 629 patients. Eur Urol 48 (4): 593-600.

Prognostic Factors in Renal Cell Carcinoma: An Evaluation of T-Stage, Histopathological Grade, p53, Ki-67, COX-2, and Her-2 Expressions

175

Guinan P et al. (1997). TNM staging of renal cell carcinoma: Workgroup No. 3. Union International Contre le Cancer (UICC) and the American Joint Committee on Cancer (AJCC). Cancer. 80: 992-993.

Guinan PD et al. (1995). Renal cell carcinoma: tumor size, stage and survival. Members of the Cancer Incidence and End Results Committee. J Urol 153: 901-903.

Hara S et al. (2002). Expression of cyclooxygenase-2 in human bladder and renal cell carcinoma. Adv Exp Med Biol 507: 123-126.

Harmen PE (1978). TNM classification of malignant tumors. Union Internationale Contre le Cancer, Geneva.

Hashimoto Y et al. (2004). Cyclooxygenase-2 expression and relationship to tumour progression in human renal cell carcinoma. Histopathology 44 (4): 353-359.

Haitel A et al. (2000). mdm2 expression as a prognostic indicator in clear cell renal cell carcinoma: comparison with p53 overexpression and clinicopathological parameters. Clin Cancer Res 6(5): 1840-4.

Herman JG et al. (1994). Silencing of the VHL tumor-suppressor gene by DNA methylation in renal carcinoma. Proc Natl Acad Sci U S A. 91 (21): 9700-9704.

Herschman HR (1996). Prostaglandin synthase 2. Biochim. Biophys Act 1299: 125-140

Hofmockel G et al. (1997). Epidermal growth factor family and renal cell carcinoma: expression and prognostic impact. Eur Urol 31 (4): 478-484.

Hofmockel G et al. (1996). Related Articles, Expression of p53 and bcl-2 in primary locally confined renal cell carcinomas: no evidence for prognostic significance. Anticancer Res 16 (6B): 3807-3811.

Hollingsworth JM et al. (2006). Rising incidence of small renal masses: a need to reassess treatment effect. J Natl Cancer Inst. 98(18):1331-1334.

Hudes G et al. ; Global ARCC Trial. (2007). Temsirolimus, interferon alfa, or both for advanced renal-cell carcinoma. N Engl J Med 356 (22): 2271-2281.

Hunt JD et al. (2005). Renal cell carcinoma in relation to cigarette smoking: meta-analysis of 24 studies. Int J Cancer. 114 (1): 101-108.

Iliopoulos O et al. (1995). Tumor suppression by the human von Hippel-Lindau gene product. Nat Med 1 (8): 822-826.

Isola J et al. (2004). Interlaboratory comparison of HER-2 oncogene amplification as detected by chromogenic and fluorescence in situ hybridization. lin Cancer Res 10 (14): 4793-4798.

Itoi T et al. (2004). Impact of frequent Bcl-2 expression on better prognosis in renal cell carcinoma patients. Br J Cancer 90 (1): 200-205.

Janzen NK et al. (2003). Surveillance after radical or partial nephrectomy for localized renal cell carcinoma and management of recurrent disease. Urol Clin North Am 30: 843-852.

Javidan J et al. (1999). Prognostic significance of the 1997 TNM classification of renal cell carcinoma. J Urol 162:1277-81.

Jayson M and Sanders H (1998). Increased incidence of serendipitously discovered renal cell carcinoma. Urology 51: 203-205.

Kanamaru H et al. (2001). Prognostic value of nuclear area index in combination with the World Health Organization grading system for patients with renal cell carcinoma. Urology 57: 257-261.

Kanamaru H et al. (1999). Immunohistochemical expression of p53 and bcl-2 proteins is not associated with sarcomatoid change in renal cell carcinoma. Urol Res 27: 169-173.

Kankuri M et al. (2001). Feasibility of Prolonged Use of Interferon-alpha in Metastatic Kidney Carcinoma. A Phase II Study. Cancer 92 (4): 761-767.

Kankuri M et al. (2006). The Association of Immunoreactive p53 and Ki-67 with T-stage, Grade, Occurrence of Metastases and Survival in Renal Cell Carcinoma. Anticancer Res 26 (5B): 3825-3833.

Kankuri-Tammilehto M et al. (2010). Prognostic Evaluation of COX-2 Expression in Renal Cell Carcinoma. Anticancer Res 30(7):3023-30.

Khan KNM et al. (2001). Expression of cyclooxygenase-2 in canine renal cell carcinoma. Vet Pathol 38: 116-119.

Kim HL et al. (2004). Using protein expressions to predict survival in clear cell renal carcinoma. Clin Cancer Res 10 (16): 5464-5471.

Kirkali Z et al. (2001). Proliferative activity, angiogenesis and nuclear morphometry n renal cell carcinoma. Int J Urol 8: 697-703.

Kovacs G et al. (1997). The Heidelberg classification of renal cell tumors. J Pathol 183: 131-133.

Lanigan D et al. (1994). A comparative analysis of grading systems in renal adenocarcinoma. Histopathology 24: 473-476.

Lam JS et al. (2005). Postoperative surveillance protocol for patients with localized and locally advanced renal cell carcinoma based on a validated prognostic nomogram and risk group stratification system. J Urol 174: 466-472.

Latif Z et al. (2002). Gene amplification and overexpression of HER2 in renal cell carcinoma. BJU Int 89 (1): 5-9.

Lebeau A et al. (2001). Her-2/neu analysis in archival tissue samples of human breast cancer: comparison of immunohistochemistry and fluorescence in situ hybridization. J Clin Oncol 19 (2): 354-363.

Linehan WM et al. (2003). The genetic basis of cancer of the kidney. J Urol 170: 2163-2172.

Lipponen P et al. (1994). Expression of proliferating cell nuclear antigen (PC10), p53 protein and c-erbB-2 in renal adenocarcinoma. Int J Cancer 57 (2): 275-280.

Lohse CM et al. (2002). Comparison of standardized and nonstandardized nuclear grade of renal cell carcinoma to predict outcome among 2,042 patients. Am J Clin Pathol 118 (6): 877-886.

Masferrer JL et al. (2000). Antiangiogenic and antitumor activities of cyclooxygenase-2 inhibitors. Cancer Res 60:1306-1311.

Masters JR (2007). Clinical applications of expression profiling and proteomics in prostate cancer. Anticancer Res 27 (3A): 1273-1276.

Matei DV et al. (2005). Synchronous collecting duct carcinoma and papillary renal cell carcinoma: a case report and review of the literature. Anticancer Res 25 (1B): 579-586.

Mathew A et al. (2002). Global increases in kidney cancer incidence, 1973-1992. Eur J Cancer Prev 11 (2): 171-178.

Maurer-Gebhard M et al. (1998). Systemic treatment with a recombinant erbB-2 receptor-specific tumor toxin efficiently reduces pulmonary metastases in mice injected with genetically modified carcinoma cells. Cancer Res 58(12): 2661-2666.

Maxwell PH et al. (1999). The tumor suppressor protein VHL targets hypoxia-inducible factors for oxygen-dependent proteolysis. Nature 399: 271-275.

May P and May E (1999). Twenty years of p53 research: structural and functional aspects of the p53 protein. Oncogene 18: 7621-7636.

Prognostic Factors in Renal Cell Carcinoma: An Evaluation of T-Stage, Histopathological Grade, p53, Ki-67,
COX-2, and Her-2 Expressions

177

McNichols DW et al. (1981). Renal cell carcinoma: long-term survival and late recurrence. J Urol 126: 17-23.

Parkin DM et al. (2003). Cancer Incidence in Five Continents Vol. VIII. The International Agency for Research on Cancer (IARC) Scientific Publication No. 155. Globocan 2002. pp.1-782.

Medeiros LJ et al. (1997). Grading of renal cell carcinoma: Workgroup No. 2. Union Internationale Contre le Cancer and the American Joint Committee on Cancer (AJCC). Cancer 80 (5): 990-991.

Mickish GH (1999). Lymphatic metastases in renal cell carcinoma. What is the value of operation and adjuvant therapy? Urologe A 38: 326-331.

Mickisch GH et al, European Organisation for Research and Treatment of Cancer (EORTC) . enitourinary Group (2001) Radical nephrectomy plus interferon-alfa-based immunotherapy compared with interferon alfa alone in metastatic renal-cell carcinoma: a randomised trial. Lancet 358 (9286): 966-970.

Minasian LM et al. (1993). Interferon alfa-2a in advanced renal cell carcinoma: treatment results and survival in 159 patients with long-term follow-up. J Clin Oncol 11: 1368-1375.

Miyata Y et al. (2003). Expression of cyclooxygenase-2 in renal cell carcinoma: correlation with tumor cell proliferation, apoptosis, angiogenesis, expression of matrix metalloproteinase-2, and survival. Clin Cancer Res 9 (5): 1741-1749.

Montemurro F et al. (2003). Safety and activity of docetaxel and trastuzumab in HER2 overexpressing metastatic breast cancer: a pilot phase II study. Am J Clin Oncol 26 (1): 95-97.

Mostofi FK and Davis CJ in Collaboration with Sobin LH and Pathologists in 6 Countries. World Health Organization (1998). Histological Typing of Kidney Tumors; in (2nd ed): International Histological Classification of Tumors. Springer 1998, Berlin Heidelberg, pp. 1-117.

Motzer RJ et al. (2002). Interferon-alfa as a comparative treatment for clinical trials of new therapies against advanced renal cell carcinoma. J Clin Oncol 20 (1): 289-296.

Motzer RJ et al. (2004). Prognostic factors for survival in previously treated patients with metastatic renal cell carcinoma. J Clin Oncol 22: 454-463.

Motzer RJ et al. (2008). Prognostic nomogram for sunitinib in patients with metastatic renal cell carcinoma. Cancer 113 (7): 1552-1558.

Motzer RJ et al.; RECORD-1 Study Group (2008). Efficacy of everolimus in advanced renal cell carcinoma: a double-blind, randomised, placebo-controlled phase III trial. Lancet 372 (9637): 449-456.

Motzer RJ et al. (2000). Effect of cytokine therapy on survival for patients with advanced renal cell carcinoma. J Clin Oncol 18 (9): 1928-1935.

Mungan MU et al. (2006). Expression of COX-2 in normal and pyelonephritic kidney, renal intraepithelial neoplasia, and renal cell carcinoma. Eur Urol 50 (1): 92-97.

Négrier S et al. (2002). Prognostic factors of survival and rapid progression in 782 patients with metastatic renal carcinomas treated by cytokines: a report from the Groupe Français d'Immunothérapie. Ann Oncol. 2002 13 (9): 1460-1468.

Négrier S et al.; For The French Immunotherapy Intergroup (2007). Medroxyprogesterone, interferon alfa-2a, interleukin 2, or combination of both cytokines in patients with metastatic renal carcinoma of intermediate prognosis: results of a randomized controlled trial. Cancer 110 (11): 2468-2477.

Nose F et al. (2002). Up-regulation of cyclooxygenase-2 expression in lymphocytic thyroiditis and thyroid tumors: significant correlation with inducible nitric oxide synthase. Am J Clin Pathol 117 (4): 546-551.

Oda H et al. (1995). Mutations of the p53 gene and p53 protein overexpression are associated with sarcomatoid transformation in renal cell carcinomas. Cancer Res 55: 658-662.

Olayioye MA et al. (2000). The ErbB signaling network: receptor heterodimerization in development and cancer. EMBO J 19 (13): 3159-3167.

Olivier M et al. (2002). The IARC TP53 database: new online mutation analysis and recommendations to users. Hum Mutat 19: 607-614.

Olumi AF et al. (2001). p53 immunoreactivity correlates with Ki-67 and bcl-2 expression in renal cell carcinoma. Urol Oncol 6: 63-67.

Paner GP et al. (2006). Immunohistochemical analysis of mucinous tubular and spindle cell carcinoma and papillary renal cell carcinoma of the kidney: significant immunophenotypic overlap warrants diagnostic caution. Am J Surg Pathol 30 (1): 13-19.

Pantuck AJ et al. (2007). Use of carbonic anhydrase IX (CAIX) expression and Von Hippel Lindau (VHL) gene mutation status to predict survival in renal cell carcinoma. Journal of Clinical Oncology, ASCO Annual Meeting Proceedings Part I. Vol 25, No. 18S: 5042.

Patard JJ et al. (2005). Prognostic value of histologic subtypes in renal cell carcinoma: a multicenter experience. J Clin Oncol 23 (12): 2763-2771.

Phuoc NB et al. (2007). Immunohistochemical analysis with multiple antibodies in search of prognostic markers for clear cell renal cell carcinoma. Urology 69 (5): 843-848.

Pinto AE et al. (2005). Prognostic biomarkers in renal cell carcinoma: relevance of DNA ploidy in predicting disease-related survival. Int J Biol Markers 20(4): 249-56.

Pyrhönen S et al. (1999). Prospective randomized trial of interferon alfa-2a plus vinblastine versus vinblastine alone in patients with advanced renal cell cancer. J Clin Oncol 17 (9): 2859-2867.

Reich NC and Levine AJ (1984). Growth regulation of a cellular tumor antigen, p53, in nontransformed cells. Nature 308: 199-201.

Repmann R et al. (2003). Adjuvant therapy of renal cell carcinoma patients with an autologous tumor cell lysate vaccine: a five-year follow-up analysis. Anticancer Res 23: 969-974.

Rini BI et al. (2011). IMA901 Multipeptide Vaccine Randomized International Phase III Trial (IMPRINT): A randomized, controlled study investigating IMA901 multipeptide cancer vaccine in patients receiving sunitinib as first-line therapy for advanced/metastatic RCC. J Clin Oncol 29: 2011.

Rini BI et al. (2010). Phase III trial of bevacizumab plus interferon alfa versus interferon alfa monotherapy in patients with metastatic renal cell carcinoma: final results of CALGB 90206. J Clin Oncol. 2010 May 1;28(13):2137-43.

Rini BI et al. (2006). Maximal COX-2 immunostaining and clinical response to celecoxib and interferon alpha therapy in metastatic renal cell carcinoma. Cancer 106 (3): 566-575.

Rioux-Leclercq N et al. (2007). Prognostic ability of simplified nuclear grading of renal cell carcinoma. Cancer 109 (5): 868-874.

Rioux-Leclercq N et al. (2000). Value of immunohistochemical Ki-67 and p53 determinations as predictive factors of outcome in renal cell carcinoma. Urol 2000: 55: 501-505.

Roberts WW et al. (2005). Pathological stage does not alter the prognosis for renal lesions determined to be stage T1 by computerized tomography. J Urol 173 (3): 713-715.

Prognostic Factors in Renal Cell Carcinoma: An Evaluation of T-Stage, Histopathological Grade, p53, Ki-67,
COX-2, and Her-2 Expressions

179

Robson CJ et al. (2002). The results of radical nephrectomy for renal carcinoma. 1969. J Urol 167 (2 Pt 2): 873-875.

Seliger B et al. (2000). HER-2/neu is expressed in human renal cell carcinoma at heterogenous levels independently of tumor grading and staging and can be recognized by HLA-A2.1 restricted cytotoxic T lymphocytes. Int J Cancer 87 (3): 345-359.

Selli C et al. (1997). Retrospective evaluation of c-erbB-2 oncogene amplification using competitive PCR in collecting duct carcinoma of the kidney. J Urol 158 (1): 245-247.

Selli C et al. (1983). Stratification of risk factors in renal cell carcinoma. Cancer 52: 899-903.

Shvarts O et al. (200).. p53 is an independent predictor of tumor recurrence and progression after nephrectomy in patients with localized renal cell carcinoma. J Urol 173: 725-728.

Signoretti S et al. (2008). Tissue-based research in kidney cancer: current challenges and future directions. Clin Cancer Res. 2008 14 (12): 3699-3705.

Skinner DG et al. (1971). Diagnosis and management of renal cell carcinoma. A clinical and pathologic study of 309 cases. Cancer 28: 1165-1177.

Slamon DJ et al. (1989). Studies of the HER2/neu protooncogene in human breast and ovarian cancer. Science 244: 707-712.

Smith WL et al. (2000). Cyclooxygenases: structural, cellular, and molecular biology. Annu Rev Biochem 69: 145-182.

Smith I et al.; HERA study team (2007). 2-year follow-up of trastuzumab after adjuvant chemotherapy in HER2-positive breast cancer: a randomised controlled trial. Lancet 369 (9555): 29-36

Sobin L and Wittekind C (2002). TNM Classification of Malignant Tumors, 6th edition. John Wiley & Sons, Inc, New York, p239.

Spanknebel K et al. (2005). Initial clinical response predicts outcome and is associated with dose schedule in metastatic melanoma and renal cell carcinoma patients treated with high-dose interleukin 2. Ann Surg Oncol 12: 381-390.

Srigley JR et al. (1997). Current prognostic factors--renal cell carcinoma: Workgroup No. 4. Union Internationale Contre le Cancer (UICC) and the American Joint Committee on Cancer (AJCC). Cancer 80: 994-996.

Sternberg CN et al. (2010). Pazopanib in locally advanced or metastatic renal cell carcinoma: results of a randomized phase III trial. J Clin Oncol 28 (6): 1061-1068. Epub 2010 Jan 25.

Stumm G et al. (1996). Concomitant overexpression of the EGFR and erbB-2 genes in renal cell carcinoma (RCC) is correlated with dedifferentiation and metastasis. Int J Cancer 20 (69): 17-22.

Störkel S et al. (1997). Classification of renal cell carcinoma: Workgroup No. 1. Union Internationale Contre le Cancer (UICC) and the American Joint Committee on Cancer (AJCC). Cancer 80: 987-989.

Störkel S et al. (1989). Prognostic parameters in renal cell carcinoma - a new approach. Eur Urol 16: 416-422.

Subbaramaiah K et al. (1996). Transcription of cyclooxygenase-2 is enhanced in transformed mammary epithelial cells.Cancer Res 56 (19): 4424-4429.

Sunela KL et al. (2009). A phase-II study of combination of pegylated interferon alfa-2a and capecitabine in locally advanced or metastatic renal cell cancer. Cancer Chemother Pharmacol.

Syrjänen K and Hjelt L (1978). Grading of human renal adenocarcinoma. Scand J Urol Nephrol 12 (1): 49-55.

Tan X et al. (2008). Global analysis of metastasis-associated gene expression in primary cultures from clinical specimens of clear-cell renal-cell carcinoma. Int J Cancer 123 (5): 1080-1088.

Thoenes W et al. (1986). Histopathology and classification of renal cell tumors (adenomas, oncocytomas and carcinomas). The basic cytological and histomorphological elements and their use for diagnostics. Pathol Res Pract 181: 125-143.

Tsui KH et al. (2000). Prognostic indicators for renal cell carcinoma. A multivariate analysis of 643 patients using the revised 1997 TNM staging criteria. J Urol 163: 1090-1095.

Tsujii M and DuBois RN (1995). Alterations in cellular adehesion and apoptosis in epithelial cells overexpressing prostaglandin endoperoxide synthase 2. Cell 83: 493-501.

Tuna B et al. (2004). Significance of COX-2 expression in human renal cell carcinoma. Urology 2004, 64(6):1116-1120.

Uchida T et al. (2002). Clinical significance of p53, mdm2, and bcl-2 proteins in renal cell carcinoma. Urology: 59: 615-620.

Usubutyn A et al. (1998). Comparison of grading systems for estimating the prognosis of renal cell carcinoma. Int. Urol. Nephrol. 30:391-397.

van Houwelingen KP et al. (2005). Prevalence of von Hippel-Lindau gene mutations in sporadic renal cell carcinoma: results from The Netherlands cohort study. BMC Cancer 5:57.

Yang JC et al. (2007). Ipilimumab (anti-CTLA4 antibody) causes regression of metastatic renal cell cancer associated with enteritis and hypophysitis. J Immunother 30 (8): 825-830.

Yang JC et al. (2003). A randomized trial of bevacizumab, an anti-vascular endothelial growth factor antibody, for metastatic renal cancer. N Engl J Med 349 (5): 427-434.

Yildiz E et al. (2004). Prognostic value of the expression of Ki-67, CD44 and vascular endothelial growth factor, and microvessel invasion, in renal cell carcinoma. BJU Int 93: 1087-1093.

Yoshimura R et al. (2004). Study of cyclooxygenase-2 in renal cell carcinoma. Int J Mol Med 13 (2): 229-233.

Zhang D et al. (1997). Vitamin E inhibits apoptosis, DNA modification, and cancer incidence induced by iron-mediated peroxidation in Wistar rat kidney. Cancer Res 57 (12): 2410-2414.

Zigeuner R et al. (2004). Value of p53 as a prognostic marker in histologic subtypes of renal cell carcinoma: a sytematic analysis of primary and metastatic tumor tissue. Urology 63: 651-655.

Zisman A et al. (2001). Re-evaluation of the 1997 TNM classification for RCC: T1 and T2 cut-off point at 4.5 cm rather than 7 cm better correlates with clinical outcome. J Urol 166: 54-58.

Zisman A et al. (2002). Mathematical model to predict individual survival for patients with renal cell carcinoma. J Clin Oncol 20: 1368-1374.

10

Treatment of Renal Cell Carcinoma in Elderly and Frail Patients

Mirjana Rajer

Institute of Oncology Ljubljana
Slovenia

1. Introduction

Renal cell carcinoma (RCC) is the most common cancer of the kidney (Motzer et.al., 1999). In the United States each year 57.000 new patients are being diagnosed with RCC resulting in 12.900 deaths (Linehan et.al., 2011). The median age at diagnosis today is 64 years and even though it represents only 3% of all cancers, the incidence is increasing steadily. With rising prevalence of some known risk factors like hypertension and population ageing, the incidence of RCC is expected to be rising even more in subsequent years. With increasing incidence of renal cell carcinoma (RCC) combined with population ageing, questions about the treatment of elderly and frail patients with RCC are becoming more and more relevant. Many of the patients with newly diagnosed RCC are in advanced age and/or have some major co-morbidities which often results in their poor performance status. Elderly or frail patients are frequently excluded from clinical trials, because the results of their treatment are often difficult to interpret. This is also true for patients with heart, lung, liver or other major co-morbidities. Excluding these patients from clinical trials leads to lack of evidence-based guidelines for their treatment and often poses to oncologists a difficult dilemma when they need to decide what treatment options to offer to patients (Scuch et.al., 2008). In the present chapter we would like to present current recommendations for diagnostics and treatment of elderly and frail patients with RCC. In the second part of the chapter results of the analysis of metastatic RCC patients treated in a single institution with emphasis on differences in the treatment between good and poor performance status patients are presented.

2. Age, performance status, co-morbidities and prognostic models

2.1 Age

Ageing is a complex process that affects every aspect of life. The US department of Health and Human Services Administration of Ageing estimates that 1 in every 8 Americans is older than 65 years. In 2006 this group represented 12,4% of the population, but by 2030 this number is expected to increase to 20%. With population ageing, incidence of all cancers is supposed to be rising in the next years and RCC is no exception (Neustadt et.al., 2008).

It is well known that the actual age is determined by physiology rather than chronology. Factors of biological aging include changes in the physical structure of the body as well as changes in the performance of motor skills and sensory awareness. These changes can lead to multiple adverse events during the hospitalisation of an elderly patient especially in the postoperative period. Delirium episodes (acute decline of attention and cognition) can occur in 15-35% of patients during hospitalisation in the postoperative period and as high as 70-78% of patients in intensive care units. Prolonged hospitalisation is also associated with falls at rate 4-10/1000 patient-days. Other common adverse events are functional decline in 32% and adverse events of drugs in 10-15% of patients (Pushkar & Govorov, 2008).

Organs have a certain capacity to resist to stress and return to normal functioning after the stress on them has passed. This concept is termed "organ reserve". This reserve diminishes with age and may explain some functional deterioration in the elderly. Organ reserve in the young is supposed to be 7-11 times greater than in the advanced age person. Declining of organ reserve with age can not be predicted properly because it is subject to individual variation. Still, it has to be taken into account in treatment decision making (Neustadt et.al., 2008).

The patient's age is incorporated in the development of treatment decision and often is an inclusion /exclusion criterion of clinical trials. For a long time it was believed that older patients may tolerate treatment less well and may develop more adverse events compared to younger patients. Consequently, many treatments were not offered to older patients only on the basis of their chronological age without any strong evidence gained from clinical trials. It is becoming more and more clear that older patients may tolerate available treatments as well as younger ones and that treatments are being equally effective in both groups. Still, not all available treatments can be given without causing harm to all patients and some prudence is needed. Evaluation of functional organ reserve, evaluation of co-morbidities and performance status is of utmost importance (Calvo et.al., 2010).

2.2 Performance status

Beside accurate diagnostics and staging of tumours, before the decision on treatment modalities, performance status needs to be assessed in all cancer patients. Importance of pre-treatment performance status evaluation has been determined on the basis of several clinical trials that confirmed its prognostic value. Performance status can be assessed based on several different scales. In oncology the most commonly used are Karnofsky scale and the ECOG score (published by Oken et al. in 1982), also named WHO or Zubrod score. Scores and their comparisons are shown in Tables1 and 2.

Percentage	Description
100%	Normal, no complaints, no signs of disease
90%	Capable of normal activity, few symptoms or signs of disease
80%	Normal activity with some difficulty, some symptoms or signs
70%	Caring for self, not capable of normal activity or work
60%	Requiring some help, can take care of most personal requirements
50%	Requiring help often, requires frequent medical care
40%	Disabled, requires special care and help
30%	Severely disabled, hospital admission indicated but no risk of death
20%	Very ill, urgently requiring admission, requires supportive measures or treatment
10%	Moribund, rapidly progressive fatal disease processes

Table 1. Karnofsky performance status scale

WHO/ECOG	Description
0	Fully active, able to carry on all predisease activities without restriction
1	Restricted in physically strenuous activity but ambulatory and able to carry out work of a light or sedentary nature. For example, light housework, office work
2	Ambulatory and capable of all self care but unable to carry out any work activities. Up and about more than 50% of waking hours
3	Capable of only limited self-care, confined to bed or chair 50% or more of waking hours
4	Completely disabled. Cannot carry on any self-care. Totally confined to bed or chair

Table 2. WHO performance status scale

Karnofsky score of 90-100% corresponds to 0 on WHO scale, 70-80% to 1, 50-60% to 2, 30-40% to 3 and 10-20% to WHO grade 4. Patient death corresponds to 0% or 5 on Karnofsky and WHO scale respectively (Pushkar & Govorov, 2008).

Poor performance status in patients with RCC can be the result of one or multiple causes leading to a heterogeneous group of patients. Causes of poor PS (> 1 WHO) may be directly connected to RCC and metastases or may be the result of co-morbidities not directly connected to cancer (e.g. cardiovascular or hepatic diseases). Causes of poor PS related to tumour may be: pain from primary tumour or metastases, pleural effusion or ascites, brain metastases, anaemia, cachexia, gastrointestinal symptoms or fatigue (Pushkar&Govorov, 2008).

In measuring PS of the patient on WHO or Karnofsky scale some caution is needed because there are some situations where assessment of patient's functional status may require more than PS values written in numbers. For example, bone metastases: involvement of pelvis, femur or spine can force the patient to become bedridden, and the evaluation of PS in those patients can be difficult. Other criticism to the PS scales is that they do not include patient's nutritional status and they don't assess cachexia. Although performance status assessed with WHO or Karnofsky scales may not always reflect the actual functional status of the patient it is a most useful tool and should be utilized before and during the treatment of all cancer patients (Shuch et.al., 2007).

2.3 Co-morbidities

Outcome of therapy is depended not only on type and tumour aggressiveness but also on functional status of the patient and co-morbidities. In predicting possible outcome in elderly patients, evaluating performance status may not be enough and a thorough evaluation of their co-morbidities and organ functional reserve is mandatory. It is estimated that five years after the diagnosis of RCC, 30% of patients die because of conditions other than RCC. There are several ways to evaluate co-morbidities like American society of anaesthesiology (ASA) score used before surgery. Even though none of them is universally accepted, they may help us to determine the functional status of the patient (Pushkar & Govorov, 2008).

Evaluation of co-morbidities is and important part in the treatment decision process; but not only that, some of them may even predict the higher risk of developing RCC. The number of patients with end stage renal disease has increased markedly and haemodialysis is the most widely used form of renal replacement therapy in the elderly. It has been demonstrated that patients on haemodialysis have a higher probability of developing RCC (Ishikawa et.al., 1990). The overall relative risk of RCC is 5-10-times higher in patients with end-stage renal failure (Levine et.al., 1992). To detect RCC early in the course of the disease, these patients should have regular urologic follow-ups. The incidence of RCC is also high in patients after kidney transplantation. Murphy reported that post-transplant patients have a 1,85 times higher risk of development of RCC that their matched controls in the general population. This higher risk was not affected by age, gender, ethnical group and time since transplantation (Pushkar & Govorov, 2008).

Neuzillet et.al. evaluated clinicopathologic characteristics and treatment outcome in 1250 RCC patients with end stage renal disease in comparison with RCC patients without end stage renal disease (ESRD). They found that ESRD patients with RCC were younger (55 vs. 62 years, p<0,01), were more frequently discovered incidentally (87% vs 44%, p<0,01), had less local and systemic symptoms and were males (76,5% vs 61,9%, p<0,01) at rate compared to RCC patients without ESRD. Tumours were detected at lower stage in patients with ESRD, had lower grade and were papillary higher in higher percentage (37% vs 7%, p<0,01) in ESRD. Interestingly, more patients with ESRD were in good performance status (ECOG 0) (76% vs 63%). Authors conclude that better tumour and patient's characteristics are the results of more abdominal imaging performed in these patients. Consequently, more incidental tumours are being diagnosed (Neuzillet et.al., 2011).

2.4 Prognostic models

In the treatment decision making process it is very important to predict the patient's survival. Patients with short predicted survival time should be evaluated carefully and best quality of life should be the primary goal of their treatment (Bukowski & Negrier, 2004).

Motzer et.al. conducted a retrospective trial to identify prognostic factors and to find predictive model of survival of patients with metastatic RCC. Pretreatment factors were evaluated. They identified five prognostic factors on the basis of which patients can be divided into three risk groups (low, intermediate or high) for which the median survival time was separated by six months. Patients with zero risk factors (low risk group) had median survival of 20 months, those with one or two risk factors (intermediate risk group), had median survival time of 10 and those with three or more risk factors (high risk group) had survival time of 4 months. The identified prognostic factors (called also Memorial Sloan Kettering prognostic factors) were (Motzer et.al., 1996):

- Lactate dehydrogenase levels > 1,5 times upper limit of normal
- Haemogloben level < lower limit of normal
- Corrected serum calcium level > 10 mg/dl (2,5mmol/l)
- Interval of less than a year from original diagnosis to the start of systemic treatment
- Karnofsky performance status < 80
- Absence of prior nephrectomy

In another trial conducted in the year 2004, Motzer evaluated survival in previously treated patients with metastatic RCC. 251 patients were included in the trial. Identified prognostic factors were:

- low (<80) Karnofsky performance status
- low haemoglobin levels
- high corrected serum calcium.

Based on these three factors he divided patients into three groups regarding their prognosis. The median survival in patients without any of the factors present was 22 months, with one factor 11,9 months and those with two or three 5,4 months. Even though his intent was to categorize patients into risk groups to better interpret the results of clinical trials, we can use this categorisation in assessing predicted survival in our every day clinical practice (Motzer et.al., 2004).

To evaluate Memorial Sloan Kettering prognostic factors, researchers at the Cleveland Clinic Taussig Center retrospectively evaluated 353 patients with metastatic RCC that were included in clinical trials between 1987 and 2002. Four of the five prognostic factors identified by Motzer were independent predictors of survival. In addition, prior radiotherapy and presence of hepatic, lung, and retroperitoneal nodal metastases were found to be independent prognostic factors. Using these expanded criteria, favorable risk is defined as zero or one poor prognostic factor, intermediate risk is two poor prognostic factors, and poor risk is more than two poor prognostic factors. Median overall survival times of these groups were 26.0, 14,4, and 7,3 months, respectively (P < ,0001) (Bukowski & Negrier, 2004, Mekhail et.al, 2005).

Different models predicting survival other than those developed by Motzer and Cleveland group have been proposed. Bamias studied prognostic factors in patients treated with sunitinib. He identified three prognostic factors: time from diagnosis to the start of sunitinib therapy, number of metastatic sites and performance status (Bamias et.al., 2010). Hudes et.al. in a trial with temsirolimus used slightly modified Motser's factors in selecting poor prognosis patients. Instead of absence of prior nephrectomy, metastases in multiple organs were included and Karnofsky performance status <70 was used (Hudes et.al., 2007).

2.5 Definitions of elderly and frail patients

Elderly population is not an uniform entity, since chronological and biological age can differ considerably (Neustadt et.al., 2008). On a basis of the observation that active oncological treatment can be outweighed by increased treatment toxicity in this patient population, age of 75 years was determined as a milestone for defining elderly patients population (Lane et.al., 2010). Frail patients are considered those in poor performance status (WHO>1) (Pushkar & Govorov, 2008). According to MSK model, patients with Karnofsky PS<80%had worse survival compared to patients with higher score (Motzer, et.al. 1996)

3. Tumour evaluation

3.1 Diagnostic procedures

In tumour evaluation, the diagnostic tests do not differ much between older and younger patient populations. In both groups CT is necessary for accurate detection of tumour and nodal extension. In patients with renal insufficiency, CT without contrast media or magnetic resonance imaging instead of CT is being performed in order to prevent further damage to kidneys by using a nephrotoxic contrast media. Abdominal ultrasound is another very useful diagnostic tool that can easily be performed in all patients regardless of their age or performance status. The role of percutaneous tumour biopsy is limited in all patients. It may be of value in frail patients or in patients with overt metastatic disease to make a diagnosis of RCC and to avoid radical nephrectomy (Pushkar & Govorov, 2008).

3.2 Differences in tumour characteristics between young and elderly patients

Renal carcinoma is the most common renal parenchymal malignancy. Most of the patients are elderly with only 3-7% of RCC occurring in patients younger than 40 years. Trials performed in patients with breast, colon and prostate carcinomas showed that younger patients have a biologically more aggressive disease that leads to worse prognosis compared to elderly patients (Denzinger et.al., 2009).

To explore this issue in RCC, Denzinger retrospectively evaluated 1042 patients that were treated between 1992 and 2005. He compared patients younger than 45 years to patients aged over 75. In a multivariate analysis lower age was associated with higher 5-years cancer specific survival (95,2% vs 72,3% p=0,009) and lower 5-y progression rate (11,3% vs 42,5% p=0,002) (Denzinger et.al., 2009). Komai et.al. also found younger age to be a favourable prognostic factor. The 5-year cancer-specific survival rate was significantly better for the younger patients than for the older patients (p = ,049). Multivariate analysis showed that age was significantly associated with cancer specific survival (Komai et. al. 2011). Similar results were obtained in a trial of Jung and co-workers on low stage RCC patients (Jung et.al., 2009). These and other trials show uniformly, that younger RCC patients have better prognosis compared to the elderly (Denzinger et.al., 2009).

Trials also uniformly showed that younger patients are more likely to have a lower disease stage, lower nuclear grade, and smaller tumor size than older patients (Denzinger et.al., 2009, Komai et.al., 2011, Jung et.al., 2009).

4. Surgical treatment of elderly and frail patients

4.1 Radical and nephron sparing surgery in localized disease

Surgical resection is effective therapy for clinically localized RCC; with options including radical nephrectomy and nephron-sparing surgery. Radical nephrectomy (RN) was for many years considered the "gold standard" in the treatment of locally advanced RCC and nephron sparing surgery (NSS) was suggested when radical nephrectomy would render the patient functionally anephric. These cases included RCC in a solitary kidney, RCC in one kidney and the other non functioning and bilateral RCC (NCCN, 2011).

In recent years nephron-sparing surgery has become more and more popular (NCCN, 2011). Several trials showed that in patients with small tumours (<7 cm) the same oncological results can be achieved with NSS compared to RN (NCCN, 2011, Leibovich et.al, 2006, Becker et.al., 2006). In the trial of Leibowich the results of 91 patients treated with NSS and 841 patients treated with RN for 4 to 7 cm RCC between 1970 and 2000 have been compared. Cancer specific survival rates at 5 years for patients treated with NSS and RN for 4 to 7 cm RCC were 98% and 86%, respectively, the difference was not statistically significant (risk ratio 1,60, 95% CI 0,50-5,12, p = 0,430). Differences were not statistically significant even when authors compared the occurrence of local relapse or distant metastases (Leibovich et.al, 2006).

Nephrectomy (radical or nephron-sparing) should be considered as part of treatment decision process in all patients with stage I-III disease fit for surgical procedure (NCCN, 2011). In elderly or poor performance status patients still amenable for surgery nephron-sparing nephrectomy rather than radical nephrectomy should be performed whenever possible (Lane et.al., 2009). In patients with decreased life expectancy and/or extensive co-morbidities, surgery represents excessive risk and other options like tumour termoablation or active surveillance should be considered (NCCN, 2011)

4.2 Cytoreductive nephrectomy in patients with metastatic disease

Multimodality treatment in patients with metastatic RCC consists of surgery combined with systemic therapy. Surgical approach consists of cytoreductive nephrectomy often combined with metastasectomy of distant metastases. This approach in cancer therapy is distinctly different from treatment of other types of cancer. The rationale for nephrectomy is multiple: enhancing the effects of systemic therapy, removing the source of distant metastases and providing additional tissue for evluation in targeted therapy (Kutikov et.al., 2010).

To assess the benefit of cytoreductive surgery in patients with poor performance status (PS WHO 2 or 3), Shuch et.al. performed a retrospective analysis of all patients who underwent CN surgery at the University of California in between 1989 and 2006. They compared the results of patients in good (WHO 0,1) with those in poor performance status (WHO 2,3). Patients with poor PS had shorter disease-specific survival compared to patients with better PS (6 months vs. 27 months). Systemic treatment in CN was administered to only 57,5% of patients in poor performance status and no objective response was seen in these patients. CN in these patients may be used only to palliate haematuria or pain, but survival benefit of CN in poor PS patients is limited. (Scuch et.al., 2008, Kutikov et.al., 2010, Pushkar & Govorov, 2008, Chouieri, 2010).

Cytoreductive surgery should be offered to patients in good performance status only. Beside these, patients with lung metastases only and those with good prognostic features benefit most from it. The role of CN in the era of targeted therapy has not been defined jet. Randomized trials are ongoing and should answer this dilemma (NCCN, 2011).

4.3 Observation and palliative surgical aproaches

Observation (so called watchful waiting or active surveillance) is a less aggressive treatment modality and should be considered as an option in elderly patients with or without major co-morbidities, especially those with small incidentally found tumours and in those with larger tumours, but very short life expectancy. For the latter, surgery represents a greater risk compared to observation alone. Kassouf et.al. demonstrated that observation is a safe option, most of the tumours observed did not show signs of growth and none of the 24 patients in the trial developed metastases during the 31.6 months of median follow-up (Pushkar & Govorov, 2008).

One question still open is whether to perform tumour biopsy to prove malignity before active therapy is delivered. In the past this approach was not frequently adopted, mainly because a lot of false negative results found and because of the fear of side effects connected to biopsy of renal mass. In recent years renal biopsy became relevant. This is due to the fact that 20% of small renal tumours are benign or have low malignant potential. Biopsy should be considered whenever some doubt exists in decision to perform surgery, minimally invasive procedures or to observe the patient (Lazzeri et.al., 2010).

Paliative nephrectomy should be considered in patients with gross haematuria or other symptoms related to primary tumour that can not be controlled by non invasive measures, like uncontrollable pain (NCCN, 2011). Moreover, it may palliate pain and treat paraneoplastic syndromes associated with metastatic RCC (Kutikov et.al., 2010).

Tumour transarterial embolisation (TAE) in RCC patients has an established role in palliative treatment. It can be used to diminish patient's suffering from pain, haematuria or paraneoplastic symptoms. It can be offered as a sole treatment option or preoperatively to diminish the blood loss during nephrectomy. Although it is considered a palliative measure, 80% of patients to whom TAE has been performed, remain disease free after the procedure (Lane et.al., 2010). TAE should be offered to patients with short life expectancy, since neovascularisation is expected to occur some time after the procedure (de Reijke et.al., 2010). Munro et.al evaluated 25 patients treated with TAE. In this survey TAE was performed in two groups of patients. The first group consisted of patients with stage IV disease (median age 73 years) and the second of mainly elderly (median age 80 years) patients stage I-III disease who were unable or unwilling to receive nephrectomy. Authors analysed the usefulness of TEA regarding symptom control, hospital stay and survival. The conclusion was that embolisation is a good treatment option for palliating symptoms derived from primary tumour in patients with advanced disease and those with localized disease and poor general condition (Pushkar & Govorov, 2008). Other palliative measures available today are cryoablation, radiofrequency ablation, high-intensity focused US; microwave thermotherapy and radiosurgery. Results with all these techniques, even if studied in trials with small included number of patients, are promising not only in terms of palliation, but also in terms of disease free and cancer related survival (Lazzeri et.al., 2010).

5. Systemic therapy of metastatic disease

Despite advances in RCC detection, still 20-30% of patients present with metastatic disease. Treatment of metastatic disease in elderly and frail patients represents a big challenge for medical oncologists. Until recently there was a widely accepted belief that the treatment may not be effective in older patients and that they may be at higher risk of developing adverse events than younger patients. Consequently, they were often excluded or inadequately represented in clinical trials. However, recent evidence indicates that available treatments may be tolerated and effective in all patients regardless of age. Metastatic RCC is a chemotherapy resistant disease and until recently treatment options of these patients were limited. With the development of targeted therapies, new treatment options became available. Yet the question of efficiency and tolerability of this agents in elderly and frail patients arose (NCCN, 2011, Scuch et.al., 2008).

5.1 Treatment with immunotherapy

Immunotherapy with interferon alfa and interlekin-2 was for a long period the cornerstone of systemic treatment of metastatic RCC. Nowadays immunotherapy is being successfully replaced by less toxic and more effective targeted therapies. Trials performed with immunotherapy have shown that patients with worse performance not only had shorter survival, but also had a decreased response rate to immunotherapy and greater frequency 3 and 4 toxicity. Decreased response to immunotherapy is supposed to be due to the fact that patients with PS>1 have a compromised immune system; immunotherapy success is clearly related to a good immune system. Nevertheless, it is difficult to determine whether the treatment is less effective because the performance status is low or whether the performance status is low because tumour is more aggressive (Pushkar & Govorov, 2008). This, together with tumour characteristics, is the reason why immunotherapy was not approved in the treatment of patients with poor performance status (Scuch et.al., 2008).

5.2 Treatment with targeted therapies

In recent years a whole new spectrum of treatments with targeted drugs became available in the treatment of metastatic RCC. These new drugs were tested to treat elderly and frail patients with promising results (Bellmunt et.al., 2011).

Sunitinib targets a number of receptor tyrosine kinases including platlet-derived growth factor receptors, vascular endothelial growth factor receptors, stem cell factor receptor, FMS-like tyrosine kinase, colony stimulating receptor and neurotropic factor receptor (NCCN, 2011). Sunitinib has established role in the treatment of metastatic RCC (Gore et.al., 2009). The efficacy and safety of sunitinib in elderly and poor prognosis patients was assessed in an expanded-access trial. Of 4371 included patients 582 (13%) had PS 2 or higher and 1418 (32%) were aged 65 or more. Results showed a 17% objective response rate in the elderly and a 9% rate in PS≥2 patients. Median progression free survival was 11,3 months (95% in elderly and 5,1 months in poor performance group). Side effects were few and tolerable. Authors concluded that sunitinib is effective and safe even in groups of patients that are supposed to tolerate treatment less well and are usually excluded from clinical trials (Gore et.al., 2009, NCCN, 2011, Calvo et.al., 2010).

Sorafenib is a small molecule that inhibits multiple tyrosine kinase receptors (NCCN, 2011). Treatment with sorafenib is considered to be equally effective in elderly and younger patients. Retrospective subgroup analysis of data from TARGET (Treatment Approach in Renal Cancer Global Evaluation) trial showed similar clinical benefit in patients aged 70 years or more compared to younger ones (83,5% in older and 84,3% in younger patients) (Calvo et.al., 2010). Incidence of adverse events were not significantly higher in elderly patients receiving sorafenib. Thus sorafenib represents an important treatment option for elderly patients with RCC (Dutcher et.al., 2010).

Temsirolimus was tested in a phase 3 trial comparing it to interferone therapy in patients with poor prognosis. Patients included in the trial had at least three of the 6 criteria for poor prognosis according to the modified MSCC. Patients were randomized to one of the three arms (temsirolimus alone, interferone alone or both treatments given together). Patients that received temsirolimus alone had longer overall survival compared to other two groups. (OS 10,9 months temsirolimus alone, 7,3 interferone, 8,4 combination). The main conclusion of this trial is that treatment with temsirolimus alone leads to moderate prolongation of survival compared to treatment with interferon in patients with poor prognosis. Based on this trial, temsirolimus is indicated in the first line of therapy in poor prognosis patients (Hudes et.al., 2009, Rejike et.al., 2010).

Bevacisumab is an recombinant humanized monoclonal antibody that binds and neutralizes circulating VEGF-A. Bevacisumab was approved by FDA for first line treatment in combination with IFN-α (NCCN, 2011). Concerns about administering bevacisumab in elderly, have been diminished by retrospective trials that showed similar efficacy and toxicity profiles compared with younger patients. Billemont et.al. presented data regarding treatment of elderly patients with all antiangiogenic therapies (sunitinib, sorafenib, bevacisumab). There were no toxic deaths, most common grade 3 or 4 were skin toxicity and mucositis. Authors conclude that antiangiogenic therapy including bevacisumab, can be administered safely to patients older than 75 years (Billemont et.al., 2010). Other retrospective trials similarly conclude that side effects, while more pronounced in the elderly, are well tolerated and not dose-limiting (Calvo, 2010).

Pazopanib is an oral VEGFR-1 and 2, PDGFR-α and β. It was approved for treatment of metastatic RCC in 2009 (NCCN, 2011). The most common side effects of pazopanib are diarrhoea, fatigue and hair depigmentation. The most worrying side effect is hepatotoxicity grade 3 present in 12% aldough fatal events are rare (0,05% of cases). Even if only 6% of patients included in the trials with pazopanib were aged > 75 years, no differences in safety and effectiveness was observed in comparison with younger ones (Calvo et.al., 2010, FDA, 2009, Bukowski, 2011).

Everolimus is an inhibitor of mTOR. It was approved for the treatment of metastatic RCC after failure of sunitinib or sorafenib in 2009 based on a phase III trial named RECORD 1 wich compared treatment with everolimus to placebo (NCCN, 2011). To assess the efficacy and safety of everolimus in elderly patients (>70 years), Hutson et.al. performed an exploratory analysis of RECORD-1 trial data. Everolimus prolonged PFS in this group of patients, compared to placebo. Some adverse events (eg, cough, diarrhea, asthenia, fatigue) were more frequent in the elderly subset vs. the overall RECORD-1 population (median age, 61 y); but this is likely related to the intrinsic characteristics of this subpopulation, given that these adverse events also were more frequent in the elderly subgroup receiving placebo (Hutson et.al., 2010).

According to the data obtained from trials published until now, most of the targeted therapies are equally effective and safe in elderly and/or frail or in young and good performance status patients. In most cases dose reduction is not necessary and some of the targeted therapies (i.e. everolimus) may even prevent worsening of renal function in transplant patients and those with multiple co-morbidities. The conclusion of multiple trials is that newer targeted drugs should be offered to elderly and/or patients with multiple co-morbidities. It can not be stressed enough that including these patients in clinical trials is mandatory (Calvo et.al., 2010).

6. Treatment with radiotherapy

In the rare case of inoperable RCC, radiotherapy can be administered with promising results. In a trial of Wersall, 58 patients with inoperable or metastatic RCC received high dose stereotactic radiotherapy (32Gy in 4 fractions, 40Gy in 4 fractions or 45Gy in 3 fractions). Partial response or stable disease was observed in 90% of patients and local control rate of 90-98% was achieved. Radiotherapy can be safely administered to elderly and frail patients and should be considered whenever radical therapy is not applicable (Wersall et.al., 2005, de Rejike et.al., 2010).

For patients with brain metastases, radiotherapy has an important role in their treatment. Using stereotactic radiotherapy similar results can be achieved as with surgical removal of brain metastases. The stereotactic radiotherapy is non-invasive, outpatient and can be applied in patients in lower PS, without worsening their condition (de Rejike et.al., 2010).

Bone metastases represent a special problem. Patients with bone metastases are often symptomatic; pathological fractures, spinal cord compression and the need for surgery are common, and nearly 80% of untreated patients experience skeletal-related events. Until recently treatment options for these patients were scarce because of the chemo and ratio-resistance of RCC. With the development of new agents like biphosphonates and targeted agents, better results in treatment of bone metastases regarding pain control and pathologic fractures can be achieved. Yuasa showed that combining radiotherapy with biphosphonates administration leads to higher objective response and less skeletal related events compared to radiation therapy alone. In administering biphosphonates caution is needed because of the renal impairment (Yuasa et.al., 2010).

7. Treatment of elderly and frail metastatic RCC patients at the Institute of Oncology Ljubljana

To explore the treatment approach in every-day practice we retrospectively evaluated T_{any} N_{any} M1 RCC patients that were treated at the Institute of Oncology Ljubljana, Slovenia, between 2006 and 2009 and for whom appropriate data were available. A patient was considered to have a metastatic disease if it was confirmed by biopsy or clear signs of metastatic disease were present on radiographic evaluation. Staging was performed by using CT imaging of thorax and abdomen. If needed other diagnostic tests were performed. Surgical procedures were done in hospitals other than Institute of Oncology. Performance status was assessed according to WHO scale. The aim was to assess possible differences in the treatment strategy decisions in good (WHO 0 or 1) versus poor (WHO>1) performance status patients.

Medical records of 368 patients were reviewed. Patients with incomplete records were excluded. Patient and tumour characteristics are presented in Table 3.

Variable	Metastatic RCC patients No=368
Male	268 (72,8%)
Female	100 (27,2%)
Median age	63.3 (34-86) years
Histology	
Clear cell	228 (62%)
Papillary	37 (10,0%)
RCC not other specified	64 (17.4%)
Sarcomatoid	26 (7,1%)
Other rare (chromophobe, collecting duct, mixed...)	13 (3,5%)

Performance status	
0	89 (24,2%)
1	108 (29,3%)
2	57 (15,5%)
3	70 (19,0%)
4	38 (10,3%)
Unknown	6 (1,6%)
Co-morbidities	
Present	93 (25,3%)
Absent	262 (71,2%)
Unknown	13 (3,5%)

Table 3. Patient and tumour caracteristics

All patients were reviewed by the multidisciplinary board that consists of an urologist, a medical oncologist and a radiation oncologist. All patients had proven metastatic disease before presentation to the board. Administered treatment is shown in Table 4.

Treatment mode	Number of patients treated (percentage)
Surgery	
Nephrectomy with radical intent (performed before metastatic disease was present)	162 (44,1%)
Cytoreductive nephrectomy	106 (28,8%)
Tumour embolisation	43 (11,6%)
Systemic therapy	
Immunotherapy	50 (13,6%)
Targeted therapy	156 (42,4%)
Watchful waiting	12 (3,3%)
Best supportive care	150 (40,0%)

Table 4. Treatment options

To establish possible differences in the decision of treatment strategy in different groups of patients, a comparison was made. All treatment decisions were made by a multidisciplinary team of oncologists on the basis of medical documentation and clinical examination of the patient by a member of the team. Comparison between groups was done with X^2 test. Differences between patients in good vs. poor performance status, patients with or without major co-morbidities and younger vs. elderly patients is shown in Table 5.

	Systemic therapy (immunotherapy or targeted therapy)	Best supportive care or observation	
Performance status			
PS 0,1	179 (90,8%)	18 (9,2%)	
PS>1	26 (15,7%)	139 (84,3%)	
			p<0,01
Co-morbidities			
Not present	160 (61%)	102 (39%)	
Present	50 (53,7%)	43 (46,3%)	
			p=0,76
Age			
< 75 years	151 (72,7%)	57 (27,3%)	
≥ 75 years	12 (7,5%)	148 (92,5)%	
			p<0,01

Table 5. Differences in treatment decisions

As expected, the patient's performance status has an important impact on treatment decision. Patients in good PS receive systemic therapy in much greater percentage of cases than patients in poor PS. Patients in poor PS are more likely to tolerate less well systemic therapy and treatment decisions in every-day practice reflects the knowledge of this fact. Defining PS, even if it is a subjective measure, is very important and should be made by an experienced clinician. Still, some patients in good PS do not get the systemic therapy and some in poor PS get it. This reflects the influence of other factors, like age of the patients and co-morbidities on treatment decisions.

The difference between treatment decisions based on co-morbidities is not clear. In our review, systemic treatment was administered to many patients with co-morbidities. An explanation for this is, that according to known data, most of the available targeted therapies are effective and safe for the majority of patients with co-morbidities. Nevertheless, half of the patients with co-morbidities present do not get the specific therapy.

With evolving results from clinical trials, new data on safety and efficacy will become available which will help clinicians in treatment decisions.

Age has a huge impact on treatment decisions. Less than 10% of metastatic RCC patients older than 75 years get systemic therapy prescribed. Prescribing targeted therapies to elderly patients still represents a challenge to clinicians. This is in accordance with the widely established tendency to believe that older patients tolerate the treatment less well and develop adverse events in higher percentage and at greater degree. Recent evidence shows that available treatments (targeted therapy) are safe and efficient in elderly as well as young patients (Calvo et.al., 2010).

8. Conclusions

Longer life expectancy together with the growing incidence of RCC has raised the number of elderly and frail patients with this malignancy. Tailoring treatment to the individual patient according to the tumour stage and patient general condition is the primary goal of treatment. Treatment options for the elderly and frail are multiple and vary in their aggressiveness. Finding the right treatment for the right patient can be a difficult task for oncologists. Improvement in all fields from surgery to targeted therapies led to broader treatment choice. The problem that remains is that often no evidence exists which treatment combination to use, since much too often these patients are excluded form clinical trials. How to encourage investigators to design clinical trials so as that these patients can be included in greater numbers, remains a difficult open question especially in large trials testing new drugs. Conducting trials addressing these populations after the drug has been approved for use in good prognosis-good performance patients deprives others of a new drug which is often well tolerable and effective.

9. References

Bellmunt, J.; Eisen, T.; Szczylk, C.; et.al. A new patient-focused approach to the treatment of metastatic renal cell carcinoma: establishing customized treatment options. *British Journal of Urology International*, Vol.107, No.8, (April 2011), pp. 1190-99, ISSN 2042-2997

Bamias, A.; Karadimou, A.; Lampaki, S.; et.al. Prognostic stratification of patients with advanced renal cell carcinoma treated with sunitinib: comparison with the Memorial Sloan-Kettering prognostic factors model. *BMC Cancer*, Vol.10, No.45, (published online February 2010), pp. 1-12, ISSN 1471-2407

Becker, F.; Siemer, S.; Humke, U.; et.al. Elective nephron sparing surgery should become standard treatment for small unilateral renal cell carcinoma: survival data of 216 patients. *European Urology*, Vol.49, No.2, (February 2006), pp. 308-13, ISSN 1871-2592

Billemont, B.; Massard, S.; Negrier, M.; et.al. Antiangiogenic treatment in elderly patients (>75 years) with metastatic RCC: Experience from the French Renal Group. Poster presented at the American Society of Clinical Oncology conference 2010.

Bukowski, RM.; Negrier, S. Prognostic factors in patients with advanced renal cell carcinoma. Development of an International Kidney Cancer Working Grup. *Clinical Cancer Research*, Vol.15, No.10, (September 2004), pp. 6310-14, ISSN 1078-0432

Bukowski, RM. Critical appraisal of pazopanib as treatment for patients with advanced metastatic renal cell carcinoma. *Cancer Management and Research,* Vol.3, (August 2011), pp. 273-85, ISSN 1179-1322

Calvo, E.; Maroto, P.; Garcia del Moro, X.; et.al. Update from the Spanish Oncology Genitourinary Group on the treatment of advanced renal cell carcinoma: focus on special populations. *Cancer metastasis review,* Vol.29 (Suppl 1) (July 2010), pp. 11-20, ISSN 0167-7659

Choueiri, TK.; Wanling, X.; Kollmansberger, C.; et.al. The Impact of cytoreductive Nephrectomy on Survival of Patients With Metastatic Renal Cell Carcinoma Receiving Vascular Endothelial Growth Factor Targeted Therapy. *The Journal of Urology,* Vol.185, No.1 (November 2010), pp. 60-6, ISSN 0022-5347

Denzinger, S.; Otto, W.; Burger, M.; et.al. Sporadic renal cell carcinoma in young and elderly patients: are the different clinicopathological features and disease specific survival rates?. *World Journal of Surgical Oncology,* Vol.5, No.16, (February 2009), pp. 5-16, ISSN 1477-7819

Dutcher, JP.; Tannir, N.; Bellmunt, J.; et.al. Experience with sorafenib and the elderly patients. *Medical oncology,* Vol.27, No.4, (December 2010), pp. 1359-70, ISSN 1357-0560

de Rejike, TM.; Bellmunt, J.; van Poppel, H.; et.al. EORTC-EU group expert opinion on metastatic renal cell cancer. *European journal of cancer,* Vol.45, No.2 (January 2009), pp. 766-73, ISSN 0959-8049

FDA   prescribing   information: http://www.accessdata.fda.gov/drugsatfda_docs/label/2009/022465lbl

Gore, ME.; Szczylik, C.; Porta, C.; et.al. Safety and efficacy of sunitinib for metastatic renal-cell carcinoma: an expanded-access trial. *The Lancet Oncology,* Vol.10, No.8 (August 2009), pp. 757-63, ISSN 1470-2045

Hudes, M.; Carducci, M.; Zomczak, M.; et.al. Temsirolimus, Interferon Alfa or Both for Advanced Renal-Cell Carcinoma. *The New England Journal of Medicine,* Vol.356, No.22, (May 2007), pp. 2271-81, ISSN 0028-4793

Hutson, TE.; Calvo, BJ.; Escudier, S.; et.al. Everolimus in elderly patients with metastatic renal cell carcinoma: An exploratory analysis of the RECORD 1 study. Poster presented at the American Society of Clinical Oncology conference, 2010

Ishikawa, I.; Saito, Y.; Shikura, N.; et.al. A ten year prospective study on the development of renal cell carcinoma in dialysis patients. *American Journal on Kidney Diseases,* Vol.16, No.5, (November 1990), pp.452-8, ISSN 0272-6386

Jung, EJ.; Lee, HY.; Kwak, C.; et.al. Young age is independent prognostic factor for cancer specific survival of low-stage clear cell renal cell carcinoma. *Urology,* Vol.73, No.1, (January 2009), pp. 1341-8, ISSN 0090-4295

Kutikov, A.; Uzzo, RG.; Caraway, A.; et.al. Use of systemic therapy and factors affecting survival for patients undergoing cytoreductive nephrectomy. *British Journal of Urology International,* Vol.106, No.2, (July 2010), pp. 218-23, ISSN 2042-2997

Komai, Y.; Fujii, Y.; Tatokoro, M.; et.al. Young age as favorable prognostic factor for cancer-specific survival in localized renal cell carcinoma. *Urology,* Vol. 77, No.4, (April 2011), pp. 847-8, ISSN 0090-4295

Lane, BR.; Abouassaly, R.; Tianning, G.; et.al. Active Treatment of Localized Renal Tumours May Not Impact Overall Survival in Patients Aged 75 Years or Older. *Cancer,* Vol.116, No.13, (July 2010), pp. 3119-26, ISSN 1097-0142

Lazzeri, M. & Guazzoni P. Early 21st Century Renal Cell Carcinoma. *Cancer*, Vol.116, No.13, (July 2010), pp. 3135-42, ISSN 1097-0142

Leibovich, BC.; Blute, ML.; Cheville, JC.; et.al. Nephron sparing surgery for appriopriately selected renal cell carcinoma between 4 and 7 cm results in outcome similar to radical nephrectomy. *The Journal of Urology*, Vol.172, No.3 (September 2004), pp. 1066-70, ISSN 0022-5347

Levine, E. renal cell carcinoma in uremic acquired renal cystic disease: incidence, detection and management. *Urologic Radiology*, Vol.13, No.2, (December 1992), pp. 203-10, ISSN 0171-1091

Linehan, WM.; Rini, AV.; Yang JC. (2011). Cancer of the kidney, In: *Cancer. Principles and Practice of Oncology*, DeVita, VT.; Lawrence, TS; Rosenberg, SA. (Ed.), 1161-91, Lipincott Williams & Wilkins, ISBN 978-1-4511-1813-1, Philadelphia, USA

Macfarlane, R.; Heng, DYC.; Xie, W.; et.al. The Impact of Kidney Function on the Outcome of Metastatic Renal Cell Carcinoma Patients Treated With Vascular Endothelial Growth Factor-Targeted Therapy. *Cancer*, (published online August 2011), pp. 1-6, ISSN 1097-0142

Mekhail, TM.; Abu-Jawde, BM.; Boumerhi, G.; et.al. Validation and extension of the Memorial Sloan-Kettering prognostic factors model for survival in patients with previously untreated metastatic renal cell carcinoma. *Journal of Clinical Oncology*, Vol.23, No.4 (February 2005), pp. 832-41, ISSN 0732-183X

Motzer, RJ.; Baick, Y.; Lawrence, W.; et.al. Prognostic Factors for Survival in Previously Treated Patients With Metastatic Renal Cell Carcinoma. *Journal of Clinical Oncology*, Vol.22, No.3 (February 2004), pp. 454-63, ISSN 0732-183X

Motzer, RJ.; Mazumdar, M.; Baick, J.; et.al. Survival and Prognostic Stratification of 670 Patients With Advanced Renal Cell Carcinoma. *Journal of Clinical Oncology*, Vol.17, No.8 (August 1999), pp. 2530-40, ISSN 0732-183X

NCCN clinical practice guidelines in oncology: Kidney cancer, Version 2 (2011): http://www.nccn.org

Neustadt, Y. and Pieczenik, S. Organ Reserve and Healthy Ageing. *Integrative Medicine*, Vol.7, No.3, (Jun/Jul 2008), pp. 50-2, ISSN 1543953X

Neuzillet, J.; Tillou, X.; Mathieu, R. Renal Cell Carcinoma (RCC) in Patients With End-Stage Renal Disease Exhibits Many Favourable Clinical, Pathologic, and Outcome Features Compared With RCC in the General Population. *European Urology*, Vol.60, No.2, (August 2011), pp. 366-73, ISSN 1871-2592

Pushkar, D. & Govorov, AV. (2008). Old and Fragile Patients, In: *Renal Cell Cancer*, J. De la Rosette, CN. Sternberg, H. van Poppel (Ed.), 353-64, Springer, ISBN 978-84628-763-3, London, England

Shuch, B.; La Rochelle, JC.; Wu, J.; et.al. Performance Status and Cytoreductive Nephrectomy. *Cancer*, Vol.113, No.6, (September 2008), pp. 1324-31, ISSN 1097-0142

Wersäll, PJ.; Blomgren, H.; Lax, I.; et.al. Extracranial stereotactic radiotherapy for primary and metastatic renal cell carcinoma. *Radiotherapy and Oncology*, Vol.77, No.1, (June 2005), pp. 88-95, ISSN 0167-8140

Yuasa, T.; Urakami, S.; Yamamoto S.; et.al. Treatment outcome and prognostic factors in renal cell cancer patients with bone metastases. *Clinical and experimental metastasis*, Vol.42, No.8, (August 2010), pp. 299-303, ISSN 0262-0898

11

Sequential Use of Targeted Therapies (TT) in Metastatic Renal Cell Cancer (mRCC): Overall Results of a Large Experience

G. Procopio, E. Verzoni, R. Iacovelli,
F. Gelsomino, M. Catanzaro and L. Mariani
'IRCCS 'Istituto Nazionale dei Tumori', Medical Oncology, Milan
Italy

1. Introduction

Renal cell carcinoma accounts for 80% of all kidney cancers -worldwide; the tumor staging at diagnosis ranges from small, low-stage tumors to more advanced neoplasms [1-5]. The survival rate has increased in recent years: nowadays, patients with localized disease have a 5-year survival >80% but in those with distant metastatic RCC, 5-year survival is <10% [6-8]. The increase in overall survival was due, at least in part, to improved surgical techniques [9,10]. Until recently cytokines (interleukin-2 or interferon-alpha), were the mainstay of systemic treatment despite low response rates and significant toxicity [11,12].

Since 2005, six targeted therapies for advanced/metastatic RCC were approved by both the FDA and EMA: three are multitargeted tyrosine kinase inhibitors (TKIs), sorafenib (SO), sunitinib (SU) and pazopanib (PZ), two are oral mTOR inhibitors, temsirolimus (TS) and everolimus (EV) and one is the anti-VEGF monoclonal antibody bevacizumab (BV), administered in combination with IFN alpha [13]. These new agents improved the progression free survival (PFS) and the overall survival (OS) in several subgroups of patients; however, expert opinion on the optimal therapeutic strategy is divided.

Two main therapeutic approaches—use of these new agents in combination or sequentially—have been studied to increase efficacy and tolerability. Sequential therapy is the current standard of care in the treatment of advanced RCC as existing combination regimens have a high incidence of adverse events without a substantial increase in efficacy. The use of sequential therapy provides a number of important advantages: patients who are refractory to one or more targeted agent(s) may benefit from treatment with a different agent; there is no/limited cross-resistance between agents and patients experiencing disease progression with one anti-angiogenic agent can subsequently benefit from treatment with another [14,15].

The results of recent phase III randomized controlled trials (RCTs) prompted the National Comprehensive Cancer Network (NCCN) and the European Association of Urology (EAU) to update their clinical practice guidelines for the treatment of metastatic RCC [16,17]. The EAU recommended SU as a first-line therapy in low- and intermediate-risk patients and concluded that SO is effective as second-line treatment after failure of cytokine therapy or in patients unfit for cytokines [18]. Clinical evidence supports the efficacy of sequential treatment with SU/SO [19]; however, the optimal sequence for SO and SU is still under debate, and additional evidence on the optimal use of sequential targeted therapies is advocated.

In this retrospective study – the preliminary results of which have been previously presented [20] - the safety and efficacy of different sequential schemes of targeted therapies, in patients with advanced/metastatic RCC were studied.

2. Methods

2.1 Patients

This retrospective study was conducted at the 'Istituto Nazionale Tumori of Milan' (National Institute of Tumors, Milan, Italy) – one of the most important Italian institutions for cancer diagnosis and treatment - between January 2004 and July 2010. Patients were patients aged ≥18 years with advanced/metastatic RCC and a life expectancy of >3 months who had been treated with antiangiogenic therapy (one or more) were eligible for enrollment in this retrospective study. Patients with Eastern Cooperative Oncology Group (ECOG) performance status (PS) of 0, 1 or 2 were included. A number of patients enrolled in this study had previously taken part in a range of prospective trials including TARGET , the EU-ARCCS , RECORD-1 , AXIS , AVOREN and ROSORC at our centre.

3. Treatment

Patients received a range of different systemic agents – SO, SU, BV, EV, TS and axitinib (AX) alone or in combination, and could have received a previous treatment with cytokines. SO was administered orally at a dose of 400 mg twice daily and SU at a daily dose of 50 mg orally with a 4 weeks on 2 weeks off schedule. BV was administered iv at 10 mg/Kg every 2 weeks in combination with Interferon-a subcutaneously, EV was administered orally at 10 mg daily continuously, TS iv weekly at 25 mg/dose and AX at 10 mg/daily orally continuously. Patients received systemic therapy until disease progression or the presence of serious adverse events.

4. Study assessments

Study assessments were conducted at baseline and once a month thereafter. Baseline characteristics were taken ≤28 days after the start of treatment. Drug safety and tolerability were assessed using the National Cancer Institute Common Terminology Criteria for Adverse Events (NCTCA version 3). Efficacy was assessed by progression-free survival (PFS) and overall survival (OS) according to the Motzer classification [21]. PFS was defined as the time from start of systemic treatment to death or disease progression whichever occurred first. Disease progression was evaluated using the Response Evaluation criteria in Solid Tumours (RECIST, version 1.0) by the treating physician. Assessments were performed monthly (every 3 weeks for patients on sunitinib, due to the schedule of administration for this drug). Patients with Bellini duct RCC were excluded from the efficacy analysis, due to the different histology of the tumor.

5. Statistical analyses

All clinical and instrumental variables and toxicity data were analyzed by descriptive statistics: mean, standard deviation, minimum, and maximum values for continuous variables, and absolute and relative frequencies for categorical variables. Curves relevant to OS (overall, Motzer and according to therapy option) were estimated by the Kaplan–Meier method and compared by means of the log-rank test. Reports of AEs were categorized according to type, severity, and outcome. A p value <0.05 was considered statistically significant.

6. Results

A total of 310 patients with metastatic RCC were observed, and followed-up for a median of 37 months (range 21–49 months). Patient characteristics at baseline are shown in **Table 1**.

Patients included in database	310	
Median age (years)	62	
Range	55–69	
Male	229	(74%)
Female	81	
ECOG PS		
0	168	(54%)
1	123	(40%)
2	19	(6%)
Histology		
Clear-cell	268	(86.4%)
Papillary	27	(8.7%)
Bellini	7	(2.2%)
Chromophobe	6	(1.9%)
Oncocytoma	1	(0.3%)
UNK	1	(0.3%)
Previous nephrectomy, %	273	(88.1%)
Fuhrman grade, %		
1	15	(5.58%)
2	93	(34.57%)
3	118	(43.87%)
4	43	(15.99%)
Missing	41	
Motzer criteria		
High	64	(20.6%)
Low	100	(32.3%)
Intermediate	146	(47.10%)
Targeted therapies %		
1	163	(52.6%)
2	113	(36.5%)
3	30	(9.7%)
4	4	(1.29%)

Number of disease sites		
1	121	(39.0%)
2	107	(34.5%)
3	67	(21.2%)
4	12	(3.9%)
5	3	(0.9%)
Sites of disease (n=599)		
Bone	88	(28.39%)
Brain	16	(5.16%)
Liver	59	(19.03%)
Lung	204	(65.81%)
Lymph nodes	119	(38.39%)
Pancreas	15	(4.84%)
Thyroid	4	(1.29%)
Other	94	(30.32%)

Table 1. Patient characteristics at baseline

Overall the majority of patients (163; 53.9%) received one treatment line with systemic agents while 113 (36.5%) received two, 30 (9.7%) received three line and four patients (1.3%) received four. One-sided analysis of variance showed that the Motzer classification/score was predictive regarding the number of therapy lines (Fisher 8.49, p<0.01) with the mean number of treatments significantly lower in the high-risk group (p<0.05) than in the low/intermediate risk groups (t-tests). Overall the majority of patients 196/310 received SO as first line followed by SU in 96 cases or SU, in 63 cases followed by SO in 13 cases). The remaining 51/310 received other systemic agents in sequence (BV, TS, AX alone or in sequence/combination with SO and SU).

Median OS was 22 months and the 5-year OS was 23.4% (95% CI 16.7, 30.0%) (**Figure 1**).

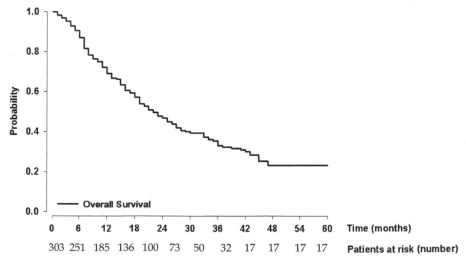

Fig. 1. Overall survival

The Motzer criteria were validated as prognostic factors in both the uni- and multi-variate analysis (p<0.001). The median and 5-year OS was 43 months and 42.8% in low-risk patients, 21 months and 15.9% in intermediate risk patients and 8 months in patients with poor risk (**Figure 2**).

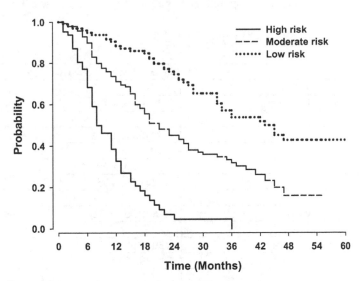

Fig. 2. Overall survival according to Motzer classification

Interestingly in both the multi- and uni-variate analysis there were no significant differences in the hazard ratios when SO+SU are compared with SU+SO and with other therapies (**Table 2, 3 and Figure 3**).

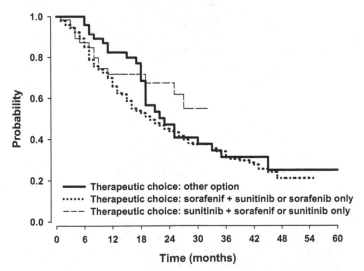

Fig. 3. Overall survival with sorafenib and sunitinib compared with other therapies

In detail, the PFS was 17 months with the specific sequence of SO+SU (9 months + 8 months) and 16 months with SU+SO (12 months + 4 months). The median PFS of first line treatment with either SO or SU was 10.5 months.

Furthermore in the multivariate overall survival analysis un-adjusted for the Motzer classification (**Table 3**) the risk was nearly 1.5 times higher in those patients who had previously been treated with cytokines compared with those who had not received cytokines (p<0.033).

	Hazard ratio (95% CI)	p
Age		
10 years increasing	0.98 (0.86; 1.11)	0.735
Sex		
Male vs. female	1.09 (0.77; 1.55)	0.635
ECOG PS		
1 vs. 0	1.69 (1.25; 2.29)	**<0.001**
2 vs. 0	2.62 (1.39; 4.95)	
Cytokine		
Yes vs. no	1.28 (0.95 ; 1.72)	0.101
Histology		
Papillary vs. clear cell	1.39 (0.85; 2.27)	0.247
Non clear cell vs. Clear cell	1.47 (0.75; 2.89)	
Nephrectomy		
Yes vs. no	0.41 (0.26; 0.65)	**<0.001**
Motzer criteria		
Intermediate vs. low risk	2.30 (1.57; 3.35)	**<0.001**
High vs. low risk	7.90 (5.07;12.31)	
Therapeutic choice		
Other option vs. Sorafenib+sunitinib	0.77 (0.51;1.17)	0.212
Sunitinib+sorafenib vs. sorafenib+sunitinib	0.69 (0.41;1.16)	

ECOG PS = Eastern Cooperative Group Performance Score

Table 2. Univariable overall survival analysis

7. Adverse events

The most commonly reported treatment-related all grade adverse events (AEs) were typical of those reported with TKIs including asthenia, hand-foot syndrome, hypertension, diarrhea, mucositis, hypothyroidism and most of these were mild or moderate in intensity (Grade 1 or 2). Overall, 61 (19.68%) patients experienced AEs Grade ≥3 (**Table 4**) and there were a total of 65 Grade ≥3 AEs, and three patients experienced a Grade 4 event (two patients receiving SU+SO had cardiac failure and one receiving SO+SU had a cardiac stroke). The percentage of patients experiencing adverse events Grade ≥3 was similar in patients treated when SO was given as in those treated first with SU then SO (18.88 and 17.46%). In those treated with other systemic therapies there was a tendency to a higher incidence of AEs (25.5%). Furthermore the nature and severity of AEs groups did not differ if SO or SU was given first.

	Adjusted for Motzer criteria		Not adjusted for Motzer criteria	
	Hazard ratio (95% CI)	p	Hazard ratio (95% CI)	p
Age				
10 years increasing	0.98 (0.85; 1.12)	0.767	0.91 (0.80; 1.04)	0.180
Sex				
Males vs. females	0.91 (0.62; 1.32)	0.611	1.09 (0.76; 1.59)	0.631
ECOG PS				
1 vs. 0	1.09 (0.78; 1.54)	0.838	1.53 (1.11; 2.12)	0.003
2 vs. 0	0.95 (0.48; 1.89)		2.42 (1.27; 4.59)	
Cytokine				
Yes vs. no	1.26 (0.91; 1.75)	0.169	1.41 (1.03; 1.94)	0.033
Histology				
Papillary vs. clear cell	1.35 (0.81; 2.24)	0.478	1.42 (0.86; 2.35)	0.285
Non clear cell vs. clear cell	1.19 (0.60; 2.39)		1.38 (0.69; 2.74)	
Nephrectomy				
Yes vs. no	0.59 (0.35; 0.98)	**0.041**	0.40 (0.24; 0.67)	**0.001**
Motzer criteria				
Intermediate vs. low risk	2.15 (1.44; 3.21)		-	
High vs. low risk	7.23 (4.42; 11.83)	**<0.001**	-	-
Therapeutic choice				
Other options vs. sorafenib+sunitinib	0.84 (0.55; 1.29)	0.388	0.85 (0.56; 1.30)	0.675
Sunitinib+sorafenib vs. Sorafenib+sunitinib	0.70 (0.40; 1.23)		0.85 (0.49; 1.47)	

ECOG PS = Eastern Cooperative Group Performance Score

Table 3. Multivariable overall survival analysis

Adverse event	N	% (N/310)
Asthenia	36	11.61
Hand-foot syndrome	13	4.19
Anemia	4	1.29
Cardiac failure	2	0.65
Hypertension	2	0.65
Mucositis	2	0.65
Abdominal pain	1	0.32
Cardiac stroke	1	0.32
Fever	1	0.32
Macroematuria	1	0.32
Nausea	1	0.32
Rash	1	0.32

Table 4. Adverse events Grade ≥3 (patients may have experienced one or more events)

8. Discussion

Despite improvements in therapy, RCC eventually progresses during therapy and other agent(s) need to be administered in an attempt to control the disease.

This large-scale retrospective analysis was carried out to investigate the effects of systemic therapy in general and in particular to compare the efficacy and safety of different sequential approaches with targeted therapies in controlling the disease progression of patients with RCC. Importantly, our results show that treatment with TKIs improves survival. In fact the median OS for patients with advanced RCC has increased from around 13 months before the introduction of TKIs to around 22 months in the last decade and the median OS of 22 months observed in the present study provides further evidence to support the importance of use of TKI in patients with advanced RCC. In addition, to our knowledge most studies have considered PFS, and not OS, as the major determinant of clinical efficacy of any sequential therapy for the treatment of RCC: our study provides new evidence on OS even in a large unselected population from a single institution. Of note, a relevant proportion of patients received sorafenib as a first-line agent, despite current recommendations suggest this molecule as a second-line treatment, and sunitinib at progression of disease. This therapeutic strategy did not result in any worsening of clinical outcomes and in a similar tolerability with respect to the other therapeutic strategies assessed. Even if this study was not designed to evaluate the feasibility of sorafenib as a first-line agent, and therefore we are unable to draw any conclusion, we believe that this finding could be of some interest in the current therapeutic scenario of RCC patients.

In addition, the Motzer criteria resulted significant prognostic factors in both the uni- and multi-variate analysis. On this basis, we suggest that these criteria should – at present - be regarded to as the most useful tool for the definition of prognosis and, as a consequence, for the optimization of therapy for every single patient.

Of note, the findings reported in the present report were obtained in a real-life scenario, on a large population of unselected patients: it has been suggested that observational trials can expand upon outcomes of randomized controlled trials, which are necessarily conducted in highly-selected patients [22].

In most patients with advanced RCC the objective of treatment is to stabilize disease and prolong survival and there is good evidence that this can be achieved with sequencing systemic agents. The use of this therapeutic approach, in fact, may determine a relevant benefit in terms of OS and quality of life, independently from the specific sequence of targeted therapies used.

Our study confirms the suitability of a TKI sequential therapy. This finding is in line with recent evidence, albeit collected in retrospective studies, which seems to support that the use of SO before SU, rather than vice versa may be more effective in extending PFS (**Table 5**). In addition, some studies suggest that SO may be associated with a more favorable safety profile than more potent SU, in terms of incidence of changes in blood counts and anemia [23,24].

The major limitations of the current study was that the sample size was not randomized and the data were collected retrospectively. In addition the study populations were very hoeterogenous with much patients received the sequence TKI followed TKI and only few cases treated with bevacizumab, everolimus, temsirolimus and axitinib.

Source	n	1st PFS (months)	2nd PFS (months)
Sorafenib→Sunitinib			
Eichelberg et al.	30	8.7	10.3
Dudek et al.	29	5.1	18.0
Porta et al.	83	9.8	8.4
Procopio et al.	50	9.5	8.3
Sablin et al.	68	6.0	6.5
Zimmerman et al.	22	11.5	5.0
Sunitinib→Sorafenib			
Dudek et al.	20	5.8	8.5
Porta et al.	87	8.3	3.7
Sablin et al.	22	5.1	3.9
VEGFi→Sorafenib			
Garcia et al	48	8.7	3.7

PFS = progression-free survival; TTP = time to progression.

Table 5. Summary of sorafenib and sunitinib sequence data (reproduced from ref 24)

In conclusion, despite the major breakthrough introduced by targeted therapies, further research is necessary to shed new lights on the most effective use of these drugs in clinical practice: in particular, the optimal sequence of TKIs has yet to be established.

Our study supports – however - the importance of TKI treatment in RCC patients to improve OS. In addition, it suggests that factors other than the specific sequence of treatment, like the Motzer classification, influence the OS in a large unselected population from clinical practice collected in a single institution. On the basis of these results and of current evidence reported in literature is now clear that there is not one therapy that will benefit all patients and treatment should be tailored to meet individual circumstances and needs. Physicians should therefore base their treatment decisions not only on data from RCTs but also on clinical experience and judgment

9. References

[1] Lindblad P. Epidemiology of renal cell carcinoma. *Scand. J. Surg.* 93(2), 88–96 (2004).
[2] Chow WH, Devesa SS, Warren JL, Fraumeni Jr JF. Rising incidence of renal cell cancer in the United States. *JAMA.* 281(17), 1628–1631 (1999).
[3] Bos SD, Mellema CT, Mensink HJ. Increase in incidental renal cell carcinoma in the northern part of the Netherlands. *Eur. Urol.* 37 (3), 267–270 (2000).
[4] Mevorach RA, Segal AJ, Tersegno ME, Frank IN. Renal cell carcinoma: incidental diagnosis and natural history: review of 235 cases. *Urology,* 39 (6), 519–522 (1992).
[5] Hock LM, Lynch J, Balaji KC. Increasing incidence of all stages of kidney cancer in the last 2 decades in the United States: an analysis of surveillance, epidemiology and end results program data. *J. Urol.* 167 (1), 57–60 (2002).
[6] Pantuck AJ, Zisman A, Belldegrun AS. The changing natural history of renal cell carcinoma. *J. Urol.*166 (5), 1611–1623 (2001).
[7] Atzpodien J, Royston P, Wandert T, Reitz M. Metastatic renal carcinoma comprehensive prognostic system. *Br. J. Cancer* 88 (3), 348–353 (2003).

[8]   Cheville JC, Lohse CM, Zincke H, Weaver AL, Blute ML. Comparisons of outcome and prognostic features among histologic subtypes of renal cell carcinoma. Am. J. Surg. Pathol. 27 (5), 612–624 (2003).

[9]   Jemal A, Tiwari RC, Murray T, et al. Cancer statistics, 2004. CA Cancer. J. Clin. 54(1), 8–29 (2004).

[10] Motzer RJ, Russo P. Systemic therapy for renal cell carcinoma. J. Urol. 163 (2), 408–417 (2003).

[11] Oudard S, George D, Medioni J et al. Treatment options in renal cell carcinoma: past, present and future. Ann. Oncol. 18 (suppl 10), 25–31 (2007).

[12] Atkins MB, Regan M, McDermott D. Update on the role of interleukin 2 and other cytokines in the treatment of patients with stage IV renal carcinoma. Clin. Cancer. Res. 10 (suppl), 6342–6346 (2004).

[13] Hutson TE. Targeted Therapies for the Treatment of Metastatic Renal Cell Carcinoma: Clinical Evidence. The Oncologist. 16 (suppl 2), 14–22 (2011).

[14] Dudek AZ, Zolnierek J, Dham A, Lindgren BR, Szczylik C. Sequential therapy with sorafenib and sunitinib in renal cell carcinoma. Cancer. 115 (1), 61–67 (2009).

[15] Motzer RJ, Escudier B, Oudard S, Hutson TE, Porta C, Bracarda S et al. Efficacy of everolimus in advanced renal cell carcinoma: a double-blind, randomised, placebo-controlled phase III trial. Lancet. 372 (9637), 449–456 (2008).

[16] National Comprehensive Cancer Network. NCCN Clinical Practice Guidelines in Oncology. Kidney Cancer. V. 2.2010. Available at http://www.nccn.org/professionals/physician_gls/PDF/kidney.pdf. Accessed March 22, 2011.

[17] Ljungberg B, Cowan N, Hanbury DC et al. European Association of Urology Guidelines on Renal Cell Carcinoma. 2010. Available at http://www.uroweb.org/gls/pdf/Renal%20Cell%20Carcinoma%202010.pdf. Accessed March 22 2011.

[18] Hutson TE, Bukowski RM, Cowey CL, Figlin R, Escudier B, Sternberg CN. Sequential use of targeted agents in the treatment of renal cell carcinoma. Crit. Rev. Oncol. Hematol. 77 (1), 48–62 (2011).

[19] Beck J,Procopio G,Bajetta E et al. Final results of the European Advanced Renal Cell Carcinoma Sorafenib (EU-ARCCS) expanded-access study: a large open-label study in diverse community settings. Ann. Oncol. 2011; Epub ahead of print.

[20] Procopio G,Verzoni E, Guadalupi V, Pietrantonio F, Salvioni R, Nicolai N, et al. Sequential use of sorafenib (So) followed by sunitinib (Su) in metastatic renal cell cancer (mRCC): a single-institution experience [abstract]. Genitourinary Cancers Symposium. Orlando, FL, February 26–28; 2009 [Abstract 319].

[21] Motzer RJ, Mazumdar M, Bacik J, Berg W, Amsterdam A, Ferrara J. Survival and prognostic stratification of 670 patients with advanced renal cell carcinoma. J. Clin. Oncol. 17 (8): 2530-40 (1999).

[22] Silverman SL. From randomized controlled trials to observational studies. Am. J. Med. 122 (2), 114-20 (2009).

[23] Grünwald V, Heinzer H, Fiedler W. Managing side effects of angiogenesis inhibitors in RCC. Onkologie 30, 519–524 (2007).

[24] Ivanyi P, Winkler T, Ganser A, Reuter C, Grünwald V. Dtsch. Arztebl. Int. 105 (13): 232–237 (2008).

Part 3

Case Reports

12

Simultaneous Nephron-Sparing Surgery and Caesarian Section for the Treatment of Renal Cell Carcinoma in Pregnancy: Case Report and Review of the Literature

Ambrosi Pertia, Laurent Managadze and Archil Chkhotua
National Center of Urology
Georgia

1. Introduction

Renal cell carcinoma (RCC) accounts for about 3% of all adult malignancies and is the most lethal urological cancer. Although extremely rare in pregnant women, it is the commonest urological neoplasm in pregnancy occurring in 1 in 1000 cases (Walker, JL., & Knight, EL., 1986). It is potentially curable with prompt diagnosis and correct management. However, treatment of the disease is a substantial challenge for both, urologist and obstetrician.

Over 70 cases of RCC in pregnancy have been reported in literature. 95% of them are clear cell type, with a poorer prognosis than the rest 5% that are chromophobe type. Women with these tumors may present at any stage of the pregnancy. Only 26% of them describe the classical triad of: loin pain, palpable mass and haematuria. The most common mode of presentation of the disease is a palpable mass (88%) and pain (50%). Haematuria implies collecting system invasion and occurs in 50% of the cases. However, haematuria in pregnant women is faint due to other possible causes, including: urinary tract infection, calculi and hydronephrosis (Pearson, GAH., & Eckford, SD., 2009). Other rare forms of presentations are: hypertension, haemolytic anaemia and hypercalcaemia (Monga, et al., 1995; Usta, IM., et al., 1998). With the advent of ultrasound there has been a change in presentation of the disease with diagnosis more frequently made incidentally during ultrasound examination performed for other reasons (Fynn, J., & Venyo, AKG., 2004).

Diagnostic evaluation of a pregnant woman with renal mass requires special consideration combining non-invasive techniques with as little radiation exposure as possible to the mother and fetus. As a first step, urine has to be sent for cytology. Abdominal CT and intravenous pyelography (IVP) are frequently used in the evaluation of non-pregnant patients and should be avoided due to the unsafe radiation exposure to fetus. Renal radionuclide scans being used to determine function of a contralateral kidney has to be replaced by Doppler scan. Ultrasonography (US) is the safest method for diagnosis of the renal mass in pregnant woman with the similar to IVP and CT sensitivity of 85% (Warshauer, DM., et al., 1988). Magnetic resonance imaging (MRI) is also suitable, due to the least radiation exposure and no harm to pregnant woman. However, it should be stressed that chest CT remains the most sensitive method for diagnosis of pulmonary metastases. The US and MRI are the investigations of choice adequately identifying, differentiating and staging the solid renal masses in pregnancy.

The management of RCC in pregnant woman should depend on tumor biology and age of gestation. Decision to operate and prevent further tumor spread should be taken in consideration of the degree of fetal maturity. The impact of surgical and adjuvant therapy on the potential for future pregnancies should be also considered.

The most frequent form of treatment of RCC in pregnancy is open or laparoscopic radical nephrectomy (RN) followed-up by spontaneous delivery (Pearson, GA., & Eckford, SD., 2009; Gnessin, E., et al., 2002; Qureshi, F., et al., 2002; Monga, M., et al., 1995; O'Connor, JP., et al., 2004; Lee, D., & Abraham, N., 2008). RN with or without termination of pregnancy (Loughlin, KR., 1995; Usta, IM., et al., 1998; Simon, I., et al., 2008), Caesarean section (CS) followed-up by RN (Stojnić, J., et al., 2009) and simultaneous RN and CS (Kobayashi, T., et al., 2000) have also been reported in the literature. There are no reports on the simultaneous nephron sparing surgery (NSS) and CS in the pregnant women.

Here we report the first case of NSS performed together with CS for the treatment of RCC in the second trimester of pregnancy. The review of the literature discussing the tretment options, timing of the surgery and multidisciplinarity of approach is also given.

2. Case history

A 33 years old female was referred to our center at 24 weeks' gestation without previous history of urological diseases and any subjective complaints. The right renal mass has been found on routine sonography. A 6X6X4.5 cm. solid tumor has been detected on MRI arising from the upper pole of the right kidney (figure 1). Regional lymph nodes were negative. Hepatic and pulmonary metastases have been excluded by abdominal and chest MRI. Renal biopsy has not been performed due to the following reasons: a) the positive predictive value of the imaging findings is so high that a negative biopsy result would not alter the management strategy; b) 10-20% of biopsies are reported to be non-conclusive; c) high risk of complications associated with biopsy (Silverman, SG., et al., 2006).

The tumor was graded according to the Padua anatomical classification and assigned the score 6. According to this score the risk of surgical complications related to the NSS was considered as low. There were no radiological signs of local extension and/or distant metastases. Clinically the tumor was staged as: T1b, N0, M0.

After extensive counseling and consultation with the obstetrician decision has been taken to postpone the operative treatment until the third trimester of gestation as recommended in the literature. The patient was followed-up by: regular urological and obstetrical checkup; sonography once per month; and weekly urinalysis, until maximal chance of fetal viability. The patient was stable without any signs of disease progression until 33rd week of gestation. After re-consulting with obstetric staff, simultaneous NSS and caesarian section was planned at this time point.

Caesarian section has been performed first under epidural anesthesia. A healthy girl weighing 2.4 kg was delivered without any surgical difficulties. The patient was intubated

Simultaneous Nephron-Sparing Surgery and Caesarian Section for the Treatment of Renal Cell
Carcinoma in Pregnancy: Case Report and Review of the Literature

211

and operation was continued with open NSS through flank incision. Enucleoresection was performed with arterial clamping and local hypothermia. Cold ischemia time was 15 min. Duration of the NSS was 115 min. Blood loss was less than 100 cc. The renal capsular defect has been covered with free peritoneal graft.

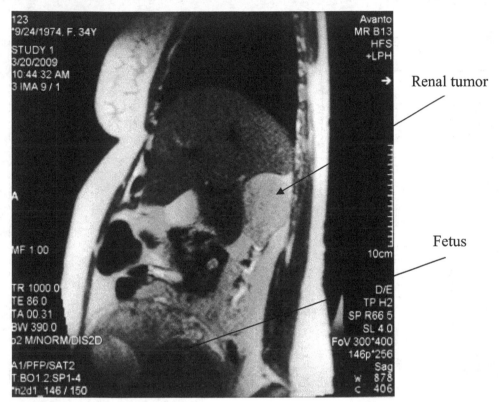

Fig. 1 MRI scan demonstrating right renal mass and the fetus

Postoperative course was uneventful for both, the mother and child. The patient made a good recovery with normal obstetric examinations. Morphology revealed clear cell RCC pT1bN0M0, grade 1. After the follow-up of 30 months the patient is doing well without any signs of the disease recurrence. The child is healthy with normal physical and mental development.

3. Discussion

RN and NSS are the treatments of choice for the patients with RCC. Oncological results and complications of the treatments are extensively evaluated showing excellent outcomes in the patients with local stages of the disease. However, management of RCC in pregnant women is extremely challenging due to the rarity and difficulty of the situation. There are several reports in the literature about the treatment of RCC at different time points of pregnancy. Table 1 describes the cases of the treatment of RCC in pregnancy reported in the literature.

Author	Year of publication	N of cases	Age of gestation at diagnosis	Stage	Treatment	Age of gestation at treatment	Pregnancy outcome
Gladman, MA., et al.	2002	2	14th and 24th weeks	T2N0Mx	RN	17th and 25th weeks	1. Spontaneous delivery at 40th weeks; 2. CS at 40th weeks
Fynn, J., Venyo, AK.	2004	1	12th week	T2N0M0	RN	24th week	CS at 24th weeks
Fazeli-Matin, S., et al.	1998	1	13th week	T2N0M0	NSS	13th week	Spontaneous delivery
Gnessin, E., et al.	2002	2	18th and 16th weeks	T1N0M0 and T2N0M0	RN	18th and 16th weeks	Spontaneous deliveries
Qureshi, F., et al.	2002	1	I trimester	T2N0MX	RN	I trimester	Spontaneous delivery
Lee, D., & Abraham, N.	2008	1	I trimester	-	Lap. nephrectomy	19th week	Spontaneous delivery
O'Connor, J., et al.	2004	1	11th week	T1N0M0	Lap. nephrectomy	19th week	Spontaneous delivery at 38 week
Simon, L., et al.	2008	1	I trimester	-	RN	I trimester	Pregnancy interruption
Pearson, GAH., Eckford, SD.	2009	1	28th week	T2	RN	CS at 34th week	CS at 32nd week
Stojnić, J., et al	2009	1	I trimester	-	RN	II trimester	CS in II trimester
Kobayashi, T., et al.	2000	1	22nd week	T2N0M0	RN	28th week	CS at 28th week

Table 1. Cases of the treatment of RCC in pregnancy reported in the literature

Simultaneous Nephron-Sparing Surgery and Caesarian Section for the Treatment of Renal Cell
Carcinoma in Pregnancy: Case Report and Review of the Literature

213

It was believed for a long time that there is no association between RCC and pregnancy. However, more recent studies discovered new facts. Lambe, M., et al. in a Swedish population-based study, found a strong association between the number of births and the risk of RCC. They have shown that the parous women were at a 40% increased risk of RCC compared to nulliparous women (Lambe, M., et al., 2002). It is known that both, normal and malignant renal cells contain oestrogen and progesterone receptors (Ronchi, E., et al., 1984). Chow, WH., et al. have shown an increased risk of RCC in pregnant women with co-existing risk factors like: parity greater than five, obesity, hypertension and diabetes (Chow, WH., et al., 1995). It has been speculated that pregnancy-associated hormonal changes, particularly high oestrogen levels, may act as promoters of malignant change by stimulating renal cell proliferation either directly or via paracrine growth factors (Concolino, G., et al., 1993). Whether these observations have any implications for the biological behavior of malignant renal cells in pregnancy is not clear, but a tendency towards immediate rather than delayed surgery seems to be appropriate. However, as neonatal survival rates increase with increasing gestation at delivery, immediate surgery at early stages of pregnancy is potentially deleterious to fetal health. Therefore, it is extremely important to define whether pregnancy has to be interrupted or allowed to continue if radical nephrectomy is carried out (Fynn, J., & Venyo, AK., 2004).

If the RCC is discovered in the first trimester, immediate surgery is recommended by majority of the authors (Loughlin, KR., 1995; Gladman, MA., et al., 2002). Whether pregnancy should be terminated at this gestation or not is debatable. The decision should be based on the patient's wishes and medical indications. It is important to consider that the risks of miscarriage and teratogenesis are high at this age, making termination a better option for some authors (Fynn, J., & Venyo, AK., 2004). Others however, disagree with this approach (Usta, IM., et al., 1998).

Management of the disease in the second trimester is more challenging. In the late second trimester surgery should be delayed to at least 28 weeks, when the fetal survival of over 90% is achievable (Loughlin, KR., 1995). In the early second trimester however, immediate surgery is recommended by some of the authors due to the low risk of the fetal loss (Fazeli-Matin, S., et al., 1998; Gnessin, E., et al., 2002; Jenkins, TM., et al., 2003).

In the third trimester the fetal lung maturity is established and immediate surgery seems convenient. It has been suggested that CS should not be performed at the time of RN as the kidney is removed through different incision (Walker, JL. & Knight, EL., 1986). If the diagnosis is made in the late third trimester the surgery can be postponed until delivery (Loughlin, KR., 1995).

In case of the metastatic disease the pregnancy should be terminated (Hendry, WF., 1997). There are no reports of patients or fetal metastases so far.

The most frequent form of treatment of RCC in pregnancy is open or laparoscopic RN followed-up by spontaneous delivery. Gladman, MA., et al. reported 2 cases of RCC diagnosed in the second trimester. RN was performed without termination of pregnancy. One patient gave birth to healthy child and the second one underwent emergency CS for fetal distress at forty weeks' of gestation (Gladman, MA., et al., 2002). Two cases of successful open RN in the second trimester have been reported by Gnessin, E., et al., Both patients gave full term spontaneous delivery to healthy children (Gnessin, E., et al., 2002).

Qureshi, F., et al. detected RCC in the first trimester. Immediate RN was performed through a thoraco-abdominal approach. The patient gave birth to a healthy infant at full term by spontaneous vaginal delivery (Qureshi, F., et al., 2002). Lee, D. & Abraham, N., and O'Connor, J., et al., reported the case of RCC discovered in the first trimester. The operation was delayed till the second trimester. Laparoscopic transperitoneal nephrectomy was performed at 19 weeks' gestation in both cases. Both patients delivered a healthy child vaginally at 39 weeks' gestation (Lee, D., & Abraham, N., 2008; O'Connor, J., et al., 2004).

Simon, I., et al. reported a rare case of Von Hippel-Lindau disease in pregnant women presented with haematuria in the first trimester. RN was carried out after pregnancy interruption (Simon, I., et al., 2008).

Pearson, GAH., & Eckford, SD., detected RCC in the third trimester of pregnancy. CS was performed at 32 weeks of gestation followed-up by RN two weeks later. The same approach has been reported by Stojnić, J., et al. (Stojnić, J., et al., 2009).

Simultaneous RN and CS has also been performed for the treatment of RCC detected in the second trimester (Kobayashi, T., et al, 2000). There are no reports on the simultaneous NSS and CS in the literature.

The data on the effect of pregnancy on long-term survival of RCC is very limited. The same is true for the effect of future pregnancies on tumor recurrence. Some authors have reported good clinical results and survival in pregnant women with RCC (Walker, JL. & Knight, EL., 1986). More data on the outcomes of different treatment options, including the effect of subsequent pregnancies on the disease recurrence are needed to answer these questions.

4. Conclusion

The management of a pregnant woman with a malignant solid renal mass should follow certain principles: 1) the welfare of the mother should be main concern, unless she wishes otherwise; 2) management of the patient has to take place in a multidisciplinary setting involving: urologist, neonatologist, obstetrician, radiologist, anaesthetist, and morphologist; 3) the standard surgical treatment of the most stages of RCC is RN or NSS; 4) timing of the surgery depends on biological behavior of the tumor and the neonatal survival rates for the different gestations; 5) In case of widespread metastatic disease, the pregnancy should probably be terminated and the woman has to be treated according to the guidelines recommended for non-pregnant patients. Here we repot the first case of NSS performed simultaneously with CS for the treatment of pregnant woman with RCC. This approach can be considered feasible in women in the second and third trimesters of pregnancy.

5. References

Concolino, G., et al. (1993). Acquired cystic kidney disease: the hormonal hypothesis. *Urology,* Vol. 41, No. 2, (February 1993), pp. 170 – 175.

Chow, W., et al. (1995). Reproductive factors and risk of renal cell carcinoma among women. *International Journal of Cancer,* 1995; Vol. 60, No. 3, (January 1995), pp.321–324.

Fazeli-Matin, S., et al. (1998). Renal and adrenal surgery during pregnancy. *Urology,* Vol. 52, No. 3, (September 1998), pp. 510 – 511.

Fynn, J., & Venyo, AK. (2004). Renal cell carcinoma presenting as hypertension in pregnancy. *Journal of Obstetrics and Gynaecology*, Vol. 24, No. 7, (October 2004), pp. 821-822.

Gnessin, E., et al. (2002). Renal cell carcinoma in pregnancy. *Urology*, Vol. 60, No. 6, (December 2002), p. 1111.

Hendry, WF. (1997). Management of urological tumours in pregnancy. *British Journal of Urology*, Vol. 80, Supplement 1, (July 1997), pp. 24 – 28.

Jenkins, TM., et al. (2003). Non-obstetric surgery during gestation: risk factors for lower birthweight. *Australian and New Zealand Journal of Obstetrics and Gynaecology*, Vol. 43, No.1, (February 2003), pp. 27 – 31.

Kobayashi, T., et al. (2000). A case of renal cell carcinoma during pregnancy: simultaneous cesarean section and radical nephrectomy. *Journal of Urology*, Vol. 163, No. 5, (May 2000), pp. 1515-1516.

Lambe, M., et al. (2002). Pregnancy and risk of renal cell cancer: a population-based study in Sweden. *British Journal of Cancer*, Vol. 86, No. 9, (May 2002), pp. 1425 – 1429.

Lee, D. & Abraham, N. (2008). Laparoscopic radical nephrectomy during pregnancy: case report and review of the literature. *Journal of Endourology*, Vol. 22, No. 3, (March 2008), pp. 517-519.

Loughlin, KR. (1995). The management of urological malignancies during pregnancy. *British Journal of Urology*, Vol. 76, No. 5, (November 1995), pp. 639-644.

Monga, M., et al., (1995). Renal cell carcinoma presenting as hemolytic anemia in pregnancy. *American Journal of Perinatology*, Vol. 12, No. 2, (March 1995), pp. 84-86.

O'Connor, JP., et al. (2004). Laparoscopic nephrectomy for renal-cell carcinoma during pregnancy. *Journal of Endourology*, Vol. 18, No. 9, (November 2004), pp. 871-874.

Pearson, GA., & Eckford, SD., Renal cell carcinoma in pregnancy. *Journal of Obstetrics and Gynaecology*, Vol. 29, No. 1, (January 2009), pp. 53-54.

Qureshi, F., et al. (2002). Renal cell carcinoma (chromophobe type) in the first trimester of pregnancy. *Scandinavian Journal of Urology and Nephrology*, Vol. 36, No. 3, pp. 228–230.

Ronchi, E., et al. (1984). Steroid hormone receptors in normal and malignant human renal tissue: relationship with progestin therapy. *Journal of Steroid Biochemistry and Molecular Biology*, Vol. 21, No. 3, (September 1984), pp. 329 – 335.

Silverman, SG., et al., (2009). Renal masses in the adult patient: the role of percutaneous biopsy. *Radiology*, Vol. 240, No. 1, (July 2009), pp. 6-22.

Simon, I., et al, (2008). Clear cell renal carcinoma presenting as a bleeding cyst in pregnancy: inaugural manifestation of a von Hippel-Lindau disease. *Clinical Nephrology*. Vol. 69, No. 3, (March 2008), pp. 224-228.

Stojnić, J., et al. (2009). Renal cell carcinoma in pregnancy: a case report. *European Journal of Gynaecological Oncology*, Vol. 30, No. 3, pp. 347-349.

Usta, IM., et al. (1998). Renal cell carcinoma with hypercalcemia complicating a pregnancy: case report and review of the literature. *European Journal of Gynaecological Oncology*, Vol. 19, No. 6, pp. 584 – 587.

Walker, JL. & Knight, EL. (1986) Renal cell carcinoma in pregnancy. *Cancer*, Vol. 58, No. 10, (November 1986), pp. 2343 – 2347.

Warshauer, DM., et al. (1988). Detection of renal masses: sensitivities and specificities of excretory urography/linear tomography, US, and CT. *Radiology*, Vol. 169, No. 2, 363–365.

Permissions

The contributors of this book come from diverse backgrounds, making this book a truly international effort. This book will bring forth new frontiers with its revolutionizing research information and detailed analysis of the nascent developments around the world.

We would like to thank Robert J. Amato, D.O., for lending his expertise to make the book truly unique. He has played a crucial role in the development of this book. Without his invaluable contribution this book wouldn't have been possible. He has made vital efforts to compile up to date information on the varied aspects of this subject to make this book a valuable addition to the collection of many professionals and students.

This book was conceptualized with the vision of imparting up-to-date information and advanced data in this field. To ensure the same, a matchless editorial board was set up. Every individual on the board went through rigorous rounds of assessment to prove their worth. After which they invested a large part of their time researching and compiling the most relevant data for our readers. Conferences and sessions were held from time to time between the editorial board and the contributing authors to present the data in the most comprehensible form. The editorial team has worked tirelessly to provide valuable and valid information to help people across the globe.

Every chapter published in this book has been scrutinized by our experts. Their significance has been extensively debated. The topics covered herein carry significant findings which will fuel the growth of the discipline. They may even be implemented as practical applications or may be referred to as a beginning point for another development. Chapters in this book were first published by InTech; hereby published with permission under the Creative Commons Attribution License or equivalent.

The editorial board has been involved in producing this book since its inception. They have spent rigorous hours researching and exploring the diverse topics which have resulted in the successful publishing of this book. They have passed on their knowledge of decades through this book. To expedite this challenging task, the publisher supported the team at every step. A small team of assistant editors was also appointed to further simplify the editing procedure and attain best results for the readers.

Our editorial team has been hand-picked from every corner of the world. Their multi-ethnicity adds dynamic inputs to the discussions which result in innovative outcomes. These outcomes are then further discussed with the researchers and contributors who give their valuable feedback and opinion regarding the same. The feedback is then collaborated with the researches and they are edited in a comprehensive manner to aid the understanding of the subject.

Apart from the editorial board, the designing team has also invested a significant amount of their time in understanding the subject and creating the most relevant covers. They scrutinized every image to scout for the most suitable representation of the subject and create an appropriate cover for the book.

The publishing team has been involved in this book since its early stages. They were actively engaged in every process, be it collecting the data, connecting with the contributors or procuring relevant information. The team has been an ardent support to the editorial, designing and production team. Their endless efforts to recruit the best for this project, has resulted in the accomplishment of this book. They are a veteran in the field of academics and their pool of knowledge is as vast as their experience in printing. Their expertise and guidance has proved useful at every step. Their uncompromising quality standards have made this book an exceptional effort. Their encouragement from time to time has been an inspiration for everyone.

The publisher and the editorial board hope that this book will prove to be a valuable piece of knowledge for researchers, students, practitioners and scholars across the globe.

List of Contributors

Kazunori Kihara, Yasuhisa Fujii, Satoru Kawakami, Hitoshi Masuda, Fumitaka Koga, Kazutaka Saito, Noboru Numao, Yoh Matsuoka and Yasuyuki Sakai
Department of Urology, Graduate School, Tokyo Medical and Dental University, Japan

Tetsuo Fujita, Masatsugu Iwamura, Shinji Kurosaka, Ken-ichi Tabata, Kazumasa Matsumoto, Kazunari Yoshida and Shiro Baba
Department of Urology, Kitasato University School of Medicine, Japan

Paul D'Alessandro, Shawn Dason and Anil Kapoor
Divison of Urology, Department of Surgery McMaster University, Hamilton, Ontario, Canada

Archil Chkhotua, Tinatin Pantsulaia and Laurent Managadze
National Center of Urology, Georgia

Mehrnaz Asadi Gharabaghi
Tehran University of Medical Sciences, Iran

Alessandro Gasbarrini and Stefano Boriani
Department of Oncologic and Degenerative Spine Surgery, Rizzoli Institute, Italy

Christiano Esteves Simões
Department of Orthopedics and Traumatology – Spine Unit, Felício Rocho Hospital, Brazil

Michele Cappuccio
Department of Orthopedics and Traumatology – Spine Surgery, Maggiore Hospital, Italy

Thean Hsiang Tan and Judith Lees
RAH Cancer Centre, Royal Adelaide Hospital, Australia

Ganesalingam Pranavan and Desmond Yip
Medical Oncology Unit, The Canberra Hospital, Australia

Desmond Yip
ANU Medical School, Australian National University, Australia

Murat Lekili
Celal Bayar University, Medical Faculty, Urology Department, Manisa, Turkey

Minna Kankuri-Tammilehto
Department of Oncology and Radiotherapy, Turku University Hospital, Finland

Mirjana Rajer
Institute of Oncology Ljubljana, Slovenia

G. Procopio, E. Verzoni, R. Iacovelli, F. Gelsomino, M. Catanzaro and L. Mariani
'IRCCS 'Istituto Nazionale dei Tumori', Medical Oncology, Milan, Italy

Ambrosi Pertia, Laurent Managadze and Archil Chkhotua
National Center of Urology, Georgia

Printed in the USA
CPSIA information can be obtained
at www.ICGtesting.com
JSHW011416221024
72173JS00004B/554